Heart Failure

NOTICE

Medicine is an ever-changing science. As new research and clinical experience broaden our knowledge, changes in treatment and drug therapy are required. The authors and the publisher of this work have checked with sources believed to be reliable in their efforts to provide information that is complete and generally in accord with the standards accepted at the time of publication; however, in view of the possibility of human error or changes in medical sciences, neither the authors nor the publisher nor any other party who has been involved in the preparation or publication of this work warrants that the information contained herein is in every respect accurate or complete, and they disclaim all responsibility for any errors or omissions or for the results obtained from use of the information contained in this work. Readers are encouraged to confirm the information contained herein with other sources. For example and in particular, readers are advised to check the product information sheet included in the package of each drug they plan to administer to be certain that the information contained in this work is accurate and that changes have not been made in the recommended dose or in the contraindications for administration. This recommendation is of particular importance in connection with new or infrequently used drugs.

Heart Failure
A Practical Approach to Treatment

William T. Abraham, MD, FACP, FACC, FAHA

Professor of Internal Medicine
Adjunct Professor of Physiology and Cell Biology
Director, Division of Cardiovascular Medicine
Deputy Director, Davis Heart and Lung Research Institute
Ohio State University
Columbus, Ohio

Henry Krum, MBBS, PhD, FRACP, FCSANZ

Professor of Medicine
Chair of Medical Therapeutics
Monash University
Director, NHMRC CCRE in Therapeutics
Departments of Epidemiology and Preventive Medicine and Medicine
Alfred Hospital, Monash University
Melbourne, Victoria
Australia

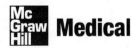 **Medical**

New York Chicago San Francisco Lisbon London Madrid Mexico City
Milan New Delhi San Juan Seoul Singapore Sydney Toronto

Heart Failure: A Practical Approach to Treatment

1 2 3 4 5 6 7 8 9 0   DOC/DOC   0 9 8 7

ISBN-13: 978-0-07-144315-9
ISBN-10: 0-07-144315-0

This book was set in Garamond by International Typesetting and Composition, Inc.
The editors were Ruth Weinberg, Christie Naglieri, and Peter J. Boyle.
The production supervisor was Catherine Saggese.
Project management was provided by International Typesetting and Composition, Inc.
RR Donnelley was printer and binder.

This book is printed on acid-free paper.

Library of Congress Cataloging-in-Publication Data

Heart failure : a practical approach to treatment / [edited by] William T. Abraham, Henry Krum.
      p. ; cm.
   Includes index.
   ISBN 978-0-07-144315-9
   1. Heart failure.   2. Heart failure—Treatment.   I. Abraham, William T.   II. Krum, Henry.
   [DNLM: 1. Heart Failure, Congestive.   2. Heart Failure, Congestive—therapy.
   WG 370 H436196   2007]
   RC685.C53H428   2007
   616.1'2906—dc22   2006038339

To our fathers:
To my late father, Coach William "Bill" Abraham, who lost the battle
to congestive heart failure after many years of good life sustained
by the therapies discussed in this book.
More than a football coach, he was a life coach
to many young men, including me.

William T. Abraham, MD, FACP, FACC, FAHA

To my late father, Joseph Krum. Persistently inspiring and inspiration to persist.

Henry Krum, MBBS, PhD, FRACP, FCSANZ

Contents

Contributors

William T. Abraham, MD, FACP, FACC, FAHA
Professor of Internal Medicine
Adjunct Professor of Physiology and Cell Biology
Director, Division of Cardiovascular Medicine
Deputy Director, Davis Heart & Lung
    Research Institute
Ohio State University
Columbus, Ohio
Devices for the Treatment of Heart Failure

**Andrew J.S. Coats, MD, MA, DM, DSc, FRACP,
FRCP, FESC, FACC, FAHA, MBA**
Deputy Vice-Chancellor (Community)
University of Sydney
Sydney, Australia
Nonpharmacologic Treatment of Heart Failure

Daniel L. Dries, MD, MPH
Assistant Professor of Medicine
Heart Failure and Transplant Program
Hospital of the University of Pennsylvania
Philadelphia, Pennsylvania
*Therapeutic Approach to Heart Failure:
    An Overview*

Maryjane Farr, MD
Director of the Richard T. Perkin Heart Failure
    Program
Weill Cornell Medical College
New York Presbyterian Hospital
New York, New York
*When to Refer Patients for Heart
    Transplantation*

Jennifer Farroni, RN, MSN, CNP
Nurse Practitioner
Heart Failure Program
Ohio State University
Columbus, Ohio
*How to Develop a Heart Failure Management
    Pathway*

David Feldman, MD, PhD
Director
Heart Failure & Cardiac Transplantation
Associate Professor of Cardiovascular Medicine
Ohio State University
Columbus, Ohio
*How to Develop a Heart Failure Management
    Pathway*

Gregg C. Fonarow, MD
Ahmanson-UCLA Cardiomyopathy Center
University of California, Los Angeles
Los Angeles, California
What Is a Heart Failure Clinic?

Alexander E. Fraley, MD, FACC
Fellow
Division of Cardiology
University of California–San Diego
San Diego, California
*How to Use Neurohormonal Antagonists
    in Heart Failure*

Gary S. Francis, MD
Cleveland Clinic Foundation
Cleveland, Ohio
Pathophysiology of Heart Failure

Mihai Gheorghiade, MD
Professor of Medicine
Associate Chief
Division of Cardiology
Northwestern University Feinberg School
    of Medicine
Chicago, Illinois
Is There Still a Role for Digitalis in Heart Failure?

Maryjane B. Giacalone, RN
Cardiology Division
Department of Medicine
Massachusetts General Hospital
Harvard Medical School
Boston, Massachusetts
*Integrating Inpatient and Outpatient Heart
    Failure Management*

Richard E. Gilbert, MBBS, PhD, FRACP
Professor of Medicine
University of Toronto
Department of Medicine
St. Michael's Hospital, Toronto
Canada and University of Melbourne
Department of Medicine St. Vincent's Hospital
Melbourne, Australia
Comorbidities and Heart Failure

Daniel J. Goldstein, MD
Surgical Director
Heart Transplantation and Mechanical Circulatory
    Support Programs
Associate Professor
Department of Cardiothoracic Surgery
Montefiore Medical Center/Albert Einstein
    College of Medicine
New York, New York
Surgical Approaches to Heart Failure

Barry H. Greenberg, MD
Professor of Medicine
Director
UCSD Heart Failure/Cardiac
    Transplantation Program
Division of Cardiology
University of California San Diego
San Diego, California
*How to Use Neurohormonal Antagonists
    in Heart Failure*

Sharon Hunt, MD
Professor
Cardiovascular Medicine
Division of Cardiovascular Medicine/CVRB
Stanford University
Stanford, California
*How to Evaluate Patients with Symptoms
    Suggestive of Heart Failure*

Mariell Jessup, MD
Professor of Medicine
Medical Director
Heart Failure and Transplant Program
Hospital of the University of Pennsylvania
University of Pennsylvania School of Medicine
Philadelphia, Pennsylvania
*Therapeutic Approach to Heart Failure:
    An Overview*

Mikhail Kosiborod, MD
Assistant Professor of Medicine, Cardiology
University of Missouri, Kansas City
Clinical Scholar
Mid America Heart Institute
Kansas City, Missouri
The Epidemic of Heart Failure

Henry Krum, MBBS, PhD, FRACP, FCSANZ
Professor of Medicine
Chair of Medical Therapeutics
Monash University
Director
NHMRC CCRE in Therapeutics
Departments of Epidemiology and Preventive
    Medicine and Medicine
Alfred Hospital, Monash University
Melbourne, Victoria
Australia
*Ancillary Pharmacological Therapies for
    Heart Failure*
Comorbidities and Heart Failure

Harlan M. Krumholz, MD, SM
Yale University School of Medicine
New Haven, Connecticut
The Epidemic of Heart Failure

Alexander Lyon, BM, BCh, MRCP
British Heart Foundation Junior Research Fellow
London, United Kingdom
What Causes Heart Failure?

Donna Mancini, MD
Medical Director for Cardiac Transplantation
Columbia University
New York Presbyterian Hospital
New York, New York
*When to Refer Patients for Heart
　Transplantation*

John J.V. McMurray, MD
Department of Cardiology
Western Infirmary, Glasgow
Scotland, United Kingdom
What Is Heart Failure?

Robert E. Michler, MD
Professor and Chairman
Department of Cardiothoracic Surgery
Co-Director
Montefiore-Einstein Heart Center
Montefiore Medical Center/Albert Einstein
　College of Medicine
New York, New York
Surgical Approaches to Heart Failure

Sara Paul, RN, MSN, FNP
Director, Heart Function Clinic
Western Piedmont Heart Centers
Hickory, North Carolina
*How to Develop a Heart Failure Management
　Pathway*

Philip A. Poole-Wilson, MD, FRCP, FMedSci
British Heart Foundation Simon Marks
　Professor of Cardiology
Department of Molecular Systems Biology
National Heart and Lung Institute
Royal Brompton Hospital
London, United Kingdom
What Causes Heart Failure

Willem J. Remme, MD, PhD
Professor of Medicine
Sticares Cardiovascular Research Institute
Rhoon, The Netherlands
*Putting It All Together: Optimizing the
　Management of Heart Failure Patients*

Joseph S. Rossi, MD
Cardiology Fellow
Northwestern University Feinberg School
　of Medicine
Chicago, Illinois
*Is There Still a Role for Digitalis in Heart
　Failure?*

Robert W. Schrier, MD
Professor of Medicine
University of Colorado School of Medicine
Denver, Colorado
How to Use Diuretics in Heart Failure Patients

Marc J. Semigran, MD
Cardiology Division
Department of Medicine
Massachusetts General Hospital
Harvard Medical School
Boston, Massachusetts
*Integrating Inpatient and Outpatient Heart
　Failure Management*

Lynne Warner Stevenson, MD. FACC
Cardiovascular Division
Brigham and Women's Hospital
Boston, Massachusetts
The Heart Failure Hospitalization

W.H. Wilson Tang, MD
Assistant Professor in Medicine
Cleveland Clinic Lerner College of Medicine
　of Case Reserve University
Cleveland, Ohio
Pathophysiology of Heart Failure

Robin J. Trupp, MSN, APRN, BC, CCRN, CCRC
Comprehensive Cardiovascular Consulting, LLC
Dublin, Ohio
PhD Student
The Ohio State University
Columbus, Ohio
Disease Management Overview

Faiez Zannad, MD, PhD, FESC
Professeur de Thérapeutique-Cardiologie
Centre d'Investigation Clinique
CIC-INSERM CHU
Hôpital Jeanne d'Arc
Toul, France
*How to Judge Disease Severity, Clinical Status,
    and Prognosis*

Michael Zembala, MD
Cardiothoracic Research Fellow
Department of Cardiothoracic Surgery
Montefiore Medical Center/Albert Einstein
    College of Medicine
New York, New York
Surgical Approaches to Heart Failure

Preface

Chronic heart failure is now finally getting the recognition it deserves as a major public health problem. Increased awareness in the medical community has been reflected by the emergence of specialist journals and meetings, specific patient resources, public awareness campaigns, and a massive increase in research activities directed toward the problem.

As part of this increase in activity to combat heart failure, numerous books have been produced that address pathophysiology, diagnostic criteria, and management principles.

However, none of these books, we believe, have directly addressed the needs of clinicians, paramedical staff, and other health-care providers. Thus, our aim with this text is to provide for busy clinicians a practical reference that is comprehensive and clinically oriented yet at the same time concise.

We discuss practical, evidence-based recommendations, with particular attention to the scientific and clinical rationale for the pharmacologic and nonpharmacologic strategies driving the current management of heart failure. We emphasize topics such as heart failure disease management programs and pathways of care, often neglected in textbooks on heart failure, because integrating these approaches is an important consideration in clinical practice.

Chapters such as "How to Evaluate Patients with Symptoms Suggestive of Heart Failure," "How to Judge Disease Severity," and simple fundamental questions such as "What Is Heart Failure?" and "What Causes Heart Failure?" best reflect the key principles guiding this textbook.

Finally, heart failure management is all about putting together the component parts available to the clinician. We provide an overview of this in our closing chapter.

We hope the readership of this book agree with the clinical utility of this text in providing a practical approach to the management of this important and now increasingly recognized condition.

William T. Abraham
Henry Krum

CHAPTER 1

What Is Heart Failure?

JOHN J. V. McMURRAY, MD

Although the designation "heart failure" is routinely used to describe a clinical syndrome recognized by physicians, the exact definition of that syndrome has proved difficult, if not impossible (Table 1-1).[1,2] Traditionally, the expression heart failure has been used by physicians to refer to a *clinical* syndrome that is a constellation of symptoms and signs, usually (but not exclusively) caused by an abnormality of the heart. Note that this traditional usage describes a symptomatic state.

Almost any abnormality of the heart can cause the syndrome of heart failure.[3] Rhythm and conduction disturbances, valvular stenosis and incompetence, pericardial and epicardial abnormalities, inherited (congenital) defects, and ventricular dysfunction can each cause heart failure. Ventricular dysfunction has been the focus of most pathophysiological and therapeutic research. It can arise from abnormalities of the myocyte, extracellular matrix, or, usually, both. Myocyte loss (due to infarction, infection, or toxic necrosis) and replacement by scar tissue leads to a reduction in contractility and ejection of blood from the ventricle, that is, predominant systolic dysfunction. Conversely, myocyte hypertrophy and associated extracellular matrix overgrowth (fibrosis) may lead to impaired ventricular filling, that is, predominant diastolic dysfunction. Rarer causes of ventricular dysfunction include disorders causing deposition of abnormal proteins within the ventricular tissue, for example, amyloid.

These diverse etiologies lead to a clinical syndrome, which, by definition, has many common features, notably dyspnea, fatigue, and sodium and water retention ("congestion").[4] Different causes may, of course, also have distinguishing features, for example, a murmur in valve disease and a bradycardia in patients with a conduction disturbance.

Central to the problem of defining and recognizing the syndrome of heart failure is the non-specificity of its cardinal clinical manifestations.[5] While that problem can be solved by appropriate investigation, the greater question is what causes those characteristic manifestations in the first place?

Previously popular and simple notions that heart failure can be equated to some measurement of cardiac function, for example cardiac output, can be quickly dispelled.[1,2] Measurements such as cardiac output may be normal (especially at rest) and patients with abnormal cardiac function (e.g., a low left ventricular ejection fraction) may be asymptomatic. Of course, patients with heart failure, unless it is advanced, are usually only symptomatic on exertion. Consequently, a widely accepted concept of heart failure is one in which the fundamental problem is inadequate delivery of blood to meet the needs of the metabolizing tissues.[1,2] Two qualifications usefully refine this construct. One is to state that this abnormal state exists despite an adequate left ventricular filling pressure.[1,2] The second identifies the problem as one of inadequate *oxygen delivery* rather than inadequate

▶ **Table 1-1** Definitions of heart failure

1933	A condition in which the heart fails to discharge its contents adequately. (Lewis.)
1950	A state in which the heart fails to maintain an adequate circulation for the needs of the body despite a satisfactory filling pressure. (Wood.)
1980	A pathophysiological state in which an abnormality of cardiac function is responsible for the failure of the heart to pump blood at a rate commensurate with the requirements of the metabolizing tissues. (Braunwald.)
1985	A clinical syndrome caused by an abnormality of the heart and recognized by a characteristic pattern of hemodynamic, renal, neural, and hormonal responses. (Poole-Wilson.)
1987	syndrome...Which arises when the heart is chronically unable to maintain an appropriately high blood pressure without support. (Harris.)
1988	A syndrome in which cardiac dysfunction is associated with reduced exercise tolerance, a high incidence of ventricular arrhythmias, and shortened life expectancy. (Cohn.)
1989	...ventricular dysfunction with symptoms.... (Anonymous.)
1993	Heart failure is the state of any heart disease in which, despite adequate ventricular filling, the heart's output is decreased or in which the heart is unable to pump blood at a rate adequate for satisfying the requirements of the tissues with function parameters remaining within normal limits. (Denolin et al.)
1994	The principal functions of the heart are to accept blood from the venous system, deliver it to the lungs where it is oxygenated (aerated), and pump the oxygenated blood to all body tissues. Heart failure occurs when these functions are disturbed substantially. (Lenfant.)
1996	Abnormal ventricular function, symptoms or signs of heart failure (past or current), and on treatment (with a favorable response to treatment). (Poole-Wilson.)
2005	(i) Symptoms of heart failure (at rest or during exercise) and (ii) objective evidence (preferably by echocardiography) of cardiac dysfunction (systolic and/or diastolic) at rest (both criteria [i] and [ii] must be fulfilled) and (iii) in cases where the diagnosis is in doubt, response to treatment directed towards heart failure.

Source: Adapted from Purcell IF, Poole-Wilson PA. Heart failure: why and how to define it? *Eur J Heart Fail.* 1999;1:7–10.

blood flow.[1,2] The importance of both these qualifications is clear. Obviously, blood flow and oxygen delivery will be inadequate, despite good pump function, when there is intravascular volume depletion and reduced oxygen carrying capacity, for example, as a result of severe hemorrhage. The paradigm of inadequate oxygen delivery despite normal filling pressure also has merit in that it allows for "high-output" syndromes of heart failure such as seen in patients with anemia, thyrotoxicosis, Paget's disease, arteriovenous shunting, and so on. It is still, however, a physiological rather than clinical definition, and measurement of inadequate delivery of oxygen to the metabolizing tissues is not easily done. More fundamentally, this construct does not explain how inadequate oxygen delivery

(if indeed that is the primary problem) is sensed by the body and how the body responds to it. It is likely that it is the responses of the body that lead to the clinical syndrome recognized by clinicians. These responses are almost certainly multiple, complex, and variable. However, one thing is certain and that is the pivotal role played by the kidney.[6] While involvement of the kidney may be a relatively late manifestation, after the cardiac injury initiating the processes leading to the clinical syndrome of heart failure, it is undeniable in the patient presenting with expansion of extracellular fluid volume and frank edema.

Before continuing to examine the body's responses in heart failure, it is worth pausing and reiterating the remarkable fact that, despite the development of hugely successful treatments for heart failure, we still do not understand two of the most fundamental processes in the development of this clinical condition, that is, the "signal" that evokes the body's response to pump dysfunction and how and where the signal (or signals) is sensed.

Returning to the responses to the failure to deliver oxygen adequately for the needs of the metabolizing tissues (assuming that is a key signal), these are protean and impossible to describe completely. Indeed, it would be true to say that almost everything measured in patients with heart failure is abnormal and very few things are completely normal.[7] Identifying the key pathophysiological responses in heart failure is difficult and the history of medicine has taught us that mechanisms thought to be important today may come to be regarded as epiphenomena by tomorrow.[7] Two attractive unifying and related hypotheses have, however, to date, stood the test of time. Harris and others proposed that heart failure can be thought of as akin to hemorrhage and the body's response is similar, that is, directed at maintaining perfusion of vital organs.[8–10] Francis, Cohn, Packer, and others focused on the array of neurohumoral abnormalities identified in heart failure, particularly those causing vasoconstriction (or perhaps, more accurately, redistribution of blood) and sodium and water retention.[11,12] Key among those are activation of the renin-angiotensin-aldosterone system (RAAS) and sympathetic nervous system (SNS) and increased release of arginine vasopressin. Of course these neuroendocrine changes also occur in response to hemorrhage where their potential benefits are obvious.[8–10] In heart failure caused by systolic dysfunction of the left ventricle at least, their sustained action is thought to be maladaptive and detrimental and that construct has probably been validated by the therapeutic success of RAAS and SNS inhibitors. This distinction between the temporary and beneficial effects of neurohumoral activation in hemorrhage and detrimental effects of sustained, long-term activation of the same in heart failure is important. It is a potential explanation, at least in part, of one other key characteristic

of the heart failure state, that is, its *progressive* nature.[13–16] In other words, patients with heart failure tend to show worsening of their condition over time, manifest as increasing symptoms hemodynamic deterioration and premature mortality. Key to the neurohumoral hypothesis is the belief that the neural, endocrine, paracrine, and autocrine systems chronically activated in heart failure indirectly (and directly) cause additional cardiac damage and pump dysfunction as well as vascular dysfunction contributing to circulatory failure. Other intercurrent cardiac events and even the metabolic, cellular, and molecular changes in the heart, per se, may also contribute to progression.[13–16]

The "hemorrhage" and "neurohumoral" hypotheses are attractive in other ways. For example, if one looks beyond the obvious vascular and renal actions of the neurohumoral pathways described, the hemorrhage hypothesis would lead one to postulate that the RAAS and SNS should also encourage coagulation (to stop bleeding), wound healing (scarring or fibrosis, for the same reason), erythropoiesis (to restore lost red blood cells and hemoglobin), and also promote anti-infective and inflammatory responses (to prevent infection as a result of breach of the skin).[17–20] Although unrecognized at the time when Harris and others were developing their hypotheses, more and more evidence has emerged that the RAAS and SNS do indeed have this wide range of effects.[17–20] Indeed, the systemic response to injury and hemorrhage is so ancient in evolutionary terms, and teleologically so fundamental to survival of the organism there are almost certainly multiple, overlapping, and redundant pathways involved.[8–10] The obvious extrapolation, if this is true, is that there may also be other therapeutic targets offering the potential success of the tools we now have to block the RAAS and SNS. Of course, this broader understanding may also help explain some of the unanticipated actions of inhibitors of the RAAS and SNS such as the anti-infarction effect of angiotensin-converting enzyme (ACE) inhibitors and the reduction in hemoglobin associated with the use of these drugs.

Although plausible and attractive, as outlined above, the hemorrhage hypothesis does not completely explain the neurohumoral picture of heart failure. We now know, for example, that blood natriuretic peptide concentrations are elevated in heart failure but reduced in hemorrhage.[21] Indeed, arguably, the heart failure state results in a neurohumoral profile more akin to sustained exertion than hemorrhage.[22]

Of course many other profound metabolic, cellular, and molecular changes occur in the heart and other tissues in heart failure, and these are not characteristic of hemorrhage where the occurrence of (and responses to) neurohumoral activation persists over a relatively short period of time compared to the patient with chronic heart failure and where the heart is fundamentally healthy.[13–15,23]

Although the neurohumoral pathways alluded to earlier clearly have powerful renal actions, which lead to sodium and water retention, it is not at all clear whether those are a complete explanation for the way in which the kidney behaves in heart failure and, despite being pivotal in the development of the key manifestations of heart failure, that is, dyspnea and edema, our understanding of the workings of the kidney in heart failure is very limited.[6,24]

While I have implied that dyspnea is directly related to sodium and water retention, I do not mean to suggest that fluid overload is its essential cause. It probably is not, though dyspnea is very likely when fluid overload is present. It may still occur in patients without clinically obvious fluid overload and its causes remain elusive, though many mechanisms have been postulated (e.g., abnormal skeletal muscle metabolic or chemoreceptor activation) and even probably disproved (e.g., raised pulmonary capillary wedge pressure).[25–27] Fatigue, the other symptom said to be characteristic of heart failure (though I am not so sure it is actually caused by heart failure), is even more mysterious in origin.[25–27]

So where are we so far with the definition of heart failure? We know it is a clinical syndrome arising from many different causes. There is an underlying cardiac abnormality (unless there is an alternative explanation such as anemia); though not all patients with the cardiac abnormality in question may have the syndrome of heart failure. The key manifestations of the syndrome are dyspnea, fatigue, and congestion, although sodium and water retention may not occur for a long period (even years) after a cardiac abnormality has been identified. We know that neurohumoral activation occurs, though the degree and extent of this may vary according to the underlying cardiac abnormality, symptom severity, and concomitant treatment.[28–30] While neurohumoral activation is important in the pathophysiology of heart failure, multiple other abnormalities are also measurable and may or may not be important. In many, if not most, patients, the kidney retains an excessive amount of sodium and water.

Modern clinical definitions of heart failure have attempted to integrate these key features. For example, the European Society of Cardiology requires (a) the presence of typical symptoms and signs; (b) evidence of a cardiac abnormality (identified by an electrocardiogram or cardiac imaging) or, alternatively, evidence of neurohumoral activation reflecting atrial or ventricular "distress," that is, elevation in concentration of a blood natriuretic peptide; and (c) if there is remaining doubt, a therapeutic response to treatment, for example, improvement in symptoms with a diuretic (Fig. 1-1).[31]

So far, I have adhered to the traditional clinical notion of heart failure as a syndrome, that is, by definition a symptomatic condition. Of course, it has been long recognized by clinicians (and experimental physiologists) that an asymptomatic (or perhaps presymptomatic) state of impaired pump function can exist and may be associated with some but not all of the characteristic abnormalities of the symptomatic state, for example, reduced functional capacity and neurohumoral activation (albeit to a lesser extent).[28] This is true for both myocardial disease (e.g., asymptomatic left ventricular systolic dysfunction after myocardial infarction) and valve disease. Whether these patients should be described as having heart failure is a moot point. Clearly they do not have a "syndrome," which,

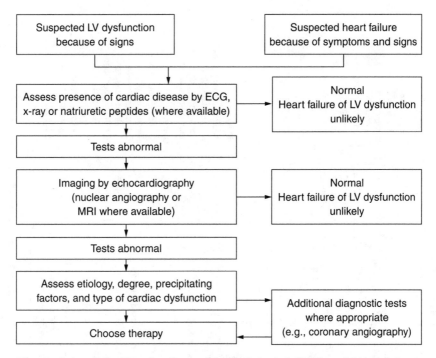

Figure 1-1 Algorithm for the modern clinical definition of heart failure. LV—left ventricular; ECG—echocardiogram; MRI—magnetic resonance imaging. (From the European Society of Cardiology requirements. Swedberg K. Task Force for the Diagnosis and Treatment of Chronic Heart Failure of the European Society of Cardiology. Guidelines for the diagnosis and treatment of chronic heart failure: executive summary (update 2005). *Eur Heart J.* 2005;26(11):1115–1140.)

by definition, requires the presence of symptoms. Perhaps there is merit in differentiating between heart failure and "symptomatic heart failure," the latter corresponding to the traditional clinical syndrome and the former a broader population including asymptomatic patients. The advantage of this expanded classification is that it highlights the opportunity to prevent (and importance of preventing) progression to the symptomatic state with all that it entails in terms of well-being, morbidity, and mortality.[32] An expanded approach of this type has been advocated in recent American College of Cardiology and American Heart Association guidelines (Fig. 1-2).[33] The potential range of cardiac

abnormalities and assessment of their severity and functional significance pose real difficulties. What degree of hypertrophy or what level of ejection fraction merits intervention, assuming those measures can even be made accurately and reproducibly? Here again, measurement of blood natriuretic peptides may act as a guide, though this is still a subject of research, and the screening for and treatment of asymptomatic cardiac disease using natriuretic peptides is not yet advocated in routine clinical practice.

In summary, to the clinician, heart failure traditionally has been recognized as a syndrome characterized by dyspnea, fatigue and congestion, caused by an abnormality of the heart, and associated with

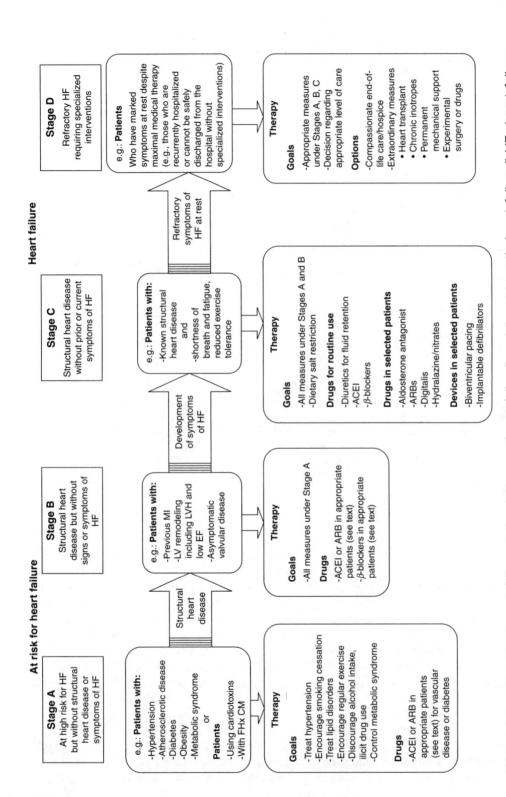

Figure 1-2 Classification of differentiating between "heart failure" and "symptomatic heart failure." HF—heart failure; LV—left ventricular; LVH—left ventricular hypertrophy; MI—myocardial infarction; EF—ejection fraction; ACEI—angiotensin-converting enzyme inhibitors; ARB—angiotensin receptor blockers; FHx CM—family history of cardiomyopathy. (From the American College of Cardiology and American Heart Association guidelines. ACC/AHA 2005 guideline update for the diagnosis and management of chronic heart failure in the adult—summary article: a report of the American College of Cardiology/American Heart Association Task Force on Practice Guidelines (writing committee to update the 2001 guidelines for the evaluation and management of heart failure), *J Am Coll Cardiol.* 2005;46(6):1116–1143).

an array of systemic pathophysiological abnormalities including, notably, neurohumoral activation and renal sodium and water retention. In many patients, an asymptomatic phase may precede development of the symptomatic syndrome and once the symptomatic state has developed, progression leading to symptomatic worsening and death is typical.

▶ REFERENCES

1. Purcell IF, Poole-Wilson PA. Heart failure: why and how to define it? *Eur J Heart Fail.* 1999;1:7–10.

2. Coronel R, de Groot JR, van Lieshout JJ. Defining heart failure. *Cardiovasc Res.* 2001;50:419–422.

3. Lip GY, Gibbs CR, Beevers DG. ABC of heart failure: aetiology. *BMJ.* 2000;320:104–107.

4. Watson RD, Gibbs CR, Lip GY. ABC of heart failure. Clinical features and complications. *BMJ.* 2000;320:236–239.

5. Davie AP, Francis CM, Caruana L, et al. Assessing diagnosis in heart failure: which features are any use? *QJM.* 1997;90:335–339.

6. Cody RJ. Sodium and water retention in congestive heart failure—the pivotal role of the kidney. *Am J Hypertens.* 1988;1:S395–S401.

7. Francis GS, Tang WH. Pathophysiology of congestive heart failure. *Rev Cardiovasc Med.* 2003;4(suppl 2):S14–S20.

8. Harris P. Congestive cardiac failure: central role of the arterial blood pressure. *Br Heart J.* 1987;58:190–203.

9. Harris P. Evolution and the cardiac patient. *Cardiovasc Res.* 1983;17:437–445.

10. Harris P. Evolution and the cardiac patient. *Cardiovasc Res.* 1983;17:313–319.

11. Francis GS, Goldsmith SR, Levine TB, et al. The neurohumoral axis in congestive heart failure. *Ann Intern Med.* 1984;101:370–377.

12. Packer M, Lee WH, Kessler PD, et al. Role of neurohormonal mechanisms in determining survival in patients with severe chronic heart failure. *Circulation.* 1987;75:IV80–92.

13. Sabbah HN, Sharov VG, Goldstein S. Programmed cell death in the progression of heart failure. *Ann Med.* 1998;30(suppl 1):33–38.

14. Francis GS. Neurohumoral activation and progression of heart failure: hypothetical and clinical considerations. *J Cardiovasc Pharmacol.* 1998; 32(suppl 1):S16–S21.

15. Poole-Wilson PA. Spirals, paradigms, and the progression of heart failure. *J Card Fail.* 1996;2:1–4.

16. Packer M. Evolution of the neurohormonal hypothesis to explain the progression of chronic heart failure. *Eur Heart J.* 1995;16(suppl F):4–6.

17. McMurray J, Dargie HJ. ACE inhibitors for myocardial infarction and unstable angina. *Lancet.* 1992;340:1547–1548.

18. Vaughan DE. Angiotensin and vascular fibrinolytic balance. *Am J Hypertens.* 2002;15:S3–S8.

19. Schnee JM, Hsueh WA. Angiotensin II, adhesion, and cardiac fibrosis. *Cardiovasc Res.* 2000;46: 264–268.

20. Suzuki Y, Ruiz-Ortega M, Lorenzo O, et al. Inflammation and angiotensin II. *Int J Biochem Cell Biol.* 2003;35:881–900.

21. Richards AM. The natriuretic peptides in heart failure. *Basic Res Cardiol.* 2004;99:94–100.

22. Milledge JS, Bryson EI, Catley DM, et al. Sodium balance, fluid homeostasis and the renin-aldosterone system during the prolonged exercise of hill walking. *Clin Sci (Lond).* 1982;62:595–604.

23. Benjamin IJ, Schneider MD. Learning from failure: congestive heart failure in the postgenomic age. *J Clin Invest.* 2005;115:495–499.

24. Ljungman S, Laragh JH, Cody RJ. Role of the kidney in congestive heart failure: relationship of cardiac index to kidney function. *Drugs.* 1990;39(suppl 4):10–21.

25. Teerlink JR. Dyspnea as an end point in clinical trials of therapies for acute decompensated heart failure. *Am Heart J.* 2003;145(suppl 2):S26–S33.

26. Clark AL, Sparrow JL, Coats AJ. Muscle fatigue and dyspnoea in chronic heart failure: two sides of the same coin? *Eur Heart J.* 1995;16:49–52.

27. Clark AL. Origin of symptoms in chronic heart failure. *Heart.* 2005 Sep 13; [Epub ahead of print].

28. Francis GS, Benedict C, Johnstone DE, et al. Comparison of neuroendocrine activation in patients with left ventricular dysfunction with and without congestive heart failure: a substudy of the Studies of Left Ventricular Dysfunction (SOLVD). *Circulation.* 1990;82:1724–1729.

29. Bayliss J, Norell M, Canepa-Anson R, et al. Untreated heart failure: clinical and neuroendocrine effects of introducing diuretics. *Br Heart J.* 1987;57:17–22.

30. Kubo SH, Clark M, Laragh JH, et al. Identification of normal neurohormonal activity in mild congestive heart failure and stimulating effect of upright posture and diuretics. *Am J Cardiol.* 1987; 60:1322–1328.

31. Swedberg K, Cleland J, Dargie H, Task Force for the Diagnosis and Treatment of Chronic Heart Failure of the European Society of Cardiology. Guidelines for the diagnosis and treatment of chronic heart failure: executive summary (update 2005). *Eur Heart J.* 2005;26:1115–1140.

32. McMurray JV, McDonagh TA, Davie AP, et al. Should we screen for asymptomatic left ventricular dysfunction to prevent heart failure? *Eur Heart J.* 1998;19:842–846.

33. Hunt SA, Abraham WT, Chin MH, et al. ACC/AHA 2005 guideline update for the diagnosis and management of chronic heart failure in the adult—summary article: a report of the American College of Cardiology/American Heart Association Task Force on practice guidelines (writing committee to update the 2001 guidelines for the evaluation and management of heart failure): developed in collaboration with the American College of Chest Physicians and the International Society for Heart and Lung Transplantation: endorsed by the Heart Rhythm Society. *Circulation.* 2005; 112:1825–1852.

CHAPTER 2

The Epidemic of Heart Failure

MIKHAIL KOSIBOROD, MD/HARLAN M. KRUMHOLZ, MD, SM

▶ INTRODUCTION

The epidemic of heart failure (HF) is perhaps one of the most important and challenging public health issues in the United States today. Recent decades have seen a dramatic rise in the number of persons who carry the HF diagnosis and the number of HF-related hospitalizations, as well as the resulting economic impact on the health-care system. Current estimates by the American Heart Association report that 5.2 million Americans have HF.[1] In addition, 600,000 incident cases and more than 1 million hospitalizations occur annually at a cost of >$33 billion.[1] If current trends in incidence and survival remain constant, studies project marked future increases in both HF prevalence and cost.[2] This review will focus on recent epidemiologic trends and will concentrate on the latest scientific contributions to the field of HF epidemiology.

▶ INCIDENCE

As background to any discussion of current trends in HF incidence, it is important to understand the limitations of the data available to researchers. No national HF surveillance system exists, and current data on HF incidence are derived primarily from cohort studies and administrative databases. Cohort studies, such as the Framingham Heart Study and Rochester Epidemiology Project, provide the most reliable information, as they include data from both inpatients and outpatients diagnosed with HF, and have the ability to apply standard validated criteria for HF diagnosis consistently over decades of follow-up. However, these cohort studies analyze relatively small homogeneous patient populations in limited geographic regions, and their findings may not reflect the experience of diverse populations across the

United States. Although large administrative database studies generally overcome these limitations by evaluating populations of patients across broad geographic regions, they have several major shortcomings as well. First, they are typically limited to patients hospitalized with HF, and do not include those diagnosed in the outpatient setting. Second, they frequently rely on administrative billing codes for HF diagnosis, which are less accurate than clinical diagnostic criteria and may substantially underestimate the number of HF-related hospitalizations.[3] Finally, administrative databases usually do not provide detailed clinical information on important clinical variables such as HF etiology and left ventricular systolic function. Nevertheless, despite their limitations, recent studies of HF incidence offer important epidemiological insights.

Data from the Framingham Heart Study indicate that HF incidence in the United States is quite high. Lloyd-Jones and colleagues demonstrated that the lifetime risk of developing HF at the age of 40 years is close to 20% in both men and women.[4] In another Framingham study of age-adjusted HF incidence trends between the 1950s and 1990s, Levy and colleagues showed an overall trend toward lower age-adjusted HF incidence during this time period that was statistically significant in women. (Table 2-1).[5] Specifically, the age-adjusted incidence decreased from 627 to 564/100,000

person-years in men (7% relative risk reduction) and from 420 to 327/100,000 person-years in women (31% relative reduction) between the periods of 1950–1969 and 1990–1999.[5] However, close analysis of the data indicates that the reduction in HF incidence actually took place between the periods of 1950–1969 and 1970–1979. In fact, it appears that no decrease in HF incidence has occurred since the 1970s.

Other studies have reported a trend of stable or even increasing age-adjusted incidence more recently. Data from the Resource Utilization Among Congestive Heart Failure (REACH) study of the Henry Ford Health System indicate that age-adjusted HF incidence cases rose slightly among women from 3.7 to 4.2 cases/1000 patients, while there was a trivial decline among men from 4.0 to 3.7 cases/1000 patients between 1989 and 1999 (neither change was statistically significant).[6] Findings of the Rochester Epidemiology Project from Olmsted County, Minnesota, show that there has been a nonsignificant increase in age-adjusted HF incidence of 4% in men and 11% in women between the periods of 1979–1984 and 1996–2000.[7]

It is somewhat surprising that the age-adjusted HF incidence has not declined in the past 20–30 years. Recent data suggest that the control of hypertension has improved in recent years.[8] Hypertension remains one of the main risk factors

▶ **Table 2-1** Temporal trends in the age-adjusted incidence of heart failure

Period	Men Incidence of heart failure (rate/100,000 person year)	Rate ratio	Women Incidence of heart failure (rate/100,000 person year)	Rate ratio
1950–1969*	627 (475–779)	1	420 (336–504)	1
1970–1979	563 (437–689)	0.87 (0.67–1.14)	311 (249–373)	0.63 (0.47–0.84)
1980–1989	536 (448–623)	0.87 (0.67–1.13)	298 (247–350)	0.60 (0.45–0.79)
1990–1999	564 (463–665)	0.93 (0.71–1.23)	327 (266–388)	0.69 (0.51–0.93)

All values were adjusted for age (<55, 55–64, 65–74, 75–84, and >85 years). Values in parantheses are 95% confidence intervals.
*This period served as the reference period.
Source: Reprinted with permission from Levy et al. *N Engl J Med.* 2002;347:1397–402, Massachusetts Medical Society.

for HF, precedes HF in >90% of patients, and has a 39% population-attributable risk of HF in men and a 59% population-attributable risk in women.[9] According to the Framingham Heart Study, the lifetime risk of HF doubles in patients with blood pressure ≥160/100 mm Hg compared with those who have blood pressure <140/90 mm Hg.[4] Data from the National Health And Nutrition Examination Survey (NHANES) showed that there were small improvements in the proportion of patients who were treated and whose hypertension was controlled (6% and 6.4%, respectively) between 1988 and 1991 and 1999 and 2000.[8]

Furthermore, recent trends in the epidemiology of myocardial infarction (MI) and coronary artery disease also suggest that age-adjusted incidence of HF should be declining. Several studies have documented better survival in patients with acute MI, such as the community-based study of patients hospitalized in Worcester, Massachusetts, that showed a decline in in-hospital mortality from 17.8% to 11.7% between the mid-1970s and 1990s.[10] However, the incidence of MI has remained unchanged during the same time period. According to data from the Rochester Epidemiology Project, the age and sex-adjusted incidence of MI experienced a nonsignificant 6% decline between 1979 and 1998.[11] The incidence of all coronary artery disease has also remained relatively stable, with a nonsignificant 9% decline between 1988 and 1998.[11] Although it has been hypothesized that better survival after MI without concomitant decline in its incidence may result in higher incidence of post-MI HF, this notion is not supported by evidence. In fact, better management of patients following MI has resulted in declining post-MI HF incidence rates (28% relative risk reduction during 1979–1994, mean follow-up 7.6 years) according to the data from Olmsted County, Minnesota.[12]

One of the key reasons for the lack of decline in age-adjusted HF incidence is the increasing prevalence of several important HF risk factors. Recent data from NHANES demonstrated that the prevalence of hypertension increased by 3.7% between 1988 and 1991 and 1999 and 2000.[8] Further, although treatment and control of

hypertension improved by 6% and 6.4%, respectively, 69% of patients still did not have adequate hypertension control.[8] Similar findings were observed in the Cardiovascular Health Study, which showed that although treatment of blood pressure improved among elderly patients, it was still suboptimal, with more than half of the patients not having adequate hypertension control.[13] Rising obesity rates may be contributing to the current lack of improvement in HF incidence as well. Data from the Framingham Heart Study indicate that the risk of developing HF in obese patients (body mass index >30) is double that of patients with normal body mass index, and after adjustment for established risk factors there is a 5–7% rise in the relative risk of HF with every 1 point increase in body mass index.[14] According to data from NHANES and the Behavioral Risk Factor Surveillance System (BRFSS), the prevalence of obesity has been rising dramatically over the last decade.[15-19] Possibly related to increased obesity rates, the prevalence of diabetes is on the rise as well.[20] Diabetes has been shown to be a significant risk factor for HF,[21] and the data from NHANES show that the control of glucose, hypertension, and hyperlipidemia remains poor among diabetic patients, and did not improve from 1988 to 2000.[22] The rising prevalence of obesity and diabetes are important contributors to the lack of improvement in age-adjusted HF incidence rates, and will likely become even more important in the near future.

Although data on the temporal trends in overall (not age-adjusted) HF incidence are lacking, incidence is likely to increase in the near future because of the aging of the American population. Data from the REACH study clearly show a dramatic increase in HF incidence with age (Fig. 2-1), with a rate as high as 40/1000 in women aged >85 years, and even higher in similarly aged men.[6] A European study from Rotterdam confirms these findings and shows that incidence rate increases with age from 1.4/1000 person-years in those aged 55–59 to 47.4/1000 person-years in those aged ≥90.[23] Thus, the rising number of elderly persons in the United States will invariably affect the

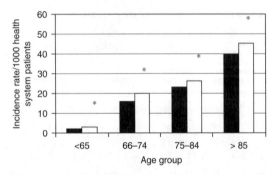

Figure 2-1   Incident cases of heart failure in men (white bars) and women (black bars) by age group in the Resource Utilization Among Congestive Heart Failure study (REACH). P < 0.0000001 for all pairwise comparisons. (Reprinted with permission from McCullough, et al. Confirmation of a heart failure epidemic: findings from the Resource Utilization Among Congestive Heart Failure (REACH) study. *J Am Coll Cardiol.* 2002;39:60–69.)

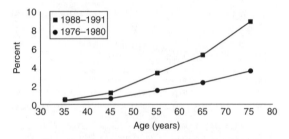

Figure 2-2   Prevalence of congestive heart failure by age, 1976–1980 and 1988–1991. (Adapted from the National Hospital Discharge Survey, National Center for Health Statistics.)

number of new HF diagnoses, even if age-adjusted incidence remains stable.

▶ PREVALENCE

There has been a marked rise in the prevalence of HF over the past 2–3 decades. The American Heart Association estimates that in 2004, 5.2 million patients had the diagnosis of HF in the United States—an increase from the 1 to 2 million estimated during the period of 1971–1975.[1] Similar to incidence, the prevalence of HF rises markedly with age. According to data from the Cardiovascular Health Study, the prevalence of HF rises from 4% in women aged 70–74 years to 14% in women aged >85 years, with a comparable marked increase among similarly aged men.[24] Comparable observations were made in the Rotterdam study from Europe, with prevalence increasing from 0.9% in subjects aged 55–64 years to 17.4% in those aged ≥85 years.[23]

Analysis of temporal trends in HF prevalence from NHANES shows dramatic increases among all age groups between the late 1970s and early 1990s, although the most rapid increase took place among the elderly (Fig. 2-2). Experience from the individual health-care systems also shows that substantial increases in HF prevalence took place during the 1990s. Data from REACH demonstrate that age-adjusted HF prevalence has increased from 3.7% to 14.3% in women and from 4.0 to 14.5/1000 patients in men during 1989–1999.[6]

Again, the aging of the American population is likely one of the important factors behind the rising prevalence rates (Fig. 2-3). The U.S. Bureau of the Census estimates that the number of persons aged >65 years has increased by nearly 4 million and the number of very elderly (those aged >85 years) increased by 1.2 million between 1990 and 2000.[25] More importantly, future projections suggest that the proportion of patients aged >60 years will increase dramatically from 16.5% in 1997 to 24.6% in 2025, with the actual number of older Americans nearly doubling from >44 million to >82.5 million during the same time period.[26] Given the higher HF prevalence in the elderly, the continuous rise in the overall numbers as well as proportion of patients with the diagnosis is likely to continue. In fact, a recent study from Scotland projects that even if the overall HF prevalence rates in the population do not increase, the aging of the population itself will cause a 17–31% increase in the number of patients with HF between 2000 and 2020.[2,27]

The other two likely contributors to the rising prevalence rates are current trends in HF

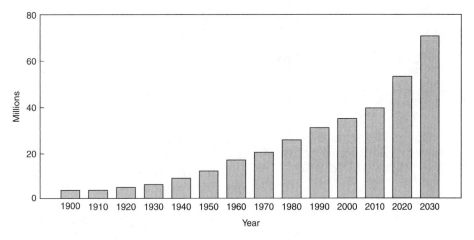

Figure 2-3   Growth of the elderly population, 1900–2030. (Adapted from the U. S. Bureau of the Census.)

incidence and mortality. As mentioned above, there is no convincing evidence that HF incidence is declining. Furthermore, the most recent data from the Framingham Heart Study and Rochester Epidemiology Project suggest that the long-term survival of HF patients has been improving over the past 2–4 decades.[5,7] With no decrease in the number of patients diagnosed each year, and better long-term survival, it is inevitable that prevalence rates will continue to climb.

► HOSPITALIZATIONS AND ECONOMIC BURDEN

The increase in HF hospitalizations has been even more dramatic than the rise in the numbers of patients with HF during the past two to three decades (Fig. 2-4). According to data from the National Hospital Discharge Survey, there was a 189% increase in the number of patients hospitalized with HF as the primary discharge diagnosis

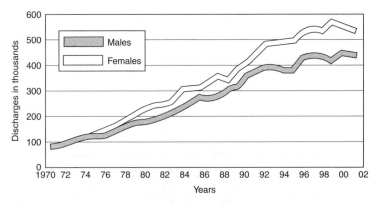

Figure 2-4   Hospital discharges for congestive heart failure by sex: United States, 1970–2002. (Adapted from the American Heart Association Heart Disease and Stroke Statistics, 2005. [update] Available at: http://www.americanheart.org/presenter.jhtml?identifier=3000090.)

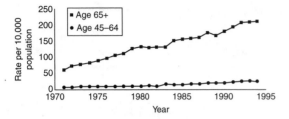

Figure 2-5 Hospitalization rates for congestive heart failure by age, 1971–1994. (Adapted from the National Hospital Discharge Survey, National Center for Health Statistics.)

between 1979 and 1999, specifically, from 377,000 to 1,088,349.[1,28] Most of the increase, once again, has been among the elderly (Fig. 2-5). This is directly translated to considerable economic impact on society; in 2005, the American Heart Association estimated that the direct cost of HF will be >25 billion dollars, with hospital charges accounting for nearly 60% of this cost.[1]

A substantial proportion of HF-related hospitalizations is accounted for by readmissions of patients previously hospitalized with HF. In one study, 44% of patients hospitalized with a primary discharge diagnosis of HF were readmitted within 6 months.[29] Economic analysis of HF-related

admissions showed that the average cost of repeat hospitalization was in excess of $7000 per patient.[30] There is also evidence that HF-related hospital readmissions are on the rise, possibly due to shorter hospital length of stay. The studies of Medicare beneficiaries with HF show a 9% increase in the odds of hospital readmission at 30 days during the period of 1993–1999.[31]

Although European countries have experienced a similar epidemic increase in HF-related hospitalizations during the late 1980s and early 1990s, recent data from Scotland suggest that the number of hospitalizations peaked in 1993–1994 and leveled off during 1995–1996 among both women and men (Fig. 2-6).[32] Similar observations were made in Canada, where the number of HF hospitalizations decreased by 7% between 1994 and 1995 and 1999 and 2000.[33] There is evidence that a similar plateau may be occurring in the United States. The National Hospital Discharge Survey indicates that the number of hospitalizations peaked in the late 1990s, and decreased to 970,000 in 2002.[1] Although the cause of this plateau is not well understood, it is possible that recent advances in HF management, including pharmacologic and disease management interventions, have decreased the number of preventable HF hospitalizations.

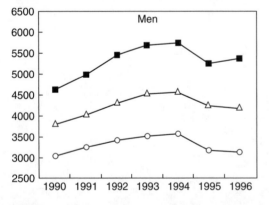

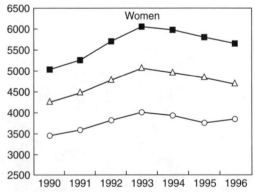

Figure 2-6 Sex-specific trends in the number of hospitalizations for heart failure as the principal diagnosis and the number of patients who contributed to these (including those with a "first ever" hospitalization), 1990–1996. ■ = total hospitalizations (principal diagnosis), Δ = number of individual patients hospitalized (principal diagnosis), and ○ = number of individual patients with a "first ever" hospitalization for heart failure (principal diagnosis). (Reprinted with permission from Stewart S, et al. *Eur Heart J.* 2001;22:209–217.)

Nevertheless, projections for trends in HF hospitalizations and associated cost are bleak. Studies from Scotland predict a 12–34% increase in HF hospitalizations by the year 2020 and in Canada the rate is expected to double by the year 2025.[2,34] Data from Canada suggest that to keep the number of new HF hospitalizations at the current level, the incidence of HF will need to decrease by 2.6% yearly.[34]

▶ OUTCOMES

Multiple studies have documented that despite recent advances in HF management, short- and long-term mortality rates remain alarmingly high. Data from the Framingham Heart Study show that age-adjusted 30-day, 1-year, and 5-year mortality in HF patients from 1990 to 1999 were 10–13%, 24–28%, and 45–59% respectively.[5] A study from the Rochester Epidemiology Project reported lower 30-day (4–6%) and 6-month (17–21%), but similar 5-year (46–50%) mortality during 1996–2000.[7] The mortality estimates from administrative database studies are even more staggering. A recent study of Medicare beneficiaries hospitalized with HF demonstrated 1-year HF mortality of nearly 32%,[31] while a report from the National Health Service in Scotland showed that the overall case-fatality rate among both inpatients and outpatients with HF during 1986–1995 was as high as 44% at 1 year and 76% at 5 years.[35]

Several recent reports have suggested that longer-term HF mortality has been improving over the past several decades. Levy and others demonstrated that 5-year mortality has declined from 70% to 59% in men, and from 57% to 45% in women between the periods of 1950–1969 and 1990–1999, an overall relative risk decrease of 32% (Table 2-2).[5] Considerable improvement in long-term HF survival was also seen in the Rochester Epidemiology Project, with a 28–52% decrease in the relative risk of long-term mortality among men between the periods of 1979–1984 and 1996–2000.[7] The relative risk reduction among women was more modest (6–33%) and not statistically significant in women aged >80 years.[7] Finally, a study of the entire HF patient population in Scotland showed that median survival improved from 1.23 to 1.64 years from 1986 to 1995.[35]

Interestingly, this improvement in long-term survival is likely contributing to the rising HF prevalence and hospitalization rates. As patients with HF live longer, and HF incidence does not decline, the total number of HF patients will rise and utilization of health-care services by these patients will be increasing. Scientific simulations and forecasts clearly show that increasing health-care utilization in the face of decreasing mortality is not a paradox, but in fact an anticipated tradeoff of lower mortality for higher morbidity, which is further compounded by the aging of the American population.[27]

▶ **Table 2-2** Temporal trends in age-adjusted mortality after the onset of heart failure among men and women aged 65–74 years of age

	30-Day Mortality		1-Year Mortality		5-Year Mortality	
	Men	Women	Men	Women	Men	Women
Period	(% [95% Confidence Interval])					
1950–1969	12 (4–19)	18 (7–27)	30 (18–40)	28 (16–39)	70 (57–79)	57 (43–67)
1970–1979	15 (7–23)	16 (6–24)	41 (29–51)	28 (17–38)	75 (65–83)	59 (45–69)
1980–1989	12 (5–18)	10 (4–16)	33 (23–42)	27 (17–35)	65 (54–73)	51 (39–60)
1990–1999	11 (4–17)	10 (3–15)	28 (18–36)	24 (14–33)	59 (47–68)	45 (33–55)

All values were adjusted for age (<55, 55–64, 65–74, 75–84, and >85 years).
Source: Reprinted with permission from Levy et al. *N Engl J Med.* 2002;347:1397–402, Massachusetts Medical Society.

Whether long-term HF mortality has continued to improve during the 1990s is less clear. Although one study of Medicare beneficiaries in Northeast Ohio showed a 14.6% relative risk decline in 1-year mortality during 1991–1997, other studies have been less convincing.[36] Although analysis of administrative data from Ontario, Canada, showed an overall trend towards lower 1-year mortality during 1992–2000, examination of the crude data from that study suggests that most of the improvement occurred between 1992 and 1993, with minimal change thereafter.[37] The study of temporal mortality trends among Medicare beneficiaries during the 1990s similarly showed a decline in 1-year mortality between 1993 and 1994, but suggested no subsequent improvement after 1994.[31] No statistically significant difference in 1-year case fatality rates could be found in the study of the Henry Ford Health System patients with HF from 1989 to 1999.[6]

Data on temporal trends in short-term HF mortality are also mixed. The above mentioned study of HF patients in Scotland showed a 17–26% relative risk reduction in 30-day HF mortality from 1986 to 1995, and the study of Medicare patients in Northeast Ohio demonstrated a 12% relative risk reduction in 30-day mortality from 1991–1997.[35,36] However, recent studies of very large patient populations in Canada and the United States did not show similar 30-day mortality improvements. The study of 77,421 patients from Ontario, Canada, did not show any trend towards better 30-day mortality either among all patients or hospitalization survivors during 1992–2000.[37] Recent analysis of 3,957,520 Medicare beneficiaries hospitalized with the primary discharge diagnosis of HF showed that there was no significant change in risk-adjusted 30-day mortality between 1993 and 1999.[31] Although most studies show a clear and significant decrease in in-hospital mortality during the 1990s (nearly 50% relative risk reduction between 1991 and 1997 in one study), this appears to be mostly explained by a dramatic decrease in the mean length of stay among the hospitalized HF patients during the same time period.[36] In fact, it appears that mortality immediately following hospital discharge

(postdischarge mortality) increased from 1991 to 1997, suggesting that although fewer patients die during hospitalizations, more HF patients die out of hospital with no overall change in short-term mortality (Fig. 2-7).[36]

Overall, it appears that although the outcomes of HF patients improved over the past several decades, recent progress has been modest at best. This is somewhat paradoxical, as some of the most dramatic advances in HF management took place during the 1990s. There are several likely explanations. The vast and rising majority of HF patients are elderly. Less than 20% of elderly HF patients fit enrollment criteria for angiotensin-converting enzyme (ACE) inhibitor and β-blocker clinical trials.[38] Due to their high burden of comorbid illness, many elderly HF patients have contraindications to these therapies. In addition, more than half have HF with preserved left ventricular systolic function, a condition in which the efficacy of ACE inhibitors and β-blockers has not been established.[39]

Recent studies of Medicare beneficiaries hospitalized with HF demonstrate that there is underuse and misuse of evidence-based therapies. Among those patients who were "ideal candidates" for ACE inhibitor and spironolactone therapies, <70% and 25%, respectively, were

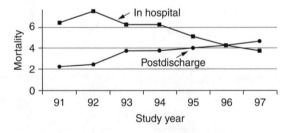

Figure 2-7 Trends in unadjusted in-hospital (■) and postdischarge (between discharge and 30 days after admission [●]) mortality rates from 1991 to 1997 for Medicare patients discharged with a principal diagnosis of heart failure from 29 hospitals participating in the Cleveland Health Quality Choice Program. All trends significant at P < 0.001. (Modified with permission from Baker, et al. *Am Heart J.* 2003;146:258–264.)

treated.[40] Data from the Cardiovascular Health Study showed that <20% of elderly patients with HF were being treated with both an ACE inhibitor and β-blocker during the 1990s.[41] Further, there is evidence that some therapies may be prescribed to patients at high risk for medication side effects. For example, nearly 31% of spironolactone prescriptions in the Medicare population were given to patients who had a major contraindication to that drug.[42]

Another possible explanation for the apparent lack of major improvement in outcomes over the past decade is that recent advances in HF management are preventing HF hospitalizations, thus resulting in an overall "sicker" population of HF patients being hospitalized over time. Since studies based on administrative data typically focus on hospitalized HF patients, apparent lack of improvement in HF outcomes could be partially due to this selection bias.

► CONCLUSION

Given the aging of the American population, no clear change in HF incidence, and improving long-term survival of patients with established HF over the last 20–30 years, the overall number of patients with HF will likely continue to increase substantially in the near future. This may have a profound effect on both the number of HF-related hospitalizations and the economic impact on the health-care system. Although further innovations in HF management and cost-saving interventions such as disease management are important, better primary HF prevention appears to be the critical factor in stemming the current HF epidemic. This will undoubtedly involve better detection and treatment of key HF risk factors, including hypertension, coronary artery disease, obesity, diabetes, and valvular disease.

► REFERENCES

1. American Heart Association. Heart Disease and Stroke Statistics—2007 Update. Available at: www.americanheart.org/presenter.jhtml?identifier=3000090. Accessed April 6, 2007.

2. Stewart S, MacIntyre K, Capewell S, et al. Heart failure and the aging population: an increasing burden in the 21st century? *Heart (British Cardiac Society)*. 2003;89:49–53.

3. Khand AU, Shaw M, Gemmel I, et al. Do discharge codes underestimate hospitalisation due to heart failure: validation study of hospital discharge coding for heart failure. *Eur J Heart Fail*. 2005;7:792–797.

4. Lloyd-Jones DM, Larson MG, Leip EP, et al. Lifetime risk for developing congestive heart failure: the Framingham Heart Study. *Circulation*. 2002;106:3068–3072.

5. Levy D, Kenchaiah S, Larson MG, et al. Long-term trends in the incidence of and survival with heart failure. *N Engl J Med*. 2002;347:1397–1402.

6. McCullough PA, Philbin EF, Spertus JA, et al. Confirmation of a heart failure epidemic: findings from the Resource Utilization Among Congestive Heart Failure (REACH) study. *J Am Coll Cardiol*. 2002;39:60–69.

7. Roger VL, Weston SA, Redfield MM, et al. Trends in heart failure incidence and survival in a community-based population. *JAMA*. 2004;292:344–350.

8. Hajjar I, Kotchen TA. Trends in prevalence, awareness, treatment, and control of hypertension in the United States, 1988–2000. *JAMA*. 2003;290:199–206.

9. Levy D, Larson MG, Vasan RS, et al. The progression from hypertension to congestive heart failure. *JAMA*. 1996;275:1557–1562.

10. Goldberg RJ, Yarzebski J, Lessard D, et al. A two-decades (1975 to 1995) long experience in the incidence, in-hospital and long-term case-fatality rates of acute myocardial infarction: a community-wide perspective. *J Am Coll Cardiol*. 1999;33: 1533–1539.

11. Arciero TJ, Jacobsen SJ, Reeder GS, et al. Temporal trends in the incidence of coronary disease. *Am J Med*. 2004;117:228–233.

12. Hellermann JP, Goraya TY, Jacobsen SJ, et al. Incidence of heart failure after myocardial infarction: is it changing over time? *Am J Epidemiol*. 2003;157:1101–1107.

13. Psaty BM, Manolio TA, Smith NL, et al. Time trends in high blood pressure control and the use of antihypertensive medications in older adults: the Cardiovascular Health Study. *Arch Intern Med*. 2002;162:2325–2332.

14. Kenchaiah S, Evans JC, Levy D, et al. Obesity and the risk of heart failure. *N Engl J Med*. 2002; 347:305–313.

15. Mokdad AH, Bowman BA, Ford ES, et al. The continuing epidemics of obesity and diabetes in the United States. *JAMA*. 2001;286:1195–1200.

16. Mokdad AH, Ford ES, Bowman BA, et al. Prevalence of obesity, diabetes, and obesity-related health risk factors, 2001. *JAMA*. 2003;289: 76–79.

17. Mokdad AH, Serdula MK, Dietz WH, et al. The spread of the obesity epidemic in the United States, 1991–1998. *JAMA*. 1999;282:1519–1522.

18. Mokdad AH, Serdula MK, Dietz WH, et al. The continuing epidemic of obesity in the United States. *JAMA*. 2000;284:1650–1651.

19. Ford ES, Mokdad AH, Giles WH. Trends in waist circumference among U.S. adults. *Obes Res*. 2003; 11:1223–1231.

20. Mokdad AH, Ford ES, Bowman BA, et al. Diabetes trends in the U.S.: 1990–1998. *Diabetes Care*. 2000;23:1278–1283.

21. He J, Ogden LG, Bazzano LA, et al. Risk factors for congestive heart failure in US men and women: NHANES I epidemiologic follow-up study. *Arch Intern Med*. 2001;161:996–1002.

22. Saydah SH, Fradkin J, Cowie CC. Poor control of risk factors for vascular disease among adults with previously diagnosed diabetes. *JAMA*. 2004;291:335–342.

23. Bleumink GS, Knetsch AM, et al. Quantifying the heart failure epidemic: prevalence, incidence rate, lifetime risk and prognosis of heart failure: the Rotterdam Study. *Eur Heart J*. 2004;25: 1614–1619.

24. Kitzman DW, Gardin JM, Gottdiener JS, CHS Research Group. Cardiovascular Health Study. Importance of heart failure with preserved systolic function in patients > or = 65 years of age. *Am J Cardiol*. 2001;87:413–419.

25. United States Department of Commerce, Economics and Statistics Administration. Bureau of the Census. The 65 years and over population: 2000. Census 2000 brief. Available at: http://www.census.gov/prod/2001pubs/c2kbr0 1-10.pdf. Accessed October 14, 2005.

26. United States Department of Commerce, Economics and Statistics Administration. Bureau of the Census. Aging of the Americas into the XXI century. Available at: http://www.census.gov/ipc/prod/ ageame.pdf. Accessed October 14, 2005.

27. Bonneux L, Barendregt JJ, Meeter K, et al. Estimating clinical morbidity due to ischemic heart disease and congestive heart failure: the future rise of heart failure. *Am J Public Health*. 1994;84:20–28.

28. Koelling TM, Chen RS, Lubwama RN, et al. The expanding national burden of heart failure in the United States: the influence of heart failure in women. *Am Heart J*. 2004;147:74–78.

29. Krumholz HM, Parent EM, Tu N, et al. Readmission after hospitalization for congestive heart failure among Medicare beneficiaries. *Arch Intern Med*. 1997;157:99–104.

30. Wexler DJ, Chen J, Smith GL, et al. Predictors of costs of caring for elderly patients discharged with heart failure. *Am Heart J*. 2001;142:350–357.

31. Kosiborod M, Lichtman JH, Heidenneich PA, et al. National trends in outcomes among elderly patients with heart failure. *Am J Med*. 2006; 119 (616):e1–e7.

32. Stewart S, MacIntyre K, MacLeod MM, et al. Trends in hospitalization for heart failure in Scotland, 1990–1996: an epidemic that has reached its peak? *Eur Heart J*. 2001;22:209–217.

33. Hall RE, Tu JV. Hospitalization rates and length of stay for cardiovascular conditions in Canada, 1994 to 1999. *Can J Cardiol*. 2003;19:1123–1131.

34. Johansen H, Strauss B, Arnold JM, et al. On the rise: the current and projected future burden of congestive heart failure hospitalization in Canada. *Can J Cardiol*. 2003;19:430–435.

35. MacIntyre K, Capewell S, Stewart S, et al. Evidence of improving prognosis in heart failure: trends in case fatality in 66 547 patients hospitalized between 1986 and 1995. *Circulation*. 2000;102:1126–1131.

36. Baker DW, Einstadter D, Thomas C, et al. Mortality trends for 23,505 Medicare patients hospitalized with heart failure in Northeast Ohio, 1991 to 1997. *Am Heart J*. 2003;146: 258–264.

37. Lee DS, Mamdani MM, Austin PC, et al. Trends in heart failure outcomes and pharmacotherapy: 1992 to 2000. *Am J Med*. 2004;116:581–589.

38. Masoudi FA, Havranek EP, Wolfe P, et al. Most hospitalized older persons do not meet the enrollment criteria for clinical trials in heart failure. *Am Heart J*. 2003;146:250–257.

39. Gottdiener JS, McClelland RL, Marshall R, et al. Outcome of congestive heart failure in elderly persons: influence of left ventricular systolic function. The Cardiovascular Health Study. *Ann Intern Med*. 2002;137:631–639.

40. Masoudi FA, Rathore SS, Wang Y, et al. National patterns of use and effectiveness of angiotensin-converting enzyme inhibitors in older patients with heart failure and left ventricular systolic dysfunction. *Circulation*. 2004;110:724–731.

41. Smith NL, Chan JD, Rea TD, et al. Time trends in the use of β-blockers and other pharmacotherapies in older adults with congestive heart failure. *Am Heart J*. 2004;148:710–717.

42. Masoudi FA, Gross CP, Wang Y, et al. Adoption of spironolactone therapy for older patients with heart failure and left ventricular systolic dysfunction in the United States, 1998–2001. *Circulation*. 2005;112:39–47.

CHAPTER 3

What Causes Heart Failure?

Alexander R. Lyon, MA, BM, BCh, MRCP/Philip A.
Poole-Wilson, MD, FRCP, FMedSci

▶ INTRODUCTION

Heart failure is a clinical entity diagnosed by doctors. The key features of the syndrome are an abnormality of the heart and the presence of symptoms, typically, tiredness and shortness of breath, which is worse on exercise. Heart failure is common, becoming more common, can be easily diagnosed, is detectable, and effective treatments are available. Death in heart failure occurs most commonly as a result of a cardiac event such as an arrhythmia (sudden death), ischemia of the heart muscle (e.g., myocardial infarction, heart attack), or decompensated heart failure. Thus the natural history of heart failure begins and ends with the heart (Fig. 3-1). But almost all of the clinical characteristics of patients with heart failure result from persistent stimulation of interacting compensatory mechanisms not just in the heart but in the peripheral circulation and body organs. The clinical manifestations and pathophysiology of heart failure should be considered as a multi-system disease.

▶ DEFINITION

The most widely quoted definition of heart failure is that heart failure is "A pathophysiological state in which an abnormality of cardiac function is responsible for the failure of the heart to pump blood at a rate commensurate with the requirements of the metabolising tissues."[1] Other early definitions have emphasized one or other

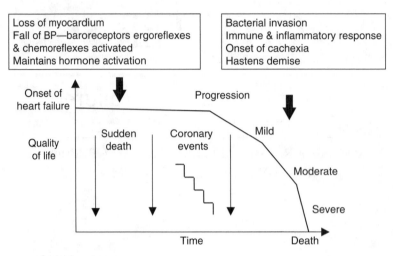

Figure 3-1   Progression of heart failure.

physiological or biochemical abnormalities. More recently, definitions have emphasized the clinical nature of heart failure, for example, "A clinical syndrome caused by an abnormality of the heart and recognized by a characteristic pattern of haemodynamic, renal, neural, and hormonal responses."[2,3] The European Society of Cardiology emphasized the need for three criteria: typical symptoms and signs, an abnormality of the heart, and preferably a response to treatment.[4] More recently the American College of Cardiology and the American Heart Association stated "Heart failure is a complex clinical syndrome that can result from any structural or functional cardiac disorder that impairs the ability of the ventricle to fill with or eject blood." A similar definition has been used in major guidelines.[5]

These recent definitions encompass the obvious central premise that a primary disease or dysfunction of the heart is present. Cardiac failure is a syndrome, not a specific disease. Management should be targeted to treat the cause as well as the spectrum of pathophysiology that comprises the syndrome. Thus, it is logical to classify the causes of cardiac failure based upon disease pathology.

▶ **DIFFERENT SYNDROMES REFERRED TO AS HEART FAILURE TO AND FUNDAMENTAL CAUSES**

A simple but clinically useful way to consider heart failure is to first make the distinction between acute heart failure, shock, and chronic heart failure (Table 3-1). Acute heart failure is synonymous with pulmonary edema and is a medical emergency. The extreme symptom of breathlessness is closely related to the elevated left ventricular pressure. Shock is a condition characterized by a low systolic blood pressure (systolic pressure <90 mm Hg), oliguria or anuria, and evidence

▶ **Table 3-1** Syndromes of heart failure

Entity	Synonym or variant
Acute heart failure	Pulmonary edema
Circulatory collapse	Cardiogenic shock (poor peripheral perfusion, oliguria, hypotension)
Chronic heart failure	Untreated, overt, congestive, undulating, treated, compensated

▶ **Table 3-2** General categories for causes of heart failure

1. Myocardial disease
2. Valve disease
3. Pericardial disease
4. Congenital heart disease
5. Arrhythmias

▶ **Table 3-4** Fundamental abnormalities in failing myocardium

1. Loss of muscle
2. Incoordinate contraction and abnormal timing of contraction
3. Extracellular
   Fibrosis, altered extracellular architecture, shape and size of ventricle, slippage of cells, fiber orientation
4. Cellular
   Change of cell structure
   Loss of intracellular matrix, hypertrophy, hyperplasia
   Change of cell function—systolic and/or diastolic
   Loss/aging of intrinsic repair mechanisms
   Molecular
      Calcium release and/or uptake
      Response of contractile proteins to calcium

of a constricted circulation such as cold periphery, sweating, and mental confusion. Chronic heart failure is a condition where persistent damage to the heart leads to a progressive state with persistent symptoms. Many adjectives are added to the term to emphasize one or other feature (Table 3-1).

The fundamental causes of heart failure are easily stated and reflect the anatomical and physiological features of the heart (Table 3-2). The most common is myocardial disease. Myocardial damage has traditionally been classified as due to one or other manifestation of coronary heart disease or as a cardiomyopathy (Table 3-3). Hypertension is commonly associated with heart failure and particularly with the progression of heart failure. But hypertension is rarely the immediate or only

cause of heart failure. Patients with hypertension often have coronary heart disease because hypertension is an important risk factor causing damage to the endothelium and promoting the development of atherosclerosis. Such classifications focus on clinical characteristics. A different approach is to consider the basic mechanisms of heart failure but that has no clinical application at present (Table 3-4).

Many words are added to the term heart failure (Table 3-5). These are often jargon. Forward and backward failure reflects old ideas on the pathophysiology of heart failure and should no longer be used. Right and left heart failure usually refer to pulmonary edema and breathlessness (left heart failure) or evidence of fluid overload such as raised venous pressure, enlarged liver, and peripheral edema (right heart failure). This jargon

▶ **Table 3-3** Myocardial causes of heart failure

Coronary artery disease	In all its many manifestations
Cardiomyopathy	Dilated (DCM) - specific or idiopathic (IDCM)
	Hypertrophic (HCM or HOCM or ASH)
	Restrictive
	ARVC
Hypertension	
Drugs	β-blockers
	Calcium antagonists
	Antiarrhythmics
Other or unknown	

DCM—dilated cardiomyopathy; IDCM—idiopathic dilated cardiomyopathy; HCM—hypertropic cardiomyopathy; HOCM—hypertropic obstructive cardiomyopathy; ASH—asymmetric septal hypertrophy; ARVC—arrhythmic right ventricular cardiomyopathy

▶ **Table 3-5** Other terms used to describe heart failure

1. Forward and backward heart failure
2. Right and left ventricular failure
3. Systolic and diastolic heart failure
4. High- and low-output heart failure

is largely nonsense, since the commonest cause of right heart failure is left heart failure; fluid retention in chronic heart failure is a consequence of retention of salt and water as a result of underperfusion of the kidney.

In recent years, a distinction has been made between systolic and diastolic heart failure. Diastolic heart failure is often referred to as heart failure with preserved ventricular function. This distinction is the source of much discussion and controversy. In simple terms, diastolic function exists when the heart remains of a normal size and systolic heart failure exists when the heart is enlarged. The old adage was that "a big heart is a bad heart." Diastolic heart failure is common in the elderly and in the presence of myocardial ischemia and hypertension.

One further distinction is of clinical importance. There exists a group of conditions where the cardiac output is greatly elevated in the presence of symptoms and signs identical to those found in heart failure (Table 3-6). This is often referred to as high-output heart failure but such a phrase is misleading as the fundamental cause is not the heart but other features of the circulation or body systems. A better terminology is to refer to these conditions as circulatory failure.

Diseases of any of the constitutive component tissues of the heart and associated great vessels can result in cardiac failure. The etiology can be approached from a reductionist perspective, starting at the whole organ and tissue level, and progressing to the cellular, subcellular, and molecular causes (proteomic and genomic), or vice versa from the expansionist perspective,

▶ **Table 3-6** Causes of circulatory failure (high-output cardiac failure)

Anemia
Thyrotoxicosis
Beriberi
Arteriovenous fistula
Cirrhosis of the liver
Paget's disease
Pregnancy
Renal cell carcinoma

starting at the molecular level, and "expanding up to the tissue and organ level."

The prevalence of the different causes varies depending upon gender, age, and geographical region. In the Caucasian population of Western Europe, the United States, and Australasia, ischemic heart disease predominates, whereas in the Afro-Caribbean population, hypertension is the commonest cause. Chagas' disease caused by the parasite *Trypanosoma cruzi* is responsible for 20% of cardiac failure in South America/Brazil,[6] but is only seen in returning travelers and immigrants from this region in European hospitals.

Coronary Heart Disease—Acute Occlusion

Coronary heart disease, consequent to atherosclerosis, is the commonest cause of heart failure in Western populations, accounting for up to 70% of cases.[7,8] The heart is critically dependent on a supply of oxygen from the coronary circulation; the adenosine triphosphate (ATP) in heart muscle will support about five beats. An acute coronary occlusion causes diastolic contractile dysfunction within 6 seconds and systolic dysfunction within 20 seconds. Intracellular acidosis develops with the switch from aerobic to anaerobic metabolism, and the intracellular accumulation of phosphate from the breakdown of creatine phosphate and ATP. Hydrogen and phosphate ions interfere directly with the contractile proteins to promote the formation of weak myofilament cross bridges. The ATP depletion reduces sarcoplasmic reticulum calcium ATPase and sodium-potassium ATPase activity. The ATP-inhibited K^+ channel opens, and triggers an efflux of potassium out of the cell (within seconds), which is subsequently amplified by reduced sodium-potassium ATPase activity. This disrupts the ionic fluxes across the sarcolemma and reduces the calcium removal from the cytoplasm during diastole, depleting the sarcoplasmic reticulum calcium stores and resulting in smaller systolic calcium transients. Lactate accumulation causes mitochondrial damage and disrupts action potential generation. The result is cardiac tissue with abnormal electrical activity, excitation-contraction coupling, and reduced contractile tension. Total occlusion of the artery leads to hemorrhagic necrosis of the myocardium supplied by the artery, leading to irreversible myocardial infarction. If the occluded coronary is reopened after an initial delay of 30 minutes or more, but before complete necrosis has developed, then the return of oxygen results in the rapid production of free radicals within 2–4 minutes of reperfusion (reperfusion injury).[9] These free radicals damage nucleic acids, cell membranes, and intracellular proteins, initiating the intracellular cascade via the p38 kinase and c-Jun N-terminal kinase pathways, activation of the caspase cascades, resulting in apoptosis and further myocardial damage (Fig. 3-2).

The wave front of infarction starts at the endocardial border and progresses to the epicardium in areas of severe ischemia. The infarcted wall becomes acutely dyskinetic (paradoxical outward movement during systole), and ventricular dilatation begins. This occurs within the constraints of the pericardium, which reaches its limits of compliance in the acute phase and exerts a constrictive effect on the acutely infarcted ventricle. The increase in left ventricular diastolic pressure after acute coronary occlusion in the dog angioplasty model can be inhibited by prior removal of the pericardium.[10]

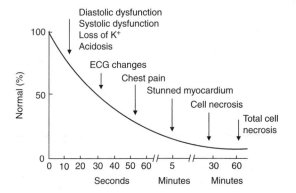

Figure 3-2 Timing of events after onset of myocardial ischemia.

Coronary Heart Disease—Left Ventricular Remodeling

Should the patient survive the acute episode of myocardial infarction, a process of left ventricular remodeling is initiated, with further architectural and structural changes to the ventricle (Tables 3-7 and 3-8). The word was first used in 1982 so as to distinguish between extension of an infarct, expansion of an infarct, and changes in distant myocardium.[11,12] Remodeling occurs in both the infarcted and remaining noninfarcted regions, further contributing to ventricular dysfunction. The extent of ventricular dysfunction depends on the size and location of the infarct, the presence of previous infarcts elsewhere in the heart, the remaining coronary supply with or without collaterals, and the involvement of other cardiac structures, which influence ventricular function such as the conducting tissue, heart valves, and pericardium.

The region of necrosis involves damaged myocytes and disruption of the extracellular matrix. Loss of type I collagen fibers and intermyocyte collagen struts occurs due to activation of matrix metalloproteinases (1, 2, and 9 predominate in the heart), and is replaced by a deposition of collagen III and IV from fibroblasts, stimulated by aldosterone and angiotensin II.[13,14] There is an overall increase in the myocardial collagen content from 5% up to 25%, but it is laid down in an irregular fashion, which disrupts the fine myocardial architecture. This allows myocyte slippage in the longitudinal direction, leading with the loss of cells and vasculature to infarct thinning and expansion.[15,16]

▶ **Table 3-7** Modish terms and concepts in coronary heart disease

1. Stunning
2. Hibernation
3. Mummified myocardium
4. Stuttering ischemia
5. Preconditioning
6. Remodeling
7. Chronic ischemia
8. Ischemic cardiomyopathy

▶ **Table 3-8** Ventricular dysfunction, stunning, hibernation, and clinical syndromes

Acute ventricular dysfunction	Immediate contractile failure (<2 minutes)	Angioplasty (PCI)
	Stunning (approximately >2 minutes <15 minutes) but before any structural change with near-normal coronary flow and dysfunction reversible	Stable or unstable angina Prinzmetal's angina Early thrombolysis Cardiac surgery
Chronic ventricular dysfunction	Early hibernation (hours but <3 months) or repetitive stunning	Unstable angina Post-infarction Silent ischemia
	Chronic hibernation (>3 months) Dysfunction with reduced coronary blood flow but reversible	Stable angina Heart failure due to coronary heart disease Aortic stenosis

PCI—percutaneous coronary intervention

This is more extensive in areas with complete absence of blood supply. The presence of collaterals, or late revascularization of the culprit vessel, reduces infarct expansion. It is more evident in anterior infarcts, and leads to an increase in left ventricular circumference up to 25% during the first week. This expansion alters the geometry of the left ventricle, with the normal ellipsoid shape progressively replaced by a more spherical shape. Sphericity indices have been used to quantify this change, based upon the ratio of the observed biplane ventricular volume divided by the volume of a theoretical ventricle with the same biplane circumference but perfectly spherical geometry. The normal human left ventricle has a sphericity index of 0.66 at end diastole and 0.55 at end systole. After anterior myocardial infarction, the sphericity index increases, with the subsequent reduction in efficiency of blood ejection from the chamber, higher filling pressures, and reduced exercise capacity.[17]

The infarction of one region of the left ventricular wall requires the remaining myocardium to compensate mechanically in order to maintain adequate cardiac output. Eccentric hypertrophy with sarcomeric replication in series occurs,[18] resulting in further increases in ventricular dimensions and compliance. The increased wall stress may stimulate the remaining noninfarcted myocardium to hypertrophy in a concentric manner, most commonly seen at the border zone of the infarct. This process starts 1–2 months after the initial infarction, and may progress for years unless a terminal cardiac event intervenes.

Transient ischemia can produce temporary reduction in contractile function, which is termed myocardial stunning (Tables 3-7 and 3-8). A definition of stunned myocardium (stunning) is mechanical dysfunction that persists after reperfusion despite the absence of irreversible damage and despite the restoration of normal or near-normal coronary flow.[19] The delayed recovery, from a few hours up to several days, occurs despite restoration of normal coronary flow in the absence of irreversible damage. At a cellular level, there is a transient increase in oxygen consumption, despite continuous impairment of mechanical function. This inefficient utilization of oxygen may represent reduced myofilament calcium sensitivity despite increases in cytosolic calcium levels, possibly due to changes in myosin ATPase activity. This is compounded by smaller degrees of free radical production, including nitric oxide-derived free radicals, which also contribute to the dysfunction of myocardial stunning. Stunning can occur in a variety of clinical settings. Early reperfusion after myocardial infarction, whether spontaneous or secondary to therapeutic thrombolysis or primary angioplasty, may salvage ischemic but noninfarcted myocardium within the territory of the culprit vessel. This is of significant importance clinically, as imaging may reveal large areas of akinetic or dyskinetic myocardium in the early post-infarct recovery period, but after allowing the stunned myocardium to recover, the long-term dysfunction may not be so severe, with the associated prognostic implications.[20] During unstable angina, and after exercise in patients with stable but critical epicardial stenoses, regional wall motion abnormalities have been demonstrated, which recover with relief of angina and/or rest.[21] The recovery time is related to the duration of angina on the treadmill or at rest, and may take over 24 hours in severe cases. Myocardial stunning is common after cardiac surgery requiring cardioplegia and cardiopulmonary bypass, due to the global myocardial ischemia generated with cessation of coronary flow.[22] This setting demonstrated that whilst inotropic agents can increase contractile function of stunned myocardium, the increase in oxygen consumption induced by the inotropic stimulation is out of proportion to the mechanical improvement. Sudden increases in myocardial oxygen consumption, such as the catecholamine surges seen in acute subarachnoid hemorrhage and pheochromocytoma patients,[23,24] create a supply-demand mismatch and can cause myocardial stunning.

Hibernating myocardium is another description of myocardial dysfunction, which has become widespread.[25] The word was first used by Diamond in 1978 when he commented, "Reports of sometimes dramatic improvement in segmental left ventricular function following coronary bypass surgery, although not universal, leaves the clear implication that ischemic noninfarcted myocardium can exist in a state of function hibernation."[26] But the term was popularized by Rahimtoola in 1985 who described it thus "A state of persistently impaired myocardial and left ventricular dysfunction at rest due to reduced coronary blood flow that can be partially or completely restored to normal if the myocardial oxygen supply/demand relationship is favorably altered, either by improving blood flow and/or

reducing demand."[27] Hibernation refers to viable myocardium, which is exposed to chronic ischemia, with hypocontractility, which is reversible on restoration of normal blood flow. As implicated by this definition, hibernation can only be diagnosed with absolute accuracy in retrospect after revascularization has been performed. In contrast to the pathology of acute occlusion described earlier, mild-moderate ischemia results in transient reduction of creatine phosphate and increase in lactate production, but by 60–85 minutes these return to near normal, and infarction does not occur, despite persistent hypoperfusion. The subsequent changes may represent an evolutionary "protective" mechanism, as fetal cardiac gene expression patterns are activated, and the chronically ischemic myocytes undergo structural cellular changes with sarcomere loss, increased abundance of glycogen granules, rough endoplasmic reticulum and mitochondria, and an increase in collagen strands.[28] These changes occur over a timescale of days to weeks, and with initially isolated functional hibernation, progressing later to structural and functional hibernation, which may be associated with wall thinning.[29]

The classical changes in left ventricular function caused by coronary artery disease and described above occur within the region supplied by the stenotic or occluded artery. Therefore, regional wall motion abnormalities can be explained by coronary disease. However, global left ventricular dysfunction without regional variation can also be caused by coronary disease. This is usually advanced three vessel disease, and may be the result of infarction, hibernation, and/or stunning. This often occurs in patients without symptoms of angina, who present with symptoms of cardiac failure. In a study of patients with global left ventricular impairment (without a history of ischemic heart disease [symptoms or documented previous history]), 52% of patients <72 years of age had coronary artery disease as defined by at least one epicardial stenosis of ≥50%.[30] Furthermore milder stenoses, which are not flow-limiting, may cause downstream myocardial dysfunction through a variety of mechanisms including cholesterol and thrombus embolism, previous occlusion and recanalization, and as regions initiating focal spasm.

Other Conditions Causing Reduced Coronary Blood Flow

Whilst atherosclerosis is the commonest form of coronary disease, many other conditions can cause heart failure by reducing coronary blood supply. These include congenital coronary anomalies, especially the interarterial anomalous left coronary artery, coronary artery fistulae, the left main stem arising from the pulmonary trunk, and the stenosed "slit-like" left main orifice. Coronary vasculitides, for example, periarteritis nodosa, Kawasaki disease, systemic lupus erythematosus (SLE), aortic dissection involving the coronary ostia or aortic valve may all cause myocardial dysfunction.

Hypertension

Hypertension is also a common cause of heart failure, accounting for 14% cases in one U.K. population-based study.[8] In the Framingham study, a 20 mm Hg increase in systolic blood pressure was associated with a 56% increased risk for developing heart failure.[31] Advances in primary care have led to a decrease in the incidence with improved detection and treatment. The majority of hypertensive patients have no specific identifiable cause, so called "essential hypertension," which places an insidious afterload strain on the heart through a variety of mechanisms including sodium and water retention, arteriolar vasoconstriction, reduced vascular compliance, faster reflection of the pulse wave from stiffer small peripheral arteries, and activation of a range of neurohormonal systems. The left ventricle demonstrates subtle abnormalities in hypertensive patients even before hypertrophy develops. These start with supranormal contraction with increased fractional shortening and wall stress. The left ventricle hypertrophies in a

concentric manner to compensate, although animal studies using gene knockout techniques have revealed that left ventricular hypertrophy (LVH) is not necessary for maintenance of adequate cardiac output in the setting of increased afterload.[32] The transcriptional changes bringing about cardiac hypertrophy occur over different timescales (Table 3-9). Therefore, pathological hypertrophy should be viewed as the first stage of hypertensive cardiac failure, although cardiac output is maintained.

Many of the molecular cascades, which induce hypertrophy, also cause myocyte apoptosis and lead to myocyte dysfunction. Angiotensin II, endothelin, the gp130 signaling family, calcineurin-mediated gene expression, stretch-induced free radical production, and the three subfamilies of the mitogen-activated protein kinase family (ERK, JNK, and p38 kinase) are all activated during development of ventricular hypertrophy, and play roles in the transformation from the hypertrophied but stable myocardium to the irreversibly damaged and dysfunctional myocardium of the failing heart.[33,34] Gap junction remodeling also occurs between hypertrophied cardiac myocytes, leading to increased dispersion of electrical activity.[35,36]

LVH causes reduced diastolic compliance, longer isovolumic relaxation time, leading to increased dependence on the atrial systole for

▶ **Table 3-9** Cardiac hypertrophy—transcriptional changes

30 minutes	Immediate early genes c-fos, c-jun, Erg-1, c-myc, Hsp70
6–12 hours	β-MHC, skeletal α-actin α-tropomyosin, ANP Na/K ATPase
12–24 hours	MLC-2, cardiac α-actin
>24 hours	Increased RNA, increased protein Increased sarcomerogenesis Increased cell size

β-MHC—β-myosin heavy chain; ANP—atrial natriuretic peptide; ATPase—adenosine tri phosphatase; RNA—ribonucleic acid ventricular filling. Acute pulmonary edema is often due to the inability to increase their end-diastolic volume (preload reserve) in response to increased preload or afterload, due to reduced compliance and relaxation. Coronary vasodilatory capacity is reduced in LVH, and hypertensives also develop atherosclerotic coronary disease. As the hypertrophy progresses, myocardial fiber shortening reduces, particularly in the midwall, and hypertrophy allows total wall shortening to be maintained despite this reduction in fiber shortening. Perivascular fibrosis spreads through the myocardium inducing myocyte necrosis as the capillary network is destroyed, and apoptosis.[37] If the hypertension remains poorly controlled, the hypertrophied ventricle progressively dilates, the wall thins, and the ventricle takes on the appearance and mechanical characteristics of the dilated failing ventricle with systolic dysfunction. The prognosis at this stage is very poor,[38] unless a significant proportion of the ventricular dysfunction can be accounted for by coexisting coronary disease amenable to revascularization. This is a dynamic process, and hypertensive cardiac failure is a good example of a disease, which progresses through various subtypes of cardiac failure (hypertrophic, dilated, diastolic, systolic), exposing the limitations of such classifications.

Valve Disease

Primary valvular disease accounts for 7% of cardiac failure cases, and the majority involves disease of the left-sided cardiac valves. Incompetence of the aortic and/or mitral valve results in a dilated ventricular phenotype, to compensate for the regurgitant volume by increasing stroke volume. This requires the development of eccentric ventricular hypertrophy to maintain the increased ventricular output. Total ventricular muscle mass is increased, although wall thickness may remain within normal limits. Initially, the dilated ventricle of the regurgitant valve can sustain the increased ventricular ejection fraction required, provided there are no coexisting threats to the myocardium,

for example, ischemic heart disease. However, the chronic strain of this increased effort eventually leads to the development of myocardial failure, with changes in excitation-contraction coupling, β-adrenoceptor expression and coupling, and interstitial fibrosis.[39] The aim of medical management is to predict this transformation in the natural history of the individual's valvular disease, in order to time valve surgery optimally.[40,41] Acute, severe regurgitation, such as that seen after papillary muscle rupture or aggressive *Staphylococcal aureus* endocarditis, cannot be tolerated and requires emergency surgery. Lesser degrees of regurgitation can be tolerated for long periods, particularly with appropriate heart failure medication, and providing arrhythmic complication do not intervene. A combination of symptom development and monitoring end-systolic diameter/volume is the most effective strategy at present; although the role of brain natriuretic peptide (BNP) monitoring in this setting has yet to be defined. Type III mitral regurgitation occurs secondary to left ventricular dilation and dysfunction, due to annular enlargement, lateral displacement of the posterior papillary muscles with resulting apical displacement of the coaptation point of the mitral valve leaflets in a tethered position.[42] These changes result in a central regurgitant jet, and this should not be confused with primary disease of the mitral valve leaflets causing mitral regurgitation. Type III mitral regurgitation responds best to treatment of the left ventricular failure, whereas the latter requires mitral valve surgery.

Aortic stenosis results in a phenotype similar to hypertensive cardiac failure, as both result in increased afterload. LVH develops initially, via the same mechanisms and with the predominant problem of diastolic filling described above. If left untreated, then the left ventricle also fails with transformation to a dilated phenotype with a reduced ejection fraction.[43] Aortic stenosis usually occurs at the level of the valve cusps, and is most commonly due to a congenital bicuspid valve in the young and middle-aged adult (6% associated with aortic coarctation), whereas atherosclerotic plaque disease on the aortic surface of the cusps is the commonest cause in the over 65 population.

With the increasing elderly population, this degenerative aortic stenosis has become the commonest valvular disease in the Western world, with between 2–9% of the population over 65 years affected.[44] Rheumatic stenosis of the aortic valve is common in the developing world, and always occurs in association with rheumatic mitral disease. Rarely, aortic stenosis occurs at a supravalvular level (Williams syndrome),[45] which can be associated with coronary anomalies, or at the subvalvular level in the left ventricular outflow tract, usually in the form of a shelf of tissue obstructing the outflow tract.

Mitral stenosis is predominantly due to rheumatic heart disease after infection with a Group A β-hemolytic *Streptococcus pyogenes*. It is common in the developing world,[46] whereas it is only seen in the surviving elderly and late middle-aged populations in the developed world. Mitral stenosis in isolation causes raised left atrial pressure, pulmonary venous and arterial hypertension, with development of right ventricular failure and atrial fibrillation.[47] However, the stenotic valve is often also regurgitant due to restricted leaflet movement, and the inflammatory pannus of rheumatic disease may extend down the chordae tendinea onto the endocardial surface of the left ventricle, both leading to left ventricular dysfunction.[48]

These principles also apply to the pulmonary and tricuspid valves, and right ventricular physiology, although the etiology of right-sided valvular disease is very different. Pulmonary hypertension, infective endocarditis, especially from intravenous drug abuse, and hospital-acquired intravenous cannulae and indwelling devices, carcinoid syndrome, rheumatic heart disease, and congenital anomalies, for example, pulmonary valve stenosis and Ebstein's anomaly, account for the majority.

Primary Disease of Cardiac Muscle—the Cardiomyopathies

Primary disease of the cardiac muscle can present in a number of guises, and previously, classification

has been based on the appearance and physiology at echocardiography (ECG) and/or cardiac catheterization, and pathological findings.[5] However, advances in molecular biology, and specifically genotyping have resulted in a reevaluation of this classification.[49] The majority of research on the disease has been presented under the traditional classification, and we will discuss the cardiomyopathies using the classical terms, and then introduce the potential future molecular classification.

In order to diagnose these conditions, it is clearly essential to exclude other causative factors such as those discussed above. However, multiple diseases can coexist and this requires assessment of the time course of the disease as a means to confirm the diagnosis. As alluded to earlier, the presence of milder, non-flow-limiting coronary disease, or a history of hypertension, may complicate the clinical scenario.

There are three basic forms of functional impairment that have been described:

1. dilated cardiomyopathy (DCM) (Table 3-10, 3-11, 3-12)
2. hypertrophic cardiomyopathy (HCM) (Table 3-13)
3. restrictive cardiomyopathy (RCM) (Table 3-14)

There are other forms of heart muscle disease, which extend this classification but are rare, such as arrhythmogenic right ventricular dysplasia, noncompacted left (or right) ventricle and catecholamine-induced myocardial stunning.

DCM is a syndrome characterized by cardiac enlargement and impaired systolic function of one or both ventricles, in the setting of normal coronary arteries, and absence of other structural or systemic causes (Table 3-10). The formal diagnosis requires the left ventricle to be dilated with the internal end-diastolic dimension (LVEDD) >2.7 m^2 of body surface area and either ejection fraction $<45\%$ or M-mode fractional shortening $<30\%$.[5] However, the normal distribution of ventricular dimension across the healthy population results in 1–2.5% of healthy individuals fitting either of these parameters.[50]

▶ **Table 3-10** Causes of dilated cardiomyopathy

Familial cardiomyopathies
Genetic cardiomyopathies
Hypertension (eventually)
Infectious causes
    Bacterial
    Fungal
    Parasitic (trypanosomiasis, toxoplasmosis,
      schistosomiasis, trichinosis)
    Rickettsial
    Spirochetal
    Viral (coxsackievirus, adenovirus, HIV)
Toxins
    Alcohol
    Cocaine
    Heavy metals (cobalt, lead, mercury)
    Carbon monoxide or hypoxia
Drugs
    Chemotherapeutic agents (bleomysin,
      doxorubicin, busulphan)
    Antibiotics and antivirals (chloroquine,
      zidovudine)
    Antipsychotics
Metabolic disorders
    Endocrine disease (diabetes mellitus)
    Nutritional deficiencies (selenium, thiamine)
    Storage disease (hemochromatosis, Refsum's
      disease, Fabry's disease)
Autoimmune and collagen vascular disease
    (sarcoidosis, SLE, rheumatoid arthritis,
    Churg-Strauss syndrome)
    Peripartum cardiomyopathy
Neuromuscular disorders (muscular dystrophies,
Friedreich's ataxia)

HIV—human immunodeficiency virus; SLE—systemic lupus erythematosus

▶ **Table 3-11** A classification of the genetic causes of heart failure affecting the cardiac myocyte

Sarcomeropathies
Cytoskeletalopathies
Laminopathies
Sarcoplasmic reticulopathies
Desmosomopathies
Mitochondrial diseases

▶ **Table 3-12** Genetic mutations linked to dilated cardiomyopathy

Sarcomeric proteins:
β-Myosin heavy chain
α-Cardiac actin
Troponin T
α-Tropomyosin
Myosin binding protein C
Sarcoplasmic reticulum proteins:
Phospholamban
Titin/myofilament anchoring proteins:
Telethonin
Titin
Sarcolemma cytoskeleton:
Dystrophin
β-Sarcoglycan
δ-Sarcoglycan
α-Dystrobrevin
Metavinculin
Emerin
Z-disk-associated proteins:
Muscle LIM protein
Desmosomal proteins
Desmoplakin
Desmin
Plakoglobin
Nuclear envelope proteins:
Lamin A/C

▶ **Table 3-13** Some genetic mutations associated with hypertrophic cardiomyopathy

Protein	Gene
β-Myosin heavy chain	MYH7
α-Myosin heavy chain	MYH6
Essential myosin light chain	MYL3
Regulatory myosin light chain	MYL2
α-Cardiac actin	ACTC
Cardiac troponin T	TNNT2
Cardiac troponin I	TNNI3
Cardiac troponin C	TNNC1
α-Tropomyosin	TPM1
Cardiac myosin binding protein C	MYBPC3
Titin	TTN
Muscle LIM protein	CRP3
Phospholamban	PLN

▶ **Table 3-14** Causes of restrictive cardiomyopathy

1. Myocardial
Infiltrative
Amyloidosis
Sarcoidosis
Gaucher's disease
Hurler's disease
Fatty infiltration
Noninfiltrative
Idiopathic restrictive cardiomyopathy
Familial restrictive cardiomyopathy
Scleroderma
Pseudoxanthoma elasticum
Diabetic cardiomyopathy
Storage
Hemochromatosis
Fabry's disease
Glycogen storage disease

2. Endomyocardial
Endomyocardial fibrosis
Hypereosinophilic syndrome
Carcinoid syndrome
Metastatic malignancy
Radiation
Drugs causing fibrotic endocarditis (serotonin, methysergide, ergotamine, busulfan)

In addition, screening of families with affected individuals frequently reveals asymptomatic relatives with borderline normal ventricular dimensions, which leads to difficulties in prognostic and therapeutic advice.

About 10% of cases of congestive cardiac failure in Western societies are due to DCM.[8] There are numerous causes of DCM (Table 3-10), but in over 50% no underlying cause is found. Whether these reflect unknown genetic mutations, previous viral myocarditis, or toxin exposure, with or without autoimmune destruction, is not known, and it is possible that an environmental insult unmasking a genetic weakness may account for a large proportion.

Whatever the etiology, the final cardiac phenotype appears to follow a common pathological pathway in response to myocardial damage. Some cases result from the progressive deterioration in ventricular muscle function with ongoing damage, whereas others result from a single episode of damage to which the ventricle responds by remodeling and hypertrophy of the remaining myocytes. The myocardium of DCM, whatever the cause, is never normal. Usually there is dilatation of all four chambers. The dilated left ventricle becomes more spherical in shape, sometimes with evidence of hypertrophy, though this is not a dominant feature. Microscopically, myocyte orientation is more tangential to the circumference, and individual myocytes are elongated with an increased cross-sectional area, but reduced intermyocyte connections and gap junction formation. Together with extensive areas of interstitial and perivascular fibrosis, the result is a disorganized tissue with abnormal contractile and relaxation properties, and heterogeneous electrical conduction.[50] DCM patients with interventricular conduction defects have significantly worse systolic function, due in part to ventricular incoordination, particularly if total isovolumic time is increased, and a worse prognosis.[51] However, the clinical course is highly varied, and particularly in the group where a single short-lived event is the sole cause, the prognosis may be excellent.

Familial linkage of DCM may account for up to 30% of cases. Mutations at 14 different chromosomal loci have been described, affecting a variety of proteins in the cardiomyocyte[52] (Tables 3-11 and 3-12). These proteins can broadly be divided into sarcomeric/myofilament proteins, titin and myofilament anchoring proteins, Z-disk-associated proteins, sarcolemmal cytoskeletal proteins, nuclear envelope proteins, and intermediate proteins linking to the extracellular matrix.[53] Familial DCM is genetically heterogeneous, and examples of all the Mendelian modes of inheritance exist, and mitochondrial inheritance has also been reported. In addition to primary cardiac mutations, genetic variance of other systems that influence development of cardiac failure are also important. The polymorphisms of the angiotensin-converting enzyme (ACE) gene have been well-characterized, and the presence of the DD genotype is associated with higher plasma ACE levels and an adverse prognostic outcome in DCM patients.[54]

A subgroup of patients with genetic causes has multisystem involvement, which may give rise to recognizable syndromes, whose genetic cause has been elucidated. Examples include Duchenne's muscular dystrophy, myotonic dystrophy, facioscapulohumeral dystrophy, Friedrich's ataxia, Naxos disease, and Carvajal syndrome (the last two representing the rare cardiocutaneous syndromes).

Postviral myocarditis represents a spectrum of patients, from those with classical fulminant viral myocarditis, whose ventricular function is observed to deteriorate during the course of their illness, through to the majority, who present with the features of DCM and a history of "recent viral illness."[55] The high background incidence of symptom complexes resembling viral prodromes in the general population added to the desire to identify a source or cause on the part of the patient may lead to significant overestimation of this disorder. Initially serological evidence of active viral infection was required, and can be demonstrated in up to 33% of nonfamilial DCM.[56] However, the viral titres are unpredictable and are dependent on the humoral immune system. Improvement in detection of viral nucleic acids, in particular by slot-blot probe hybridization and polymerase chain reaction (PCR), has demonstrated the persistence of viral particles in cardiomyocytes after viral myocarditis in patients who subsequently develop DCM.[57] Replicative activity of these viral particles is not a necessity, and their mere presence can induce DCM in patients with activated immune systems. The enteroviruses are the commonest culprit, and myosin shares approximately 40% of its amino acid sequence with the coxsackie B3 viral capsid protein.[58] This provides a potent autoimmune trigger, which may also occur in response to cardiac protein epitopes exposed during membrane disruption in the acute phases of viral myocarditis. Interaction with the cellular and humoral immune systems is critical, and some DCM patients have abnormalities of the various components of the immune system. Predisposition to

unregulated activation following the appropriate viral trigger may unify the viral and immunological hypotheses causing the continuing damage and deterioration of the myocardium.

The worldwide human immunodeficiency virus (HIV) epidemic has created a new category of DCM. There are a variety of cardiac complications of HIV infection and its treatment, but left ventricular enlargement and dysfunction has been demonstrated in 15% of patients, with a further 4% having isolated right ventricular impairment.[59] DCM is strongly associated with markers of advanced disease, including CD4 count of <100 cells/mL, and the presence of an HIV-related encephalopathy. The underlying etiology is multifactorial, including direct myocyte infection by HIV, myocarditis secondary to opportunistic infections, autoimmune cardiac damage, nutritional deficiencies, and cardiotoxicity from both HIV therapy and illicit intravenous drug abuse (if the cause of HIV infection).

A variety of toxins can damage the myocardium. The degree of exposure, both in dose and temporal course, together with the potency of the toxin, will determine the level of myocardial damage. Excess alcohol consumption leads to a form of DCM, and is the underlying cause in 3% cases.[60] Alcohol may cause myocardial damage by various mechanisms. Ethanol and its metabolites acetaldehyde and acetate have a direct toxic effect of cardiomyocytes.[61] This can cause an acute myocardial depression when ingested in large quantities, raising blood ethanol levels >1000 mg/L. Over the chronic course of excess consumption, requiring >80 g/day for >5 years, ethanol impairs excitation-contraction coupling, contractile protein and sarcolemmal function, with reduced myofibrillary protein synthesis. Like other forms of DCM, the hearts of chronic alcoholics with dilated ventricles show an excess of collagen and interstitial fibrosis. Left ventricular dilatation or dysfunction is detectable in up to 30% of chronic alcoholics, but unlike many of the other causes of DCM, these changes are reversible if abstinence is initiated early in the course of the excess consumption. In addition to the direct effects, alcohol can cause cardiac failure through a variety of other means. Thiamine deficiency associated with poor nutritional intake is common in alcoholics and causes heart failure in beriberi syndrome.[62] Alcohol predisposes to atrial fibrillation and hypertension, both of which can result in heart failure. Certain toxic substances can be present in various alcoholic beverages. For example, an outbreak of DCM in Canada was traced to an excess of cobalt contaminating the brewing of a popular beer.[63,64] Finally, chronic alcoholism leads to profound cognitive impairments including Korsakoff's psychosis and dementia,[65] which will result in alcoholics being less compliant with their heart failure medication, whatever the cause.

Acute cocaine abuse can cause direct myocardial depression, in addition to the ischemia induced by coronary vasospasm.[66] There are reports of DCM in chronic cocaine abusers, and there is a synergistic toxic effect of taking cocaine and alcohol together, with the cometabolite cocaethylene also a potent dopamine reuptake inhibitor, which is more lethal than cocaine alone in animal models.[67] Various other drugs of abuse, including amphetamines, 3,4-methylenedioxymethamphetamine (MDMA) (ecstasy), organic solvents (toluene, kerosene, gasoline, acrylic paint sprays), and organic nitrites (e.g., amyl nitrite) have been associated with myocardial dysfunction and heart failure.

A variety of prescribed drugs have cardiac side effects, and in particular cardiotoxicity resulting in a DCM phenotype.[68] The commonest culprits are the anthracycline-derived chemotherapy agents for a variety of solid and hematological malignancies.[69] Soon after their introduction, late cardiac failure was reported in up to 30% patients who had received >500 mg/m^2 of doxorubicin (Adriamycin). Despite limiting doses to <450 mg/m^2 and excluding patients with preexisting cardiac dysfunction on screening ECG, up to 3% of patients still develop anthracycline-induced DCM. The presentation is highly variable and although the cardiac failure develops a median of 3 months after a dose of anthracycline chemotherapy, case reports presenting decades later are in the literature. The mechanism of toxicity is uncertain, and may

involve free radical production and uncoupling of mitochondrial ATP synthesis by doxorubicin binding to cardiolipin in cardiac mitochondrial membranes. Trastuzumab (Herceptin) is a novel monoclonal antibody against erythroblastic leukemia viral oncogene homolog 2 (ErbB2), a coreceptor for neuroregulin signaling, and an effective chemotherapeutic agent in the treatment of breast cancer. It was initially introduced as a second-line agent to anthracyclines, but 7% of patients treated developed cardiomyopathy.[70] The protective mechanism of ErbB2 signaling in the heart is still to be elucidated,[71] and trials of trastuzumab monotherapy are also ongoing, but it is accepted that it lowers the threshold of anthracycline-induced cardiotoxicity. Likewise, Paclitaxel also amplifies the effect of anthracycline toxicity, up to 14% of patients receiving dual chemotherapy in a trial for metastatic breast cancer.[72] Radiation therapy can rarely cause late ventricular systolic dysfunction, though modern techniques including dose fractionation and computerized blocking to reduce cardiac exposure have now limited its incidence.

Peripartum cardiomyopathy is a form of DCM, which must meet the following criteria: (1) the development of cardiac failure in the last 4 weeks of pregnancy or within 5 months of delivery, (2) absence of other causes of cardiac failure, (3) absence of recognizable heart disease prior to the final 4 weeks of the pregnancy, (4) DCM criteria for left ventricular dysfunction.[73] This definition attempts to exclude preexisting but undiagnosed DCM, which will become symptomatic during pregnancy prior to the final 4 weeks of the third trimester. There is a varied course, with up to 50% cases reversible on macroscopic imaging criteria. However, it is more common in subsequent pregnancies, and is associated with other complications of pregnancy such as older maternal age, multiple pregnancy, and preeclampsia.

Uncontrolled tachycardia, predominantly atrial fibrillation, is now recognized as a cause of left ventricular dilation and failure in a pattern mimicking DCM. It has been called tachycardia-induced cardiomyopathy, and generally requires heart rates of >120 beats/min to be present for at least 3 months.[74] The continuous excess metabolic demand creates an insidious oxygen supply-demand mismatch, and the ventricular dysfunction is reversible once adequate rate control has been established. As the alternative clinical diagnosis is arrhythmia driven by the primary DCM, the diagnosis can only be made in retrospect after rate control has allowed the ventricle to recover. However, is it likely that this subtype of cardiac failure can be superimposed on other causes of left ventricular dysfunction, emphasizing the importance of rate control in heart failure patients.

Hypertrophic Cardiomyopathy

Hypertrophic cardiomyopathy (HCM) is a relatively common cardiac condition, affecting 1 in 500 of the general population.[75] It is characterized by the presence of cardiac hypertrophy with a hyperdynamic left ventricle, in the absence of the other causes of LVH, systemic hypertension or aortic stenosis, or of magnitude beyond that expected by mild forms of these conditions. The hypertrophy is typically asymmetrical, although concentric HCM does occur, and the usual diagnostic cutoff is a wall thickness of ≥15 mm. However, genotype-phenotype correlations demonstrate that almost any wall thickness is compatible with the presence of an HCM mutation. The interventricular septum is predominantly affected, but advances in imaging technology have revealed a variety of other forms including isolated midventricular, apical, and right ventricular HCM. In addition to causing heart failure, many forms predispose to malignant ventricular arrhythmias, and HCM is the commonest cause of sudden death in the young adult population.[76]

In patients with significant septal or midventricular hypertrophy, obstruction of the left ventricular ejection may occur. This usually involves the left ventricular outflow tract, and results from the systolic anterior movement of the mitral valves leaflets leading to midsystolic contact with the septum. This causes a dynamic obstruction, and may be persistent (detectable in every cardiac cycle), labile (variable) or latent, but provocable by exercise, standing, postectopic response, the Valsalva maneuver, or amyl nitrite inhalation. The presence or absence of a gradient is important as it has prognostic significance, although the magnitude of the gradient does not.[77] In addition, the treatment options are different in obstructive disease.

Mitral valve regurgitation, caused by the systolic anterior movement, concomitant mitral valve prolapse, anterior mitral valve leaflet (AMVL) damage from repeated traumatic contact with the septum, and/or involvement of the papillary muscles in the fibrotic disease process, also exacerbates heart failure in HCM patients.

The hypertrophied left ventricle is hyperdynamic with good systolic function early in disease, often with generation of high intraventricular pressures in obstructive disease. However, the left ventricle in HCM has reduced compliance, and is dependent on atrial systole for adequate filling. These diastolic abnormalities are independent of the degree or geometry of the hypertrophy, suggesting a more widespread microscopic disease process. The increased atrial pressures required lead to atrial distension and enlargement, and significant deterioration accompanies conversion of rhythm to atrial fibrillation. Progressive myocardial fibrosis from ischemia and myocyte degeneration eventually leads to wall thinning and progressive dilatation of the left ventricle in a subgroup of HCM patients, and if they survive free of malignant arrhythmias, then they can convert from a hypertrophic to a dilated left ventricular phenotype with severe systolic dysfunction and outflow obstruction disappears.[78]

Apical HCM was first described in the Japanese population in the 1970s, but is now increasingly recognized globally.[79] It characteristically presents with chest pain in the young adult with anterior T-wave inversion in addition to voltage criteria for LVH. Ventriculography reveals a spade-shaped left ventricle at end diastole and the diagnosis is confirmed by cardiac magnetic resonance (MR). The prognosis with apical HCM is better than other forms.

Fifty percent of patients have demonstrable genetic causes (Table 3-13), which are predonichantly transmitted in a Mendelian autosomal dominant inheritance.[80] All the mutations known to cause HCM affect 1 of 13 genes, all which encode sarcomeric proteins involved in the structure, regulation and contraction of the thick and thin filaments. Over 200 different mutations have been found, with varying degrees of penetrance, even for the same mutation within a family cohort. This genetic heterogeneity added to the clinical heterogeneity ranging from benign to malignant forms with a high rate of sudden death, varying ages of presentation, and symptom profiles leads unfortunately to the current scenario where identifying the mutant protein does not have sufficient positive or negative predictive power for prognosis. The link between genotype and pathophysiology is not clearly elucidated, and most cases show significant myocyte disarray, with disruption of myocardial bundles into a characteristic whorled pattern. Some myocytes are hypertrophied but otherwise appear normal, whereas others have grossly disorganized intracellular architecture. Extensive fibrosis is evident, and abnormal intramural coronary arteries with wall thickening and lumen reduction are present.

Restrictive Cardiomyopathy

The third group of cardiomyopathies is the restrictive cardiomyopathies (Table 3-13).[81,82] The main feature of restrictive cardiomyopathy is abnormal diastolic function. The ventricular walls become rigid and noncompliant, usually due to either an infiltrative or fibrotic pathology. This impedes ventricular filling leading to high atrial pressures with associated atrial distension, and the characteristic tall, peaked "restrictive" E wave on transmitral and/or transtricuspid Doppler ECG. It is important to recognize that the term restrictive when applied to transmitral filling represents abnormally high atrial pressure with rapid early filling, which may occur in many other conditions causing heart failure, and the diagnosis of restrictive cardiomyopathy depends upon exclusion of these other causes, certain characteristic features, and identification of the cause. Depending upon the underlying pathology, the ventricles are either normal size or only slightly enlarged due to thickening of the ventricular wall. This increased thickness is due to infiltrative deposits or fibrosis, and not myocyte hypertrophy. Systolic function may initially appear normal, but usually deteriorates as the disease advances.

The causes of restrictive cardiomyopathy compromise a variety of conditions listed in Table 3-13. The main causes vary according to geographical location. In Europe, United States, and Australasia, cardiac amyloid is the commonest form of RCM whereas in the equatorial regions of Africa, the Indian subcontinent, and parts of South America, endomyocardial fibrosis (EMF) is one of the commonest overall causes of cardiac failure. The commonest causes will be briefly discussed.

Amyloidosis is a heterogeneous collection of systemic disorders, which are characterized by the extracellular deposition of autologous proteins, which form twisted sheets of β-pleated fibrils in various tissues including the heart. A simple stratification of these conditions is as follows:

1. A small excess in synthesis of a normal protein results in slow deposition, which takes decades to develop, for example, wild-type transthyretin giving rise to "senile amyloidosis."
2. A significant excess of a normal protein results in rapid deposition and a faster clinical time course presenting at a younger age. Various mutations of transthyretin have been described, and this form is familial amyloidosis, inherited in an autosomal dominant fashion, and is more common in the Afro-Caribbean population.
3. A rapid synthesis of an abnormal protein, for example, the immunoglobulin light chain produced by the plasma cells of multiple myeloma, traditionally referred to as amyloid light-chain (AL) amyloidosis.
4. The slower synthesis of an abnormal protein, such as the acute phase reactant Serum amyloid A, which accumulates in chronic inflammatory conditions such as rheumatoid arthritis and tuberculosis.

Sheets of the β-pleated fibrils deposit between myocardial fibers and may occur in the ventricles, atria, on the cardiac valves, and in the aortic and coronary artery walls. The classical presentation is with heart failure dominated by right-sided findings, low voltage complexes on the ECG, and a characteristic appearance on ECG of granular, speckled, or sparkling myocardium, which is thick, but does not thicken during systole.[83] The thickening may be nonuniform and resemble HCM, and the characteristic restrictive transmitral filling pattern is present. In the absence of systemic evidence of multiple myeloma, endomyocardial biopsy may confirm diagnosis demonstrating the presence of cardiac amyloid on Congo red staining, and a typical appearance on cardiac MR with a characteristic pattern of global subendocardial late enhancement coupled with abnormal myocardial and blood-pool gadolinium kinetics has been described.[84]

Fabry's disease, also known as angiokeratoma corporis diffusum universale, has recently been identified as a common cause of cardiomyopathy with features of HCM and RCM.[85] It is an X-linked disorder due to lysosomal α-galactosidase A deficiency, leading to the intracellular accumulation of glycosphingolipids (especially globo-triaosyl-ceramide), which causes increased ventricular wall thickness, restrictive diastolic filling, conduction tissue disease, and abnormalities of the mitral valve.[86] Endomyocardial biopsy may reveal low α-galactosidase A activity. The skin and kidneys may also be involved.

Sarcoidosis is a granulomatous disorder of unknown etiology, which may involve the myocardium in up to 5% patients. This leads to stiffening of the ventricular myocardium, conduction abnormalities, ventricular arrhythmias, and rarely myocardial infarction due to coronary involvement. The commonest cardiac problem in sarcoidosis is right ventricular failure secondary to the diffuse pulmonary fibrosis seen in advanced cases.[87]

EMF occurs in equatorial regions as noted earlier, with the highest incidence in Uganda, Rwanda, and Nigeria.[81] There is extensive fibrosis, particularly affecting the endocardium, and involves the inflow tracts of the right and/or left ventricles, often involving the atrioventricular valves and subvalvular apparatus. Both apices are also frequently affected. Combined right and left ventricular involvement occurs in 50% cases, with 40% left-sided, and the remaining 10% right-sided. Endocardial fibrosis acts as a substrate for intracavity thrombus formation, leading to cavity obliteration, pulmonary and systemic emboli. The underlying etiology is not known, and the presence of eosinophilia in some, but not all, series has led to speculation of an eosinophil-triggered damage, perhaps initiated by parasitic infection. However, this has not been confirmed. Eosinophils release a number of molecular mediators, which are toxic to the myocardium, and patients with marked eosinophilia may develop endomyocardial involvement. This is most striking in patients with the hypereosinophilic syndrome (Löffler's endocarditis), who have persistent eosinophilia of >1500/mm^3. The circulating eosinophils invade the endocardium, release their toxins (e.g., eosinophil cationic protein), and trigger an intense myocarditis and endocarditis.[88] Mural thrombosis and fibrosis may result, and coronary artery involvement may lead to superimposed myocardial ischemia.

The above pathological categories are a useful classification to approach the broad clinical entity of cardiac failure. In the clinical scenario, patients present with variable constellations of symptoms, signs, and findings, and cardiac failure has been divided into a variety of categories as described above. Patients' symptoms are highly subjective, and are based on both cardiac and noncardiac factors such as muscle tone, anemia, concomitant respiratory or renal disease, cultural and society issues, and there is no significant correlation between symptom severity and objective measurements of cardiac function, although there is some value in prognostic determination.

The authors advocate the practical approach of subclassification based upon the clinical time course and etiology (Tables 3-1, 3-2, 3-3). However, as molecular and genetic diagnostic techniques improve and become more widely available, newer classification may become based on the particular protein, which is affected.

There is already a move to rename familial HCM and DCM in this way, with the new categories listed in Table 3-9. Finally the development of the field of stem cell biology has revealed new insights into cardiac physiology. The demonstration of resident cardiac stem cells with mitotic activity in the adult human heart,[89] and the possible derivation of cardiac cells during repair from circulating bone marrow-derived cells,[90,91] has disbanded the view of the heart as a postmitotic organ of fixed cell number. This dynamic turnover appears to decrease with age, and we believe that the development of cardiac failure is in part due the overwhelming of the aging, inadequate repair processes by the insults of acquired heart disease, which are far greater than those experienced previously in evolution when the repair systems were created and selected. The supplementation of these reparative processes with novel cellular and molecular therapies may hopefully swing the balance away from cardiac failure, whatever its label or cause.

► REFERENCES

1. Martin WH, Berman WI, Buckey JC, et al. Effects of active muscle mass size on cardiopulmonary responses to exercise in congestive heart failure. *J Am Coll Cardiol.* 2002;14:683–694.

2. Lee KS, Marwick TH, Cook SA, et al. Prognosis of patients with left ventricular dysfunction, with and without viable myocardium after myocardial infarction: relative efficacy of medical therapy and revascularization. *Circulation.* 1994;90: 2687–2694.

3. Mulligan IP, Fraser AG, Lewis MJ, et al. Effects of enalapril on myocardial noradrenaline overflow during exercise in patients with chronic heart failure. *Br Heart J.* 1989;61:23–28.

4. Task FM, Swedberg K, Writing Committee, et al. Guidelines for the diagnosis and treatment of chronic heart failure: executive summary (update 2005): the Task Force for the Diagnosis and Treatment of Chronic Heart Failure of the European Society of Cardiology. *Eur Heart J.* 2005;1;26(11):1115–1140.

5. Hunt SA, Abraham WT, Chin MH, et al. ACC/AHA 2005 Guideline Update for the Diagnosis and Management of Chronic Heart Failure in the Adult: a report of the American College of Cardiology/ American Heart Association Task Force on Practice Guidelines (Writing Committee to Update the 2001 Guidelines for the Evaluation and Management of Heart Failure): Developed in Collaboration with the American College of Chest Physicians and the International Society for Heart and Lung Transplantation: Endorsed by the Heart Rhythm Society. *Circulation.* September 20, 2005;112(12):e154–e235.

6. Mendez GF, Cowie MR. The epidemiological features of heart failure in developing countries: a review of the literature. *Int J Cardiol.* 2001;80(2–3):213–9.

7. McDonagh TA, Morrison CE, Lawrence A, et al. Symptomatic and asymptomatic left-ventricular systolic dysfunction in an urban population. *Lancet.* September 20, 1997;350(9081):829–33.

8. Cowie MR, Wood DA, Coats AJS, et al. Incidence and aetiology of heart failure: a population-based study. *Eur Heart J.* March 2, 1999;20(6): 421–8.

9. Zweier JL, Talukder MAH. The role of oxidants and free radicals in reperfusion injury. *Cardiovasc Res.* May 1, 2006;70(2):181–90.

10. Applegate RJ. Load dependence of left ventricular diastolic pressure-volume relations during short-term coronary artery occlusion. *Circulation.* February 1991;83(2):661–73.

11. Hutchins GM, Bulkley BH. Infarct expansion versus extension: two different complications of acute myocardial infarction. *Am J Cardiol.* 1982;65:1446–1450.

12. McKay RG, et al. Left ventricular remodeling after myocardial infarction: a corollary to infarct expansion. *Circulation.* 1986;74:693–702.

13. Kim HE, Dalal SS, Young E, et al. Disruption of the myocardial extracellular matrix leads to cardiac dysfunction. *J Clin Invest.* 2001;106(7): 857–66.

14. Johar S, Cave AC, Narayanapanicker A, et al. Aldosterone mediates angiotensin II-induced interstitial cardiac fibrosis via a Nox2-containing NADPH oxidase. *FASEB J.* July 1, 2006;20(9):1546–8.

15. Olivetti G, Capasso JM, Sonnenblick EH, et al. Side-to-side slippage of myocytes participates in ventricular wall remodeling acutely after myocardial infarction in rats. *Circ Res.* 1990;67: 23–34.

16. D'Armiento J. Matrix metalloproteinase disruption of the extracellular matrix and cardiac dysfunction. *Trends Cardiovasc Med.* April 2002; 12(3):97–101.

17. Mitchell GF, Lamas GA, Vaughan DE, et al. Left ventricular remodeling in the year after first anterior myocardial infarction: a quantitative analysis of contractile segment lengths and ventricular shape. *J Am Coll Cardiol.* May 1992; 19(6):1136–44.

18. Kramer CM, Rogers WJ, Park CS, et al. Regional myocyte hypertrophy parallels regional myocardial dysfunction during post-infarct remodeling. *J Mol Cell Cardiol.* September 1998;30(9):1773–8.

19. Bolli R, Marban E. Molecular and cellular mechanisms of myocardial stunning. *Physiol Rev.* April 1, 1999;79(2):609–34.

20. Bolli R. Why myocardial stunning is clinically important. *Basic Res Cardiol.* July 1998;93(3): 169–72.

21. Gerber BL, Wijns W, Vanoverschelde JL, et al. Myocardial perfusion and oxygen consumption in reperfused noninfarcted dysfunctional myocardium after unstable angina : direct evidence for myocardial stunning in humans. *J Am Coll Cardiol.* December 1999;34(7):1939–46.

22. Anselmi A, Abbate A, Girola F, et al. Myocardial ischemia, stunning, inflammation, and apoptosis during cardiac surgery: a review of evidence. *Eur J Cardiothorac Surg.* March 2004;25(3):304–11.

23. Kono T, Morita H, Kuroiwa T, et al. Left ventricular wall motion abnormalities in patients with subarachnoid hemorrhage: neurogenic stunned myocardium. *J Am Coll Cardiol.* 1994;24(3): 636–40.

24. Takizawa M, Kobayakawa N, Uozumi H, et al. A case of transient left ventricular ballooning with pheochromocytoma, supporting pathogenetic role of catecholamines in stress-induced cardiomyopathy or takotsubo cardiomyopathy. *Int J Cardiol.* January 2, 2007;114(1):E15–E17.

25. Vanoverschelde JL, Melin JA. The pathophysiology of myocardial hibernation: current controversies and future directions. *Prog Cardiovasc Dis.* 2001;43:387–398.

26. Diamond GA, Forrester JS, deLuz PL, et al. Post-extrasystolic potentiation of ischemic myocardium by atrial stimulation. *Am Heart J.* 1978;95: 204–209.

27. Rahimtoola SH. A perspective on the three large multicenter randomized clinical trials of coronary bypass surgery for chronic stable angina. *Circulation.* 1985;72:V123–V135.

28. Vanoverschelde JL, Melin JA. The pathophysiology of myocardial hibernation: current controversies and future directions. *Prog Cardiovasc Dis.* March 2001;43:387–98.

29. Depre C, Kim SJ, John AS, et al. Program of cell survival underlying human and experimental hibernating myocardium. *Circ Res.* August 20, 2004;95(4):433–40.

30. Fox KF, Cowie MR, Wood DA, et al. Coronary artery disease as the cause of incident heart failure in the population. *Eur Heart J.* 2001;22:228–236.

31. Haider AW, Larson MG, Franklin SS, et al. Systolic blood pressure, diastolic blood pressure, and pulse pressure as predictors of risk for congestive heart failure in the Framingham Heart Study. *Ann Intern Med.* January 7, 2003; 138(1):10–6.

32. Esposito G, et al. Genetic alterations that inhibit in vivo pressure-overload hypertrophy prevent cardiac dysfunction despite increased wall stress. *Circulation.* 2002;105:85–92.

33. Sugden PH. Signalling pathways in cardiac myocyte hypertrophy. *Ann Med.* 2001;33:611–622.

34. Spragg DD, Leclercq C, Loghmani M, et al. Regional alterations in protein expression in the dyssynchronous failing heart. *Circulation.* 2003; 108:929–932.

35. Teunissen BE, Jongsma HJ, Bierhuizen MF. Regulation of myocardial connexins during hypertrophic remodelling. *Eur Heart J.* November 2004;25(22):1979–89.

36. Peters NS, Green CR, Poole-Wilson PA, et al. Reduced content of connexin43 gap junctions in ventricular myocardium from hypertrophied and ischemic human hearts. *Circulation.* September 1993;88(3):864–75.

37. Diez J, Gonzalez A, Lopez B, et al. Mechanisms of disease: pathologic structural remodeling is more than adaptive hypertrophy in hypertensive heart disease. *Nat Clin Pract Cardiovasc Med.* April 2005;2(4):209–16.

38. de Carvalho Frimm C, Soufen HN, Koike MK, et al. The long-term outcome of patients with hypertensive cardiomyopathy. *J Hum Hypertens.* February 17, 2005;19(5):393–400.

39. Ishihara K, Zile MR, Kanazawa S, et al. Left ventricular mechanics and myocyte function after correction of experimental chronic mitral regurgitation by combined mitral valve replacement and preservation of the native mitral valve apparatus. *Circulation.* 1992;86:II16–II25.

40. ACC/AHA 2006 Guidelines for the Management of Patients With Valvular Heart Disease: A Report of the American College of Cardiology/American Heart Association Task Force on Practice Guidelines (Writing Committee to Revise the 1998 Guidelines for the Management of Patients

With Valvular Heart Disease): Developed in Collaboration With the Society of Cardiovascular Anesthesiologists: Endorsed by the Society for Cardiovascular Angiography and Interventions and the Society of Thoracic Surgeons. *Circulation.* August 1, 2006;114(5):E84–E231.

41. Borer JS, Bonow RO. Contemporary approach to aortic and mitral regurgitation. *Circulation.* November 18, 2003;108(20):2432–8.

42. Amigoni M, Meris A, Thune JJ, et al. Mitral regurgitation in myocardial infarction complicated by heart failure, left ventricular dysfunction, or both: prognostic significance and relation to ventricular size and function. *Eur Heart J.* February 1, 2007;28(3):326–33.

43. Otto CM. Valvular aortic stenosis: disease severity and timing of intervention. *J Am Coll Cardiol.* June 6, 2006;47(11):2141–51.

44. Otto CM, Lind BK, Kitzman DW, et al. The cardiovascular HS: association of aortic-valve sclerosis with cardiovascular mortality and morbidity in the elderly. *N Engl J Med.* July 15, 1999;341(3):142–7.

45. Eroglu AG, Babaoglu K, Oztunc F, et al. Echocardiographic follow-up of children with supravalvular aortic stenosis. *Pediatr Cardiol.* November 2006;27(6):707–12.

46. Essop MR, Nkomo VT. Rheumatic and nonrheumatic valvular heart disease: epidemiology, management, and prevention in Africa. *Circulation.* December 6, 2005;112(23):3584–91.

47. Chambers J. The clinical and diagnostic features of mitral valve disease. *Hosp Med.* February 2001;62(2):72–8.

48. Gaasch WH, Folland ED. Left ventricular function in rheumatic mitral stenosis. *Eur Heart J.* July 1991;12(Suppl B):66–9.

49. Maron BJ, Towbin JA, Thiene G, et al. Contemporary definitions and classification of the cardiomyopathies: An American Heart Association Scientific Statement From the Council on Clinical Cardiology, Heart Failure and Transplantation Committee; Quality of Care and Outcomes Research and Functional Genomics and Translational Biology Interdisciplinary Working Groups; and Council on Epidemiology and Prevention. *Circulation.* April 11, 2006;113(14):1807–16.

50. Davies MJ, McKenna WJ. Dilated cardiomyopathy: an introduction to pathology and pathogenesis. *Br Heart J.* 1994;72:S24.

51. Duncan AM, Francis DP, Henein MY, et al. Limitation of cardiac output by total isovolumic time during pharmacologic stress in patients with dilated cardiomyopathy: activation-mediated effects of left bundle branch block and coronary artery disease. *J Am Coll Cardiol.* January 1, 2003;41(1):121–8.

52. Burkett EL, Hershberger RE. Clinical and genetic issues in familial dilated cardiomyopathy. *J Am Coll Cardiol.* April 5, 2005;45(7):969–81.

53. Kostin S, Hein S, Arnon E, et al. The cytoskeleton and related proteins in the human failing heart. *Heart Fail Rev.* October 2000;5(3):271–80.

54. Raynolds MV, Bristow MR, Bush EW, et al. Angiotensin-converting enzyme DD genotype in patients with ischaemic or idiopathic dilated cardiomyopathy. *Lancet.* October 30, 1993;342 (8879):1073–5.

55. Mason JW. Myocarditis and dilated cardiomyopathy: an inflammatory link. *Cardiovasc Res.* October 15, 2003;60(1):5–10.

56. Caforio ALP, Mahon NJ, Tona F, et al. Circulating cardiac autoantibodies in dilated cardiomyopathy and myocarditis: pathogenetic and clinical significance. *Eur J Heart Fail.* August 2002;4(4):411–7.

57. Bowles NE, Richardson PJ, Olsen EG, et al. Detection of Coxsackie-B-virus-specific RNA sequences in myocardial biopsy samples from patients with myocarditis and dilated cardiomyopathy. *Lancet.* May 17, 1986;1(8490):1120–3.

58. Cunningham MW, Antone SM, Gulizia JM, et al. Cytotoxic and viral neutralizing antibodies crossreact with streptococcal M protein, enteroviruses, and human cardiac myosin. *Proc Natl Acad Sci.* February 15, 1992;89(4):1320–4.

59. Prendergast BD. HIV and cardiovascular medicine. *Heart.* July 1, 2003;89(7):793–800.

60. Piano MR. Alcoholic cardiomyopathy: incidence, clinical characteristics, and pathophysiology. *Chest.* 2002;121(5):1638–50.

61. Zhang X, Li SY, Brown RA, et al. Ethanol and acetaldehyde in alcoholic cardiomyopathy: from bad to ugly en route to oxidative stress. *Alcohol.* April 2004;32(3):175–86.

62. Naidoo DP. Beriberi heart disease in Durban: a retrospective study. *S Afr Med J.* August 15, 1987;72(4):241–4.

63. Keen WW. Quebec beer-drinker's cardiomyopathy. *JAMA.* December 25, 1967;202(13):1145.

64. Alexander CS. Cobalt-beer cardiomyopathy: a clinical and pathologic study of twenty-eight cases. *Am J Med*. October 1972;53(4):395–417.

65. Thomson AD, Marshall EJ. The natural history and pathophysiology of Wernicke's encephalopathy and Korsakoff's psychosis. *Alcohol Alcohol*. March 1, 2006;41(2):151–8.

66. Lange RA, Hillis LD. Cardiovascular complications of cocaine use. *N Engl J Med*. August 2, 2001;345(5):351–8.

67. Hearn WL, Rose S, Wagner J, et al. Cocaethylene is more potent than cocaine in mediating lethality. *Pharmacol Biochem Behav*. June 1991;39(2):531–3.

68. Yeh ETH, Tong AT, Lenihan DJ, et al. Cardiovascular complications of cancer therapy: diagnosis, pathogenesis, and management. *Circulation*. June 29,;109(25):3122–31.

69. Singal PK, Iliskovic N. Doxorubicin-induced cardiomyopathy. *N Engl J Med*. September 24, 1998;339(13):900–5.

70. Smith KL, Dang C, Seidman AD. Cardiac dysfunction associated with trastuzumab. *Expert Opin Drug Saf*. September 2006;5(5):619–29.

71. Crone SA, Zhao YY, Fan L, et al. ErbB2 is essential in the prevention of dilated cardiomyopathy. *Nat Med*. May 2002;8(5):459–65.

72. Martin M, Lluch A, Ojeda B, et al. Paclitaxel plus doxorubicin in metastatic breast cancer: preliminary analysis of cardiotoxicity. *Semin Oncol*. October 1997;24(5 Suppl 17):S17.

73. Sliwa K, Fett J, Elkayam U. Peripartum cardiomyopathy. *Lancet*. August 19, 2006;368(9536):687–93.

74. Khasnis A, Jongnarangsin K, Abela G, et al. Tachycardia-induced cardiomyopathy: a review of literature. *Pacing Clin Electrophysiol*. July 2005;28(7):710–21.

75. Maron BJ, McKenna WJ, Danielson GK, et al. American College of Cardiology/European Society of Cardiology Clinical Expert Consensus Document on Hypertrophic Cardiomyopathy. A report of the American College of Cardiology Foundation Task Force on Clinical Expert Consensus Documents and the European Society of Cardiology Committee for Practice Guidelines. *Eur Heart J*. November 2003;24(21):1965–91.

76. Ho CY, Seidman CE. A contemporary approach to hypertrophic cardiomyopathy. *Circulation*. June 20, 2006;113(24):E858–E862.

77. Maron MS, Olivolto I, Betocchis S, et al. Effect of left ventricular outflow tract obstruction on clinical outcome in hypertrophic cardiomyopathy. *N Engl J Med*. 2003;348:295–303.

78. Cregler LL. Progression from hypertrophic cardiomyopathy to dilated cardiomyopathy. *J Natl Med Assoc*. 1989;81:820,824–826.

79. Sakamoto T. Apical hypertrophic cardiomyopathy (apical hypertrophy): an overview. *J Cardiol*. 2001;37 (Suppl 1):161–78.

80. Richard P, Charron P, Carrier L, et al. Hypertrophic cardiomyopathy: distribution of disease genes, spectrum of mutations, and implications for a molecular diagnosis strategy. *Circulation*. May 6, 2003;107(17):2227–32.

81. Sliwa K, Damasceno A, Mayosi BM. Epidemiology and etiology of cardiomyopathy in Africa. *Circulation*. December 6, 2005;112(23):3577–83.

82. Hancock EW. Cardiomyopathy: differential diagnosis of restrictive cardiomyopathy and constrictive pericarditis. *Heart*. September 1, 2001;86(3):343–9.

83. Falk RH. Diagnosis and management of the cardiac amyloidoses. *Circulation*. September 27, 2005;112(13):2047–60.

84. Maceira AM, Joshi J, Prasad SK, et al. Cardiovascular magnetic resonance in cardiac amyloidosis. *Circulation*. January 18, 2005;111(2):186–93.

85. Sachdev B, Takenaka T, Teraguchi H, et al. Prevalence of Anderson-Fabry disease in male patients with late onset hypertrophic cardiomyopathy. *Circulation*. March 26, 2002;105(12):1407–11.

86. Pieroni M, Chimenti C, de Cobelli F, et al. Fabry's disease cardiomyopathy: echocardiographic detection of endomyocardial glycosphingolipid compartmentalization. *J Am Coll Cardiol*. April 18, 2006;47(8):1663–71.

87. Doughan AR, Williams BR. Cardiac sarcoidosis. *Heart*. February 1, 2006;92(2):282–8.

88. Janin A. Eosinophilic myocarditis and fibrosis. *Hum Pathol*. May 2005;36(5):592–3.

89. Beltrami AP, Barlucchi L, Torella D, et al. Adult cardiac stem cells are multipotent and support myocardial regeneration. *Cell*. September 19, 2003;114(6):763–76.

90. Quaini F, Urbanek K, Beltrami AP, et al. Chimerism of the transplanted heart. *N Engl J Med*. January 3, 2002;346(1):5–15.

91. Orlic D, Kajstura J, Chimenti S, et al. Bone marrow cells regenerate infarcted myocardium. *Nature*. April 5, 2001;410(6829):701–5.

CHAPTER 4

Pathophysiology of Heart Failure

GARY S. FRANCIS, MD W. H./WILSON TANG, MD

► INTRODUCTION

Heart failure is defined differently by various authors (see Chap. 1), but for the clinician, it is fundamentally a complex clinical syndrome, and not a stand-alone diagnosis. Like anemia or renal failure, it has many causes and etiologies. Although the pathophysiology is to some extent dependent on the etiology, there are many common features regardless of the underlying cause and there are always some underlying structural abnormalities. The clinical symptoms include shortness of breath and fatigue, either at rest or during exertion. In advanced cases, there is usually evidence of salt and water retention.

This chapter will deal with pathophysiologic mechanisms that contribute to the development and progression of signs and symptoms of heart failure. In general, heart failure implies structural disease of the heart with functional consequences to the circulation. It causes signs and symptoms in patients, and can theoretically occur from any form of heart disease. Hypertension, coronary artery disease, valvular heart disease, and cardiomyopathy are leading causes of heart failure in the Western world (see Chap. 3). Heart failure should be distinguished from circulatory failure, which occurs when a component of the circulation impedes circulatory homeostasis, such as excessive circulating volume from acute renal failure. In such cases, the heart itself may be structurally and functionally normal, so that the term "circulatory failure" may be preferred by some. Heart failure may also occur in patients with acute infective endocarditis when the heart is suddenly overloaded with acute aortic regurgitation, at least in the early stages. Myocardial performance may be normal in such settings, but the heart is structurally and functionally abnormal because of sudden valvular insufficiency. These multiple variations and various terminologies have added some confusion as to what really constitutes heart failure. For purposes of this chapter, heart failure is a clinical syndrome (i.e., there are signs and symptoms) with some underlying structural heart disease.

▶ ADAPTIVE RESPONSES OF THE MYOCARDIUM IN HEART FAILURE

The heart has many short-term adaptations to offset a perceived reduction in myocardial performance or excessive hemodynamic load. The use of the Frank-Starling mechanism allows increased preload or enhanced end-diastolic volume to sustain cardiac performance, both under normal conditions and during heart failure. The sympathetic nervous system is activated, thus increasing the force of contraction of the heart and the heart rate. The sympathetic nervous system, among other mechanisms, also facilitates the activation of the renin-angiotensin-aldosterone system (RAAS), which operates to restore circulating volume (if it is reduced) and protect blood pressure (if it is falling), thereby maintaining perfusion of vital organs mainly via physiologic effects of angiotensin II. The heart under chronic "siege" can also increase its own mass, with or without chamber dilatation, to augment the number of contractile filaments.[1] The increase in myocardial mass and remodeling of the heart occurs over a prolonged period of time (usually months to years), while activation of the Frank-Starling mechanism, the sympathetic nervous system, and the RAAS occur nearly instantaneously. Together, these mechanisms converge to allow the heart to physiologically adapt to impaired function and perverse loading conditions.[2] Circulatory homeostasis and cardiac output can be maintained despite a reduced ejection fraction. These adaptive myocardial responses allow blood pressure to be protected and allow the development of clinical overt heart failure to be forestalled.

Release of counter-regulator peptides from the heart such as natriuretic peptides may also aid the failing heart by promoting peripheral vasodilation, natriuresis and diuresis, and by offsetting activation of the sympathetic nervous system and the RAAS.[3] These adaptive responses are evolutionary remnants that have provided a survival advantage long before heart failure was ever a threat. They continue to provide short-term and some long-term adaptation in patients with heart failure.

Index Event—How Does Heart Failure Start?

Heart failure has a beginning, and this is often referred to as the "index event." This event may be clinically obvious, such as the sudden loss of large amounts of contractile tissue, as might occur in the setting of an acute myocardial infarction (AMI). Or, the index event might be insidious, such as the development of poorly treated hypertension, the gradual development of aortic stenosis, aortic insufficiency, or mitral insufficiency. In some cases, the index event might go undiagnosed, such as the onset of lymphocytic infiltrative myocarditis or amyloid heart disease. Or, the index event might be clinically silent, such as the expression of mutant gene or genes that eventually lead(s) to hypertrophic or dilated cardiomyopathy. Recognizing, defining, and understanding the index event is very important in grasping how the heart failure will likely evolve, the pace at which it will worsen, the prognosis, and the appropriate treatment. To say the patient has "heart failure" is not enough. The etiology, mechanism of onset, and progression should be considered in all cases. Physicians should make an attempt to know where the patient is in the natural history of the syndrome, and how the process is unfolding over time. That being said, in the "real world," many patients with heart failure do not have an obvious underlying cause identified, despite extensive evaluation (Chap. 7).

▶ MALADAPTIVE RESPONSES OF THE MYOCARDIUM IN HEART FAILURE

Eventually, if the mass of poorly or noncontracting myocardial tissue is sufficiently large, or if the loading conditions are very adverse, the heart will fail. The cardiac output will progressively fall, the arterial-mixed venous oxygen difference may widen, and the kidneys begin to retain salt and water. Concomitant with these changes, the patient may become progressively more symptomatic with shortness of breath, fatigue, and "congestion." These changes may wax and wane, can take days or years to express themselves, and can sometimes be remarkably attenuated with proper treatment. The pace at which the natural history of heart failure unfolds is highly variable and depends on many extrinsic factors (diet, response to medications, compliance of drug therapy, etc.) as well as intrinsic factors (gene expression, age, severity of index event, etc.) that often lie beyond the control of the physician. This is why it has been so difficult to predict prognosis in individual patients. Nevertheless, it is always worth considering the underlying mechanisms of how each individual patient arrived at the point that the physician first sees them. In a sense, heart failure represents adaptations that have "gone awry," or fail to curb the relentless progression of the syndrome.

▶ HOW ADAPTATIONS IN HEART FAILURE GO WRONG

Most of the adaptations that occur in patients with heart failure evolved for short-term benefit, such as to allow "fight or fright" (the sympathetic nervous system), to ward off hemodynamic compromise from blood loss (sympathetic nervous system and RAAS), or severe dehydration (RAAS). As rudimentary life-forms gradually moved from the salty oceans to land, those who evolved mechanisms to conserve salt and water (such as the RAAS) ensured themselves a distinct survival advantage in a relatively salt and water-poor environment. The evolution of the sympathetic nervous system also ensured survival in the face of imminent danger in a very hostile environment by protecting blood pressure, promoting hemostasis, and increasing heart rate, awareness and the ability to escape the hostile environment. These are very old evolutionary steps, perhaps some 600 million years old that were never powerful enough to ward off the ultramodern scourge of coronary heart disease, myocardial infarction, hypertension, valvular heart disease, and heart failure. Thus, although they may still be adaptive in the early stages of heart failure, they ultimately become very counterproductive, contributing importantly to the pathophysiology of the heart failure as myocardial dysfunction progressively worsens. This transition from adaptive to maladaptive activation of the sympathetic nervous system and RAAS, and from early structural changes in the heart and vasculature to progressive organ dysfunction, best characterizes the pathophysiology of heart failure. Ultimately, there is the release of a host of potentially detrimental neurohormones and cytokines, more perverse loading conditions, a change in the size and shape of the heart, ineffective attempts at maintaining circulatory homeostasis, and multiorgan failure.

The Frank-Starling Mechanism

Simply stated, the Frank-Starling mechanism refers to the fact that the energy of contraction is a function of the muscle fiber length. The end-diastolic volume regulates the work of the heart. The sarcomere length in normal dog hearts at the midwall of the left ventricle averages 2.1 μm at end diastole, and 1.8 μm at end systole. Although Starling believed that a descending pressure-volume limb occurred in the canine heart, this is in reality not likely. Mitral valve incompetence occurs at very high left ventricular (LV) distending pressures, resulting in mitral regurgitation and a decrease in cardiac output. In skeletal muscle, there is a descending limb, as there is a diminishing overlap of thick and thin filaments with increasing muscle length. Such is not the case with the heart, where there is a narrow optimal length of sarcomeres at 2.2 μm. Stretching beyond that point may diminish LV performance.

Patients with heart failure have a blunted Starling relationship at rest and during exercise, so that for any degree of stretching of the myocardium due to elevated end-diastolic volume, there is less incremental change in the contractile state of the myocardium.[4] In heart failure, ventricular function curves cannot be elevated to normal ranges by the adrenergic overdrive, probably in part because the failing heart is relatively deplete of tissue norepinephrine as well as β_1-receptor density. Even during exercise, the ventricular function curve's upward movement is blunted. Patients with progressive heart failure continue to use their day-to-day Starling forces to drive forward flow, but their ability to respond to increased end-diastolic volume is clearly diminished. They manifest less "cardiac reserve" when called upon to increase myocardial contractility.

Distribution of Cardiac Output and the Role of the Peripheral Vasculature

There is usually increased vascular tone in patients with more advanced heart failure. This crude attempt to maintain perfusion pressure in the face of a falling blood pressure also occurs in the setting of hypovolemia, which is a much older biological phenomenon than heart failure. Volume depletion has had many millions of years to allow for favorable mutations to counteract the problem. Those species that were able to adjust to a paucity of salt and water in the environment evolved systems that conserve salt and volume, thus enhancing perfusion to vital organs in order to survive. The sympathetic nervous system and the RAAS serve this purpose. Of some interest,

they also appear to be activated in patients with very early LV dysfunction even prior to the development of symptoms.[5]

Blood flow is also redistributed in patients with heart failure, with more relative flow being directed towards vital organs such as the brain, heart, and splanchnic beds despite an overall reduction in cardiac output. Skeletal muscle flow is also increased at rest in heart failure, while renal blood flow is reduced. Reflex control mechanisms are altered in a complex manner to help facilitate redistribution of flow. Baroreceptor reflexes are impaired, so there is less bradycardia during a rise in arterial pressure. There may also be some structural changes in the vessel walls, thus reducing vascular compliance. The sodium content of the vascular wall may be increased, contributing to arterial stiffening and increased thickness of the vascular wall.

The response to hyperemia is blunted in heart failure, and exercise-induced vasodilation is also clearly attenuated. This is at least in part due to peripheral vascular endothelial dysfunction common to the heart failure condition. Some of the vasodilator response can be restored by administering L-arginine, a precursor to endothelium-derived nitric oxide (NO). There may be impaired expression of NO synthase in the peripheral vasculature of patients with heart failure, whereas inducible NO synthase may be increased in the myocardium, leading to diminished myocardial responsiveness to catecholamines. Therefore, NO's role in the heart failure syndrome is very complex, and may be quite discordant in the peripheral vasculature and heart muscle.[6] The level of myocardial NO in the failing heart has been a point of controversy. Increased expression of inducible NO synthase has been observed in failing myocardium.[7] NO may mediate the effects of inflammatory cytokines (e.g., tumor necrosis factor-α [TNF-α]) on β-adrenergic receptor function, making the heart less responsive to catecholamines. It may also act to facilitate apoptosis. Its role in the syndrome of heart failure is not yet very clear, but it likely has some role that remains poorly defined.

Taken together, these changes in cardiac output distribution, altered reflexes, and impaired conductance of flow are probably adaptive in off-setting a low cardiac output. Redistribution of blood flow to more vital organs likely offers an additional survival advantage. However, over time such "adaptive" responses may worsen renal function, impair exercise tolerance, and favor tissue and circulatory congestion. While we know that the RAAS is activated in response to dehydration, diuretics, a low-sodium diet, and a hyponatremic perfusate to the macula densa of the kidney, we still do not clearly understand what activates the sympathetic nervous system in patients with heart failure. However, activation of the sympathetic nervous system has long been associated with a poor prognosis, and likely plays a predominant role in the long-term pathophysiology of heart failure along with prolonged activation of the RAAS.[8,9] Many of the changes observed in the size, shape, and geometry of the heart itself in the syndrome of the heart failure are likely related to excessive sympathetic stimulation and heightened RAAS activity, which act as growth factors to promote myocyte hypertrophy.[10]

Ventricular Remodeling

When the heart is under perverse loading conditions, whether it is volume or pressure overload, it responds with myocyte hypertrophy. Pure volume overload tends to elongate the cardiac cell due to new sarcomeres being laid down in series, so-called eccentric hypertrophy. Pure pressure overload leads to an increase in cell size due to the generation of new sarcomeres being laid down in a parallel fashion, so-called concentric hypertrophy.[11] The length of the sarcomeres does not change, but because of more sarcomeres per cell, the size of the cell increases. The typical mammalian myocyte may be 130–160 μm long, but lengths up to 400 μm can be observed in specimens taken fresh from diseased hearts in patients undergoing heart transplantation for severe chronic heart failure.[12] Although there is the possibility that some cardiac myocytes may undergo cellular division, this is unusual. For the most part, the cardiac

myocyte responds to altered loading conditions by changing its size and shape. This in turn leads to a change in the size and shape of the heart, so-called myocardial "remodeling." The regulation of how the altered pressure or volume signal is transduced in such a way as to specify eccentric or concentric hypertrophy is still poorly understood, but different gene patterns are involved for each phenotype.[13] In heart failure, there is often a hybrid of both eccentric and concentric hypertrophy, with length usually being disproportionately affected. It is the convergence of abnormal loading conditions and neurohormone release that contributes to myocyte hypertrophy, thus leading to increase LV mass (essentially an adaptive response). However, as the LV chamber relentlessly dilates, systolic wall stress may increase, thus impairing LV systolic function, and hastening the transition from left ventricular hypertrophy (LVH) to heart failure.

In chronic coronary disease, a relative volume overload may develop, stimulating the remaining viable cardiac myocytes to elongate, producing an eccentric type of hypertrophy. However, acute ischemia and myocardial infarction themselves stimulate myocyte hypertrophy directly, and often a hybrid of concentric and eccentric hypertrophy is observed in patients with ischemic cardiomyopathy. The elongation of the cardiac myocyte is associated with chamber dilation, though clearly other mechanisms come into play in the cardiac dilative process, including possibly cell dropout (apoptosis and necrosis) and "slippage" of myocytes away from proper alignment.[14]

LV mass is increased nearly equally in both pressure- and volume-overloaded hearts. Wall thickness is greater in pressure-overloaded hearts, but is also sufficiently thickened in volume-overloaded hearts to counterbalance the increased radius, so that the ratio of wall thickness and chamber radius can be kept normal. This is important, for if wall thickness fails to keep pace with increased radius, wall systolic stress will increase and myocardial performance will diminish. It appears as though myocardial hypertrophy develops in a manner that maintains systolic stress within normal limits. The wall thickening, at least early in heart failure, can be looked upon as a way to maintain myocardial performance by maintaining systolic wall stress. When the LV chamber size continues to dilate, wall thickness may be insufficient and clinical decompensation can occur. The changes in the geometry of the heart are critical to the eventual transition from increased LV mass to overt heart failure. The structural changes define the chronic progression of the heart failure syndrome (Fig. 4-1). The large, dilated heart is far less economical, and more likely to have serious (sometimes fatal) dysrhythmias than hearts with no structural changes, and severe dyssynchrony (electrical and mechanical) is more common.

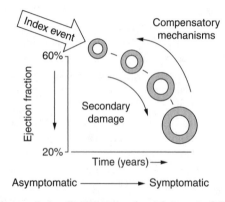

Figure 4-1 Pathogenesis of heart failure. Heart failure begins after an index event produces an initial decline in pumping capacity of the heart. Following this initial decline in pumping capacity of the heart, a variety of compensatory mechanisms are activated. While these neurohormonal systems are able to restore cardiovascular function to maintain asymptomatic status, the sustained activation of these systems can lead to secondary end-organ damage within the ventricle over time, with worsening left ventricular (LV) remodeling and subsequent cardiac decompensation. As a result of worsening LV remodeling and cardiac decompensation, patients undergo the transition from asymptomatic to symptomatic heart failure. (From Mann DL. Mechanisms and models in heart failure: a combinatorial approach. *Circulation.* 1999;100: 999–1008. With permission from Lippincott Williams & Wilkins).

Cardiomyopathy is the byproduct of long-standing adverse loading conditions, unrelenting neurohormonal stimulation, increased production of matrix metalloproteinases (MMPs), and enhanced cell dropout due to apoptosis and necrosis of cardiac myocytes. Of course, the myocytes themselves may demonstrate intrinsically reduced contractile strength, but this has been difficult to study. Cells isolated from their in situ milieu to undergo in vitro studies may not be truly representative of in vivo myocytes. Nevertheless, alterations in calcium excitation-contraction coupling, β-adrenergic receptor coupling to downstream proteins, myosin adenosine triphosphatase (ATPase) activity, and other regulatory proteins have been repeatedly demonstrated to be abnormal in heart failure. However, the quantitative contribution that each of these changes make to altered organ function has been elusive, and probably varies depending on the conditions under which the studies are done.

Alterations in Interstitial Matrix

In addition to an increase in myocyte size, there is increased collagen deposition within the heart as heart failure progresses. Both reactive and replacement collagen deposition are noted.[15] The ratio of fibroblasts to cardiac myocytes is roughly 4:1 in human hearts. Heart failure tends to "activate" fibroblasts to produce more collagen. Increased deposition of collagen tends to make the chamber stiff, thus altering the pressure/volume relation in diastole. LV filing may be impaired. For any given left ventricular end-diastolic volume (LVEDV), there may be a greater incremental change in corresponding pressure, thus raising pulmonary capillary wedge pressure under certain conditions. This becomes an even greater problem for patients with severe hypertrophy and small LV chambers, as often observed in heart failure with preserved LV systolic function. The increased synthesis of collagen is probably related to activation of fibroblasts by angiotensin II, aldosterone, and altered stress/strain forces on the heart (Fig. 4-2).

The heart's interstitial matrix is rich in types I and III fibrillar collagen. Type III collagen provides a weave of struts that probably helps align

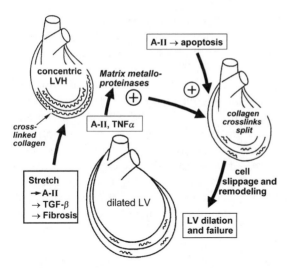

Figure 4-2 Proposed role of angiotensin II and matrix metalloproteinases in the progression from concentric left ventricular (LV) hypertrophy to dilated cardiomyopathy. Primary stimulus to increased collagen is pictured as stretch-induced formation of angiotensin II (A-II), which both promotes growth and stimulates fibrosis via transforming growth factor-β (TGF-β). Metalloproteinases stimulated by angiotensin II and tumor necrosis factor-α (TNF-α)- split collagen cross-link with cell slippage and LV dilation. Angiotensin II-induced apoptosis further promotes remodeling. (From Opie LH. Cellular basis for therapeutic choices in heart failure. *Circulation.* 2004;110:2559–2561. With permission from Lippincott Williams & Wilkins.)

the myocytes properly. There has been a long-standing assumption that MMPs are active in heart failure and may sever these struts, thus allowing the myocytes to be "pulled apart," so-called myocyte slippage.[16] If this is so, it is likely that this mechanism could contribute to chamber dilation. Likewise, the activity of tissue inhibitors of metalloproteinases (TIMPs), a family of proteins that normally inhibit MMPs, may be decreased in the myocardium of patients with heart failure, thus facilitating the action of MMPs to degrade collagen struts and produce myocyte slippage.

Despite the reduction or dissolution of collagen struts normally present to align myocytes,

the quantity of myocardial interstitial collagen may increase in heart failure and thus contribute to diastolic dysfunction.[17] Muscle and chamber stiffness is overall increased, which has important consequences for LV filling pressure and its relation to LVEDV.

Myocyte Loss

Both reduction in LV performance and LV remodeling may be related to cell dropout or myocyte loss. Myocardial necrosis occurs, either localized as in AMI, or diffuse as seen in dilated cardiomyopathy or toxic cardiomyopathy. In contrast to necrosis, apoptosis is a genetically programmed type of cell death unassociated with inflammation or release of troponin, eventuating in phagocytosis of the remnants of the cardiac myocytes. Both types of cell death occur in heart failure, but the quantitative contribution they make to the remodeling process or cardiac dysfunction cannot be easily measured. The amount of apoptosis seems to be highly variable in various studies, but certainly could contribute to myocardial dysfunction in some cases.

▶ TRANSITION FROM INCREASED CELL MASS TO HEART FAILURE

As the heart gradually adapts to the perturbed circulatory homeostasis of early heart failure, the LV mass increases and there may be insufficient capillary density to properly energize some cardiac myocytes. Myocardial contractility, as measured by Vmax, is diminished, and there is a decline in isometric force development and shortening velocity. Eventually, the amount of wall thickness needed to normalize systolic wall stress may be insufficient and myocardial performance further declines. Abnormalities of important cellular proteins that regulate Ca^{2+} exchange, excitation-contraction coupling, and force-frequency relation can be measured. However, it is not always clear if these are primary or secondary abnormalities. Nevertheless, altered excitation-contraction may be phenotypically expressed as a dyssynchronously contracting ventricle with associated electrocardiographic bundle branch block. Such patients may be greatly benefited by cardiac resynchronization therapy (i.e., biventricular pacing).[18] Abnormal proteins exist and likely contribute to reduced myocardial performance and dyssynchrony. β-Receptor density is reduced, presumably in part due to excessive local concentration of norepinephrine, and there appears to be an unhinging of the membrane bound β-receptors from the Gs proteins, and a tighter coupling to the Gi proteins, thus attenuating the response to excessive norepinephrine on the heart. This is presumably an evolutionary conserved protective effect, thus preventing lethal overstimulation of the heart by catecholamines. The net result, however, is a likely reduction in myocardial reserve, as might be needed during exercise.

The transition from adaptive increases in myocardial mass to maladaptive changes leading to overt heart failure is complex and as yet not fully understood. Nevertheless, the observations of the excessive sympathetic drive and unrelenting activity of the RAAS has led investigators toward the development of β-adrenergic blocking drugs and drugs that block the RAAS, therapies proven to be the cornerstones of treatment.

Altered Myocardial Energetic in Heart Failure

Coronary blood flow at rest is often normal in patients with heart failure, but has been found to be reduced in some patients with dilated cardiomyopathy and in some with ischemic cardiomyopathy. Capillary density may be reduced as LV mass increases. Patients with LVH typically demonstrate reduced coronary reserve, a feature consistent with diminished hyperemic response common to many vascular beds in the setting of heart failure. Coronary blood flow may also diminish to match reduced contractile state, a condition referred to as "hibernating myocardium." Importantly, hibernating but viable myocardium may improve with revascularization.[19]

There has been controversy as to whether myocardial oxidative phosphorylation is abnormal in heart failure. Myocardial failure in the setting of abnormal loading conditions may be associated with an inability of the mitochondria to keep pace with the needs of the contractile apparatus, the so-called "energy-starved" heart proposed by Katz and colleagues.[20] Reductions in creatine phosphorylation and creatine kinase activity have been proposed, and may account for the abnormal PCr/ATP (Phosphocreatine/Adenosine triphosphate) ratio noted on nuclear magnetic resonance spectroscopy in some failing human hearts. A reduction in high-energy phosphates in the failing heart may ultimately reduce the hydrolysis of ATP, thereby reducing the amount of available energy for contraction.

Other Peptides and Inflammatory Cytokines

There is a host of neurohormones, peptides, and cytokines that are found to be increased in the syndrome of heart failure. Some may simply be markers of disease or epiphenomena, and others such as arginine vasopressin (AVP), brain natriuretic peptide (BNP), endothelin (ET), and TNF-α may play some pathophysiologic role. A number of novel strategies have been designed to block these counterproductive neurohormones (AVP, ET, and TNF-α inhibitors) or augment the counter-regulatory ones (BNP).[21] To date, such strategies have been largely unsuccessful in improving survival, but such therapeutic agents often provide short-term improvement in hemodynamics and in renal function. Only β-adrenergic blockers and RAAS blockers have consistently improved long-term survival.

Diastolic and Systolic Heart Failure

Patients with systolic heart failure tend to have impaired emptying of the end-diastolic volume and impaired diastolic filling of the ventricle, whereas patients with diastolic heart failure have preserved systolic emptying of the ventricle, but often pronounced impairment of LV filling. The LV chamber tends to dilate in systolic heart failure to accommodate a low ejection fraction, whereas patients with preserved systolic function and heart failure tend to have normal or even small LV chamber size. Diastolic heart failure is characterized by LVH and a stiff chamber with impaired relaxation. Controversy remains regarding the definition of so-called "diastolic heart failure" and what the core lesion might be.[22] Clinicians should be aware, however, that the two conditions (i.e., systolic and diastolic heart failure) often coexist and are indistinguishable at the bedside. They generally respond to the same therapies, suggesting that they share some common pathophysiologic features.

▶ SUMMARY

Heart failure is a complex clinical syndrome characterized by underlying structural heart disease and/or cardiac dysfunction. The patients complain of dyspnea and fatigue, either at rest or with exertion. Virtually any form of heart disease can eventually lead to heart failure, so the etiologic basis is vast. Unifying features include activation of the sympathetic nervous system, heightened activity of the RAAS, and LV remodeling. Neurohormonal activation is a rapidly responding process that restores circulatory homeostasis in the short term, but over time contributes importantly to the pathogenesis of heart failure. LV remodeling is also adaptive in the early stages of heart failure, but ultimately is an inefficient mechanism for maintaining homeostasis. Multiple mechanisms also contribute to the pathogenesis of heart failure, providing many potential therapeutic options.

▶ REFERENCES

1. Konstam MA, Udelson JE, Anand IS, et al. Ventricular remodeling in heart failure: a credible surrogate endpoint. *J Card Fail.* 2003;9:350–353.

2. Cohn JN, Ferrari R, Sharpe N. Cardiac remodeling—concepts and clinical implications: a consensus paper from an international forum on cardiac remodeling: behalf of an International Forum on Cardiac Remodeling. *J Am Coll Cardiol.* 2000;35:569–582.

3. Woods RL. Cardioprotective functions of atrial natriuretic peptide and B-type natriuretic peptide: a brief review. *Clin Exp Pharmacol Physiol.* 2004;31:791–794.

4. Schwinger RH, Bohm M, Koch A, et al. The failing human heart is unable to use the Frank-Starling mechanism. *Circ Res.* 1994;74:959–969.

5. Francis GS, Benedict C, Johnstone DE, et al. Comparison of neuroendocrine activation in patients with left ventricular dysfunction with and without congestive heart failure: a substudy of the Studies of Left Ventricular Dysfunction (SOLVD). *Circulation.* 1990;82:1724–1729.

6. Champion HC, Skaf MW, Hare JM. Role of nitric oxide in the pathophysiology of heart failure. *Heart Fail Rev.* 2003;8:35–46.

7. Haywood GA, Tsao PS, von der Leyen HE, et al. Expression of inducible nitric oxide synthase in human heart failure. *Circulation.* 1996;93:1087–1094.

8. Cohn JN, Levine TB, Olivari MT, et al. Plasma norepinephrine as a guide to prognosis in patients with chronic congestive heart failure. *N Engl J Med.* 1984;311:819–823.

9. Francis GS, Cohn JN, Johnson G, The V-HeFT VA Cooperative Studies Group. Plasma norepinephrine, plasma renin activity, and congestive heart failure: relations to survival and the effects of therapy in V-HeFT II. *Circulation.* 1993;87:VI40–V148.

10. Hunter JJ, Chien KR. Signaling pathways for cardiac hypertrophy and failure. *N Engl J Med.* 1999;341:1276–1283.

11. Carabello BA. Concentric versus eccentric remodeling. *J Card Fail.* 2002;8:S258–S263.

12. Gerdes AM, Kellerman SE, Moore JA, et al. Structural remodeling of cardiac myocytes in patients with ischemic cardiomyopathy. *Circulation.* 1992;86:426–430.

13. Calderone A, Takahashi N, Thaik CM, et al. Pressure- and volume-induced left ventricular hypertrophies are associated with distinct myocyte phenotypes and differential induction of peptide growth factor mRNAs. *Circulation.* 1995;92:2385–2390.

14. Kajstura J, Leri A, Castaldo C, et al. Myocyte growth in the failing heart. *Surg Clin North Am.* 2004;84:161–177.

15. Weber KT. Fibrosis in hypertensive heart disease: focus on cardiac fibroblasts. *J Hypertens.* 2004;22:47–50.

16. Spinale FG, Gunasinghe H, Sprunger PD, et al. Extracellular degradative pathways in myocardial remodeling and progression to heart failure. *J Card Fail.* 2002;8:S332–S338.

17. Burlew BS, Weber KT. Cardiac fibrosis as a cause of diastolic dysfunction. *Herz.* 2002;27:92–98.

18. Abraham WT, Fisher WG, Smith AL, et al. Cardiac resynchronization in chronic heart failure. *N Engl J Med.* 2002;346:1845–53.

19. Ceconi C, La Canna G, Alfieri O, et al. Revascularization of hibernating myocardium: rate of metabolic and functional recovery and occurrence of oxidative stress. *Eur Heart J.* 2002;23:1877–1885.

20. Katz AM. Is the failing heart energy depleted? *Cardiol Clin.* 1998;16:633–44, viii.

21. Tang WH, Francis GS. Novel pharmacological treatments for heart failure. *Expert Opin Investig Drugs.* 2003;12:1791–1801.

22. Kawaguchi M, Hay I, Fetics B, Kass DA. Combined ventricular systolic and arterial stiffening in patients with heart failure and preserved ejection fraction: implications for systolic and diastolic reserve limitations. *Circulation.* 2003; 107:714–720.

CHAPTER 5

How to Judge Disease Severity, Clinical Status, and Prognosis

FAIEZ ZANNAD, MD, PhD, FESC

▶ INTRODUCTION

A noncomprehensive list of factors that can assess the severity of heart failure (HF) and are related to outcomes in patients with chronic heart failure (CHF) include age; gender; ethnicity; etiology; comorbidity; New York Heart Association (NYHA class); exercise capacity; peak VO_2; poor qua- lity of life; low body weight; left bundle branch block (LBBB); atrial fibrillation; nonsustained, sustained, and inducible ventricular tachycardia (VT); prolonged PR and QRS duration; T-wave alternans; QT dispersion; low heart rate variability; depressed baroreflex sensitivity; history of HF hospitalization; resuscitated death; hyponatremia; hypokalemia; raised serum creatinine and blood urea nitrogen (BUN); transaminases; bilirubin and urates; anemia; neuroendocrine activation; high serum brain natriuretic peptide (BNP); low left ventricular ejection fraction (LVEF); diastolic function parameters; raised serum levels of markers of extracellular matrix metabolism; viable myocardium; and central hemodynamic parameters.[1]

The above list of many predictive variables reflects the difficulties in choosing which prognostic variables to use for clinical purposes. This situation has been described by Jay Cohn as "Poverty amidst a wealth of variables." Indeed, it appears that no single prognostic indicator is perfect.[2,3]

Prognostic stratification should differ in relation to the goal and must be useful for making therapeutic decisions. It may also be used for clinical trial design and more specifically for optimization of the risk level of the enrolled patient population, which is the main determinant of the trial population sample size.

Prognostic analyses have been predominantly carried out on populations with left ventricular systolic dysfunction (LVSD). Therefore, the following overview is mainly focused on prognostication in such patients. Much less data are available for HF with preserved systolic function.[4]

It must also be recognized that causal disease as well as comorbid conditions can strongly impact outcomes such as coronary etiology and diabetes.[5-7] In addition, among demographic characteristics, advanced age, as one may expect, and Black ethnicity are consistently reported to negatively influence outcome.[8]

Nearly all predictors of prognosis are influenced by treatment, which can modify their prognostic weight over time. The influence of etiology, comorbidity, age, and ethnicity will not be discussed in this overview.

▶ SYMPTOMS, FUNCTIONAL STATUS, AND THE SEVERITY OF HEART FAILURE

New York Heart Association Classification

Using the NYHA classification and clinical judgment, patients may be classified into Class I–IV or alternatively into asymptomatic, mild, moderate, or severe. However, mild symptoms do not mean minor cardiac dysfunction. Indeed it should be emphasized that there is a poor relationship between symptoms and the severity of cardiac dysfunction or prognosis.[9,10]

Exercise Testing

Dyspnea and fatigue are the two main causes of limitation of functional capacity in patients with CHF; therefore, it makes sense to assess the severity of the disease by measuring its influence on exercise capacity.

Recommendations for exercise testing in HF patients have been released by the Working Group on Cardiac Rehabilitation and Exercise Physiology and the Working Group on Heart Failure of the ESC.[11]

Exercise capacity has proven to be a strong determinant of the risk profile in CHF. Oxygen uptake is a more stable and reliable measure of exercise tolerance than exercise time. A peak VO_2 <10 mL/kg/min identifies high risk and a peak VO_2 >18 mL/kg/min identifies low-risk patients.

Values between these cutoff limits define a zone of medium-risk patients without further possible stratification by VO_2.[11] Change of VO_2 over time and following optimized therapy is more relevant than absolute values at one single assessment. A markedly reduced and continuously declining exercise capacity in patients with optimized therapy should warrant intensifying therapeutic management and is an indication for heart transplant.[11,12]

In patients with serious limitation of functional capacity, submaximal testing with the 6-minute walk test has been shown to provide useful prognostic information when walking distance is <300 m.[13,14] However, the value of the 6-minute walk test has been established using mainly clinical trial databases and is unclear in the clinical setting. Cutoff values of VO_2 = 14 mL/kg/min and distance walked in 6 minutes of 300 m are used for indicating heart transplantation, although this has never been properly validated.

Quality of Life

Although quality of life as measured by appropriate questionnaires (the Minnesota Living with Heart Failure, the SF-36, and the Kansas City Cardiomyopathy Questionnaire) may be associated with prognosis, it is not used in the context of classification of severity.[15-17]

History of HF Hospitalization

The significant morbidity associated with HF is reflected in hospital readmission rates, which are higher than those observed for acute myocardial infarction. Estimates of risk of death or readmission vary, but the largest randomized trial in patients hospitalized with decompensated HF found the 60-day mortality rate to be 9.6% and the combined 60-day mortality or readmission rate to be 35.2%.[18] The Euro Heart Failure Survey program found that 24% of patients with HF were readmitted within 12 weeks of discharge.[19] Additionally, in a population-based survey in London, United Kingdom, 50% of patients with a new diagnosis of HF were subsequently hospitalized at least once over a period of 19 months.[20] History of HF hospitalization is associated with a very high risk of mortality. Mortality rate reported by the Euro Heart Failure Survey (13% mortality at 12 weeks) is probably an underestimation.[19] Prospective cohorts report 1-year mortality as high as 40%.[21,22]

► ELECTROCARDIOGRAM

A normal electrocardiogram (ECG) may rule out LVSD (negative predictive 90%).[23-26] LBBB and/or wide QRS are associated with LVSD and poor outcome.[27]

QRS duration may guide the use of resynchronization therapy.[28] Atrial fibrillation or flutter and ventricular arrhythmia may be recorded using simple ECG. These arrhythmias are more frequent in severe left ventricular (LV) dysfunction, and are associated with poor outcome.

Asymptomatic ventricular arrhythmias on ambulatory electrocardiographic monitoring do not identify specific candidates for antiarrhythmic or device therapy. Contrary to findings from the GESICA trial, nonsustained VT was not found to be a specific predictor of mortality in a multivariate analysis of the CHF-STAT and PROMISE studies.[29,30]

In patients with symptomatic arrhythmias, Holter monitoring may detect and characterize atrial and ventricular arrhythmias, which could be causing or exacerbating symptoms of HF, and guide antiarrhythmic therapy.

Other parameters derived from Holter monitoring are those assessing heart rate variability. Heart rate variability is reduced in HF as a consequence of depressed autonomic balance.[31-33] Time and frequency domain measures of heart rate variability correlate with clinical and hemodynamic measures of severity, and are independently associated with survival.[30,31,34-37] However, so far, there has been no validation of specific management strategies based on heart rate variability assessment.

▶ LEFT VENTRICULAR FUNCTION

Left Ventricular Ejection Fraction

The most important measurement of ventricular function is LVEF for distinguishing patients with cardiac systolic dysfunction from patients with preserved systolic function. In asymptomatic patients with LVSD, EF is an important prognostic marker for the development of manifest HF and death.[38,39] Low EF with or without symptoms is the single risk factor considered as the basis for initiating treatment with angiotensin-converting enzyme (ACE) inhibitors.[40] Low EF in symptomatic patients is an formal indication for β-blocker and angiotensin receptor blocker therapy.[41,42] Patients with low EF that remain symptomatic on ACE inhibitor and β-blocker therapy should receive an aldosterone receptor blocker.[43] Low EF in patients with ischemic CHF is an indication for an implantable cardioverter defibrillator (ICD), and a low EF and wide QRS in patients receiving optimal medical therapy is an indication for ICD with resynchronization therapy.[28] Therefore, LVEF is the single most useful prognostic factor, because it is the basis of important therapeutic decisions. Although reproducibility of LVEF assessment with single photon emission computed tomography (SPECT) is better than with echocardiography, it is echo LVEF that is most extensively used for therapeutic decisions.

Diastolic Function

Staging of diastolic dysfunction may be performed during a routine echocardiographic examination assessing transmitral blood flow velocities and mitral annular velocities. Three abnormal left ventricular filling patterns have been described corresponding to mild, moderate, and severe diastolic dysfunction, respectively.[44,45] Mild diastolic dysfunction is characterized by a reduction of peak transmitral E-velocity and an increase in the atrial-induced (A) velocity. Therefore, the E/A ratio is reduced and usually <1. In moderate diastolic dysfunction,

E/A ratio and E-deceleration time may be normal. Only tissue Doppler imaging may depict reduced peak E velocity.[45] Patients with severe diastolic dysfunction have a pattern of "restrictive filling," with a short isovolumic relaxation time (IVRT), an elevated peak E-velocity, a short E-deceleration time, and a markedly increased E/A ratio.[46-49]

Beyond these distinctive patterns, a restrictive filling pattern, characterized by short transmitral E-deceleration time (115–150 milliseconds) and increased E/A flow velocity ratio (>1.5–2), is associated with increased mortality.[50,51]

Although assessment of diastolic function may be clinically useful in determining prognosis in HF patients, so far there is no prospective validation of therapeutic management strategies based on the assessment of diastolic function.

Other Measurements of Cardiac Function

Ventricular volume changes over time, and the onset or worsening of mitral regurgitation have important decisional implications because it should lead to further diagnostic investigations and/or intensification of therapy.[52,53]

Other measurements include fractional shortening, myocardial performance index, and left ventricular wall motion index.[54-57] Cardiac magnetic resonance imaging is a highly accurate and reproducible technique for the assessment of left and right ventricular volumes and function.[58,59]

▶ MYOCARDIAL VIABILITY

Although this is controversial, results of nonrandomized trials in ischemic CHF indicate that revascularization can improve clinical status and survival in patients with hibernating myocardium.[60-62]

Therefore, in patients with CHF and coronary artery disease, exercise or pharmacological stress echocardiography may be useful for detecting ischemia as a cause of reversible or persistent dysfunction and in determining the viability of akinetic myocardium.[63,64] Viable myocardium (stunned or nontransmural infarction) has preserved flow reserve and sustained contractile improvement. Hibernating myocardium has blunted flow reserve and a biphasic contractile response.

Cardiac magnetic resonance imaging after an injection of gadolinium can identify areas of delayed hyperenhancement in areas of stunning or hibernation.[65,66]

▶ RISK OF SUDDEN DEATH

A review of the measures of risk of sudden arrhythmic death has been reported by Huikuri and others.[67] Several observational studies have shown that low EF predicts both sudden and nonsudden cardiac death.[68,69] MADIT II SCD-HeFT showed that ICDs reduce mortality among patients with an EF 30% with ischemic HF.[70] SCD-HeFT has shown that in Class II or III CHF patients with EF <35%, simple shock ICD may decrease mortality.[71] The COMPANION trial has shown that ICD combined with resynchronization with biventricular pacing decreases mortality in patients with EF <35% and ECG measured QRS duration >120 milliseconds.[28]

Resuscitated sudden death, when it occurs out of context of an acute ischemic event, is a strong predictor of recurrence of sudden death and warrants implantation of an ICD.[72]

Electrical programmed stimulation is useful only in patients with low EF and nonsustained VT. Patients with nonsustained VT, low EF, and inducible VT benefit from ICD therapy, according to two randomized trials.[72–74] Sustained VT warrants antitachycardia ICD implantation.

The majority of other variables occasionally reported to be associated with the risk of sudden death in observational and case-control studies have not received a prospective validation and are not included in therapeutic strategy algorithms. Therefore, this is an area where prognostication is most needed. A large number of patients may be implanted with an ICD, which would never fire for a life-threatening arrhythmia. Robust and reliable risk factors may limit the implantation of ICDs to patients who would need it most.

▶ HEMATOLOGY AND BIOCHEMISTRY

Anemia

A growing body of literature from observational databases and clinical trials suggests that anemia is an independent risk factor for adverse outcomes in patients with HF.

Anemia has recently been recognized as an important comorbid condition and potentially novel therapeutic target in patients with HF. It is common in CHF patients, with a prevalence ranging from 4% to 55% depending on the population studied. Lower hemoglobin (Hb) is associated with greater disease severity, and higher hospitalization and mortality rates.

Multiple potential mechanisms of interaction exist between anemia and the clinical syndrome of CHF, including hemodilution, inflammatory activation, renal insufficiency, and malnutrition. Although correction of anemia appears to be an attractive therapeutic approach, it is still unclear whether it is useful. Multiple ongoing studies will provide data on the balance of risks and benefits of anemia treatment in chronic HF.[5,75]

Kidney Function

Kidney function has a significant impact on clinical outcomes of patients with congestive heart failure. Impaired renal function, whether mild or severe, is an independent predictor of a worse prognosis.[76,77] CHF patients with elevated serum creatinine levels of 1.5–2 mg/dL have a 41% higher death rate, and those with a glomerular filtration rate (GFR) of <44 mL/min have a threefold increase in mortality.[78,79]

Renal function may be a primary determinant of disease progression in patients with HF, rather than simply being a marker of the severity of underlying disease.

Renal function is an independent prognostic indicator of mortality, possibly due to the direct effects of renal dysfunction on survival. The fluid retention resulting from failing kidneys may lead to neurohormonal activation, ventricular dilatation, and arrhythmias. In addition, electrolyte and metabolic abnormalities—hematologic effects and consequences on the immune system that commonly occur in renal failure—could conceivably lead to a worse outcome. Renal dysfunction may also prevent the use of medications known to improve clinical outcome and survival such as ACE inhibitors.[80]

Preserving or improving kidney function in patients with CHF is one of the major unmet needs in CHF management and an area where research should be intensified. The majority of clinical trials that have led to our current evidence-based management excluded patients with renal failure. Therefore, apart from the usual recommendation of caution of use of a number of drugs, there is no specific guideline of management based on the presence of renal failure in patients with CHF.

Serum Sodium

Serum sodium concentration is a powerful predictor of cardiovascular mortality. Although hyponatremia is thought to be an indicator of the level of stimulation of the renin-angiotensin system (RAS), it is among the most consistent prognostic factor in advanced HF,[81] even in the contemporary patients receiving RAS inhibitor therapy.

▶ NEUROENDOCRINE EVALUATIONS

Natriuretic Peptides

An excellent recent overview has summarized the role of BNP in HF.[82] BNP and N-terminal probrain natriuretic peptide (NT-proBNP) have considerable prognostic potential, although evaluation of their role in treatment decision and monitoring remains to be determined.

Several clinical and epidemiological studies have demonstrated a direct relationship between increasing plasma concentrations of BNP (and its precursor NT-proBNP) and decreasing cardiac function.[83–85] There is also evidence that their elevation in CHF patients with preserved systolic function can indicate that diastolic dysfunction is present.[86,87]

In patients at high risk for developing new HF, an elevated atrial natriuretic peptides (ANP) was 85% sensitive and 66% specific for the development of a subsequent HF episode during 1 year of follow-up.[88] A Framingham community study has shown that a strategy of combining EF and BNP (or NT-proBNP) improved risk stratification beyond using either alone.[89]

Elevated ANP and BNP have been shown to be predictive of poor long-term survival and of sudden cardiac death.[90–94] In those with elevated BNP, rate-corrected QT interval was a strong and independent predictor of total mortality, as well as sudden death mortality.[95]

Change in BNP is also useful to predict clinical outcomes. A decrease in BNP during treatment was associated with fewer adverse events after discharge for acutely decompensated HF.[96] Outpatients with the greatest increase in BNP despite therapy had the poorest outcome.[97]

At present, the relative merits of the available assays for BNP and NT-proBNP, the value of BNP for therapeutic decision making and in monitoring therapy are important areas for continuing investigation. The natriuretic peptide assays commercially available are fluorescence or radioimmunoassay for BNP, and electrochemiluminescent assay for NT-proBNP. In general, the plasma BNP concentration rises with age and may be slightly higher in women than in men. A suggested "normal" range for BNP is 0.5–30 pg/mL (0.15–8.7 pmol/L) and 68–112 pg/mL (8.2–13.3 pmol/L) for NT-proBNP.[98]

Neuroendocrine Evaluations Other than Natriuretic Peptides

In large cohorts of patients, there is good evidence that circulating levels of noradrenaline, renin, angiotensin II, aldosterone, vasopressin, endothelin-1, and adrenomedullin are related to the severity and prognosis of HF, but in individual patients these predictors are inaccurate and difficult to interpret. Degree of neurohormonal activation cannot guide treatment with renin-angiotensin and aldosterone inhibitors.

▶ SCORING AND PROGNOSTIC ALGORITHMS

An interesting prognostic approach can lie in integrated strategies based on an initial screening of patients of different disease severity and then the application of specific algorithms to selected subjects.[95] A review of prognostic algorithms has been reported by Bouvy and others.[99] None is widely accepted for routine use in HF. Available prognostic algorithms are usually limited because they are mainly derived prospectively from nonrepresentative cohorts or clinical trial databases. Very few have received a formal external validation in independent prospective cohorts.

▶ ACUTE HEART FAILURE SYNDROMES

In acute heart failure syndromes (AHFS), predictive models for mortality and rehospitalization can aid clinical decision making. Patients at low risk could potentially be treated and discharged from the hospital early, whereas those at high risk may benefit from intensive specialized care.

In this setting, stratification based on the degree of neurohormonal activation and the severity of LVSD become less discriminant.[6] Central hemodynamic patterns (pulmonary capillary pressure and right ventricular function) are relatively more important.[100–102] Invasive hemodynamic monitoring variables by means of a pulmonary arterial catheter may be useful to monitor therapy and for decision making in patients with AHFS not responding promptly to appropriate treatment and when it must be decided whether to use ventricular assistance or replacement therapies.[6,103]

Three main prognostic indicators are emerging as most important in AHFS. These include myocardial injury (quantified by troponin), renal dysfunction (as measured by increases in serum creatinine or BUN, and decreases in serum sodium), and hemodynamic congestion (as measured by increased pulmonary capillary wedge pressure [PCWP] or BNP/NT-proBNP). While previous research has largely focused on correction of altered hemodynamics (e.g., increasing cardiac output), new data suggest that the above three factors may be more important for long-term prognosis as well as for therapeutic targets. While current standard therapies may improve symptoms (e.g., diuretics), they may worsen renal function. Similarly, while some positive inotropes may improve hemodynamics (increase cardiac index), they may promote myocardial injury.

Several observational studies have shown that 30–50% of patients hospitalized with AHFS have detectable plasma levels of cardiac troponin at the time of admission in the absence of an acute coronary event. These patients have a two-fold increase in 60-day postdischarge mortality and a three-fold increase in the rehospitalization rate during the same time period.[104]

The severity of renal dysfunction in hospitalized patients with AHFS provides important prognostic information for in-hospital and postdischarge mortality. Aggravated renal dysfunction (defined as ≥25% increase in serum creatinine concentration to ≥2 mg/dL) occurs in at least 20–30% of patients undergoing intensive treatment for HF.[105] The development of worsening renal function is associated with an increased risk of death, a significantly longer length of stay, and higher in-hospital cost.[106] Impaired renal function also increases the likelihood of readmission after discharge from hospitalization for HF.[107,108] A1 adenosine antagonism might preserve renal function while simultaneously promoting natriuresis during treatment for HF and is currently under clinical investigation.[109]

Approximately 20% of patients hospitalized with AHFS and systolic dysfunction have hyponatremia (serum sodium <136 mEq/L), and these patients have a twofold increase in in-hospital and postdischarge mortality, and a 30% increase in the combined readmission or mortality rate.[110,111] Vasopressin antagonist therapy (such as Tolvaptan) is being tested with the aim of improving postdischarge outcomes in patients with AHFS.[112] Though Tolvaptan initiated for acute treatment in AHFS patients did not have an effect on long-term moratality or heart failure morbidity,[113] it did relieve acute symptoms.[114]

▶ CONCLUSION

It is likely that different sets of variables will prove useful in different settings. In primary care, it is important to be able to stratify risk on the basis of simple, readily available clinical or laboratory variables to identify patients who should be referred for specialist advice. Serum BNP monitoring may emerge as a useful tool in this setting. Meanwhile, primary care physicians rely mainly on functional capacity, signs, and symptoms.

For the specialists, prognostic variables are required to direct the intensity of therapy. The main selection criteria in clinical trials were symptoms, NYHA class, LVEF and, in some trials, history of recent hospitalization for HF. Therefore, only these variables are prognostic factors strongly validated and widely accepted and applied in evidence-based patient management.

In more advanced HF, prognostic stratification may guide the need for or urgency of device therapy and/or surgery, including transplantation. Peak VO$_2$ and the 6-minute walk test are among the most used assessments for the management of transplant waiting list. They should also be recommended as decision tools for indicating cardiac resynchronization therapy in patients with optimized drug therapy. VT inducibility during ventricular programmed stimulation is useful (only) in patients with asymptomatic VT, in order to direct ICD indication.

New validated information and more integrated approaches may offer, in the future, prognostic algorithms that are more robust prognostication in HF. Genomics and proteomics may offer novel disease markers and risk (or protecting) factors. However, to date, no tests can overcome the clinical judgment in grading risk and guiding therapy in HF patients.

▶ REFERENCES

1. Cowburn P, Cleland J, Coats A, et al. Risk stratification in chronic heart failure. *Eur Heart J.* 1998;19:696–710.
2. Cohn J. Prognostic factors in heart failure: poverty amidst a wealth of variables. *J Am Coll Cardiol.* 1989;14:571–572.
3. Eichhorn E. Prognosis determination in heart failure. *Am J Med.* 2001;110:S14–S36.
4. Gustafsson F, Torp-Pedersen C, Brendorp B, et al. Long-term survival in patients hospitalized with congestive heart failure: relation to preserved and reduced left ventricular systolic function. *Eur Heart J.* 2003;24:863–870.
5. Felker G, Shaw L, O'Connor C. A standardized definition of ischemic cardiomyopathy for use in clinical research. *J Am Coll Cardiol.* 2002;39:210–218.
6. Nohria A, Tsang S, Fang J, et al. Clinical assessment identifies hemodynamic profiles that predict outcomes in patients admitted with heart failure. *J Am Coll Cardiol.* 2003;41:1797–1804.
7. Dries D, Sweitzer N, Drazner M, et al. Prognostic impact of diabetes mellitus in patients with heart failure according to the etiology of left ventricular systolic dysfunction. *J Am Coll Cardiol.* 2001;38:421–428.
8. Pulignano G, Del Sindaco D, Tavazzi L, et al. Clinical features and outcomes of elderly outpatients with heart failure followed up in hospital cardiology units: data from a large nationwide cardiology database (IN-CHF Registry). *Am Heart J.* 2002;143:45–55.
9. Marantz P, Tobin J, Wassertheil-Smoller S, et al. The relationship between left ventricular systolic function and congestive heart failure diagnosed by clinical criteria. *Circulation.* 1988;77:607–612.
10. Van den Broek S, Van Veldhuisen D, De Graeff P, et al. Comparison between New York Heart Association classification and peak oxygen consumption in the assessment of functional status and prognosis in patients with mild to

moderate chronic congestive heart failure secondary to either ischemic or idiopathic. *Am J Cardiol.* 1992;70:359–363.

11. Working Group on Cardiac Rehabilitation and Exercise Physiology and Working Group on Heart Failure of the European Society of Cardiology: Recommendations for exercise testing in chronic heart failure patients. *Eur Heart J.* 2001;22:37–45.

12. Mancini D, Eisen H, Kussmaul W, et al. Value of peak exercise oxygen consumption for optimal timing of cardiac transplantation in ambulatory patients with heart failure. *Circulation.* 1991;83:778–786.

13. Guyatt G, Sullivan M, Thompson P, et al. The 6-minute walk: a new measure of exercise capacity in patients with chronic heart failure. *CMAJ.* 1985;132:919–923.

14. Bittner V, Weiner D, Yusuf S, et al. Prediction of mortality and morbidity with a 6-minute walk test in patients with left ventricular dysfunction. *JAMA.* 1993;270:1702–1707.

15. Rector T, Cohn J, Pimobendan Multicenter Research Group. Assessment of patient outcome with the Minnesota Living with Heart Failure questionnaire: reliability and validity during a randomized, double-blind, placebo-controlled trial of pimobendan. *Am Heart J.* 1992;124:1017–1025.

16. McHorney C, Ware J, Raczek A. The MOS 36-Item Short-Form Health Survey (SF-36): II. Psychometric and clinical tests of validity in measuring physical and mental health constructs. *Med Care.* 1993;31:247–263.

17. Green C, Porter C, Bresnahan D, et al. Development and evaluation of the Kansas City Cardiomyopathy Questionnaire: a new health status measure for heart failure. *J Am Coll Cardiol.* 2000;35:1245–1255.

18. Cuffe M, Califf R, Adams K J, et al. Short-term intravenous milrinone for acute exacerbation of chronic heart failure: a randomized controlled trial. *JAMA.* 2002;287:1541–1547.

19. Cleland J, Swedberg K, Follath F, et al. The EuroHeart Failure survey programme— a survey on the quality of care among patients with heart failure in Europe. Part 1: patient characteristics and diagnosis. *Eur Heart J.* 2003; 24:442–463.

20. Cowie M, Fox K, Wood D, et al. Hospitalization of patients with heart failure: a population-based study. *Eur Heart J.* 2002;23:877–885.

21. Zannad F, Cohen-Solal A, Desnos M, et al. Clinical and etiological features, management and outcomes of acute heart failure: the EFICA cohort study. *Eur Heart J.* 2002;4 (Suppl):579.

22. Zannad F, Briançon S, Juillière Y, et al. Incidence, clinical and etiologic features, and outcomes of advanced chronic heart failure: the EPICAL Study. Epidemiologie de l'Insuffisance Cardiaque Avancee en Lorraine. *J Am Coll Cardiol.* 1999;33:734–42.

23. Rihal C, Davis K, Kennedy J, et al. The utility of clinical, electrocardiographic, and roentgenographic variables in the prediction of left ventricular function. *Am J Cardiol.* 1995;75:220–223.

24. Gillespie N, McNeill G, Pringle T, et al. Cross sectional study of contribution of clinical assessment and simple cardiac investigations to diagnosis of left ventricular systolic dysfunction in patients admitted with acute dyspnoea. *BMJ.* 1997;314:936–340.

25. Mosterd A, de Bruijne M, Hoes A, et al. Usefulness of echocardiography in detecting left ventricular dysfunction in population-based studies (The Rotterdam Study). *Am J Cardiol.* 1997;79:103–104.

26. Badgett R, Lucey C, Mulrow C. Can the clinical examination diagnose left-sided heart failure in adults? *JAMA.* 1997;277:1712–1719.

27. Baldasseroni S, Opasich C, Gorini M, et al. Left bundle-branch block is associated with increased 1-year sudden and total mortality rate in 5517 outpatients with congestive heart failure: a report from the Italian network on congestive heart failure. *Am Heart J.* 2002;143:398–405.

28. Bristow M, Saxon L, Boehmer J, et al. Cardiac-resynchronization therapy with or without an implantable defibrillator in advanced chronic heart failure. *N Engl J Med.* 2004;350:2140–2150.

29. Doval H, Nul D, Grancelli H, et al. Nonsustained ventricular tachycardia in severe heart failure. Independent marker of increased mortality due to sudden death. GESICA-GEMA Investigators. *Circulation.* 1996;94:3198–3203.

30. Teerlink J, Jalaluddin M, Anderson S, et al. Ambulatory ventricular arrhythmias in patients with heart failure do not specifically predict an increased risk of sudden death. PROMISE (Prospective Randomized Milrinone Survival Evaluation) Investigators. *Circulation.* 2000;101:40–46.

31. Nolan J, Flapan A, Capewell S, et al. Decreased cardiac parasympathetic activity in chronic heart failure and its relation to left ventricular function. *Br Heart J.* 1992;67:482–485.

32. Malik M, Camm A. Heart rate variability: from facts to fancies. *J Am Coll Cardiol.* 1993;22: 566–568.

33. Hohnloser S, Klingenheben T, Zabel M, et al. Intraindividual reproducibility of heart rate variability. *Pacing Clin Electrophysiol.* 1992;15: 2211–2214.

34. Mortara A, La Rovere M, Signorini M, et al. Can power spectral analysis of heart rate variability identify a high risk subgroup of congestive heart failure patients with excessive sympathetic activation? A pilot study before and after heart transplantation. *Br Heart J.* 1994;71:422–430.

35. Panina G, Khot U, Nunziata E, et al. Role of spectral measures of heart rate variability as markers of disease progression in patients with chronic congestive heart failure not treated with angiotensin-converting enzyme inhibitors. *Am Heart J.* 1996;131:153–157.

36. Brouwer J, Van Veldhuisen D, Man in 't Veld A, The Dutch Ibopamine Multicenter Trial Study Group. Prognostic value of heart rate variability during long-term follow-up in patients with mild to moderate heart failure. *J Am Coll Cardiol.* 1996;28:1183–1189.

37. Ponikowski P, Anker S, Chua T, et al. Depressed heart rate variability as an independent predictor of death in chronic congestive heart failure secondary to ischemic or idiopathic dilated cardiomyopathy. *Am J Cardiol.* 1997;79:1645–1650.

38. Lewis E, Moye L, Rouleau J, et al. Predictors of late development of heart failure in stable survivors of myocardial infarction: the CARE study. *J Am Coll Cardiol.* 2003;42:1446–1453.

39. Zornoff L, Skali H, Pfeffer M, et al. Right ventricular dysfunction and risk of heart failure and mortality after myocardial infarction. *J Am Coll Cardiol.* 2002;39:1450–1455.

40. Flather M, Yusuf S, Kober L, ACE-Inhibitor Myocardial Infarction Collaborative Group. Long-term ACE-inhibitor therapy in patients with heart failure or left-ventricular dysfunction: a systematic overview of data from individual patients. *Lancet.* 2000;355.

41. Beta-Blocker Evaluation of Survival Trial Investigators: A trial of the beta-blocker bucindolol in patients with advanced chronic heart failure. *N Engl J Med.* 2001;344:1659–1667.

42. Poole-Wilson P, Swedberg K, Cleland J, et al. Comparison of carvedilol and metoprolol on clinical outcomes in patients with chronic heart failure in the Carvedilol Or Metoprolol European Trial (COMET): randomised controlled trial. *Lancet.* 2003;362:7–13.

43. Pitt B, Zannad F, Remme W, et al. The effect of spironolactone on morbidity and mortality in patients with severe heart failure. Randomized Aldactone Evaluation Study Investigators. *N Engl J Med.* 1999;341:709–717.

44. Appleton C, Hatle L, Popp R. Relation of transmitral flow velocity patterns to left ventricular diastolic function: new insights from a combined hemodynamic and Doppler echocardiographic study. *J Am Coll Cardiol.* 1988;12:426–440.

45. Sohn D, Chai I, Lee D, et al. Assessment of mitral annulus velocity by Doppler tissue imaging in the evaluation of left ventricular diastolic function. *J Am Coll Cardiol.* 1997;30:474–480.

46. Thomas J, Choong C, Flachskampf F, et al. Analysis of the early transmitral Doppler velocity curve: effect of primary physiologic changes and compensatory preload adjustment. *J Am Coll Cardiol.* 1990;16:644–655.

47. Myreng Y, Smiseth O, Risoe C. Left ventricular filling at elevated diastolic pressures: relationship between transmitral Doppler flow velocities and atrial contribution. *Am Heart J.* 1990;119:620–626.

48. Flachskampf F, Weyman A, Guerrero J, et al. Calculation of atrioventricular compliance from the mitral flow profile: analytic and in vitro study. *J Am Coll Cardiol.* 1992;19:998–1004.

49. Little W, Ohno M, Kitzman D, et al. Determination of left ventricular chamber stiffness from the time for deceleration of early left ventricular filling. *Circulation.* 1995;92: 1933–1939.

50. Rihal C, Nishimura R, Hatle L, et al. Systolic and diastolic dysfunction in patients with clinical diagnosis of dilated cardiomyopathy: relation to symptoms and prognosis. *Circulation.* 1994;90:2772–2779.

51. Giannuzzi P, Temporelli P, Bosimini E, et al. Independent and incremental prognostic value of Doppler-derived mitral deceleration time of early filling in both symptomatic and asymptomatic patients with left ventricular dysfunction. *J Am Coll Cardiol.* 1996;28: 383–390.

52. St John S, Lee D, Rouleau J, et al. Left ventricular remodeling and ventricular arrhythmias after myocardial infarction. *Circulation.* 2003;107: 2577–2582.

53. Koelling T, Aaronson K, Cody R, et al. Prognostic significance of mitral regurgitation and tricuspid regurgitation in patients with left ventricular systolic dysfunction. *Am Heart J.* 2002;144:524–529.

54. Hoglund C, Alam M, Thorstrand C. Atrioventricular valve plane displacement in healthy persons: an echocardiographic study. *Acta Med Scand.* 224:557-62, 1988.

55. Tei C, Ling L, Hodge D, et al. New index of combined systolic and diastolic myocardial performance: a simple and reproducible measure of cardiac function—a study in normals and dilated cardiomyopathy. *J Cardiol.* 1995;26:357–366.

56. Berning J, Steensgaard-Hansen F. Early estimation of risk by echocardiographic determination of wall motion index in an unselected population with acute myocardial infarction. *Am J Cardiol.* 1990;65:567–576.

57. Willenheimer R, Israelsson B, Cline C, et al. Simplified echocardiography in the diagnosis of heart failure. *Scand Cardiovasc J.* 1997;31:9–16.

58. Bellenger N, Davies L, Francis J, et al. Reduction in sample size for studies of remodeling in heart failure by the use of cardiovascular magnetic resonance. *J Cardiovasc Magn Reson.* 2000;2:271–278.

59. Grothues F, Moon J, Bellenger N, et al. Interstudy reproducibility of right ventricular volumes, function, and mass with cardiovascular magnetic resonance. *Am Heart J.* 2004;147:218–223.

60. Cleland J, Pennell D, Ray S, et al. Myocardial viability as a determinant of the ejection fraction response to carvedilol in patients with heart failure (CHRISTMAS trial): randomised controlled trial. *Lancet.* 2003;362:14–21.

61. Pasquet A, Robert A, D'Hondt A, et al. Prognostic value of myocardial ischemia and viability in patients with chronic left ventricular ischemic dysfunction. *Circulation.* 1999;100:141–148.

62. Udelson J, Bonow R. Radionuclide angiographic evaluation of left ventricular diastolic function. In: Gaasch WH, LeWinter M (eds): *Left ventricular diastolic dysfunction and heart failure.* Malvern, USA, Lea & Febiger,1994:167–191.

63. Pierard L, Lancellotti P, Benoit T. Myocardial viability: stress echocardiography vs nuclear medicine. *Eur Heart J.* 1997;18:D117–D123.

64. Williams M, Odabashian J, Lauer M, et al. Prognostic value of dobutamine echocardiography in patients with left ventricular dysfunction. *J Am Coll Cardiol.* 1996;27:1332–1339.

65. Al-Saadi N, Nagel E, Gross M, et al. Noninvasive detection of myocardial ischemia from perfusion reserve based on cardiovascular magnetic resonance. *Circulation.* 2000;101:1379–1383.

66. Kim R, Wu E, Rafael A, et al. The use of contrast-enhanced magnetic resonance imaging to identify reversible myocardial dysfunction. *N Engl J Med.* 2000;343:1445–1453.

67. Huikuri H, Makikallio T, Raatikainen M, et al. Prediction of sudden cardiac death: appraisal of the studies and methods assessing the risk of sudden arrhythmic death. *Circulation.* 2003;108:110–115.

68. The Multicenter Post Infarction Research Group: Risk stratification and survival after myocardial infarction. *N Engl J Med.* 1983;309: 331–336.

69. Bigger J, Fleiss J, Kleiger R, The Multicenter Post-Infarction Research Group. The relationships among ventricular arrhythmias, left ventricular dysfunction, and mortality in 2 years after myocardial infarction. *Circulation.* 1984;69:250–258.

70. Moss A, Zareba W, Hall W, Multicenter Automatic Defibrillator Implantation Trial II Investigators. Prophylactic implantation of a defibrillator in patients with myocardial infarction and reduced ejection fraction. *N Engl J Med.* 2002;346:877–883.

71. Bardy G, Lee K, Mark D, et al. Amiodarone or an implantable cardioverter-defibrillator for congestive heart failure. *N Engl J Med.* 2005;352:225–237.

72. The Antiarrhythmic Versus Implantable Defibrillators (AVID) Investigators: A comparison of antiarrhythmic-drug therapy with implantable defibrillators in patients resuscitated from near-fatal ventricular arrhythmia. *N Engl J Med.* 1997; 337:1576–1583.

73. Moss A, Hall W, Cannom D, Multicenter Automatic Defibrillator Implantation Trial Investigators. Improved survival with an implanted defibrillator in patients with coronary artery disease at high risk for ventricular arrhythmia. *N Engl J Med.* 1996;335:1933–1940.

74. Buxton A, Lee K, Fisher J, Multicenter Unsustained Tachycardia Investigators. A randomized study of the prevention of sudden

death in patients with coronary artery disease. *N Engl J Med*. 1999;341:1882–1890.

75. Anand I, McMurray J, Whitmore J, et al. Anemia and its relationship to clinical outcome in heart failure. *Circulation*. 2004;110:149–154.

76. Girbes A, Van Veldhuisen D, De Kam P, et al. Renal function is the most important determinant of survival in patients with severe congestive heart failure. *JACC*. 1998;31:154A.

77. Maggioni A, DiGregorio L, Gorini M, et al. Predictors of 1 year mortality in 2086 outpatients with congestive heart failure: data from Italian Network on Congestive Heart Failure. *Am Coll Cardiol*. 1998;31:218A.

78. Dries D, Exner D, Domanski M, et al. The prognostic implications of renal insufficiency in asymptomatic and symptomatic patients with left ventricular systolic dysfunction. *J Am Coll Cardiol*. 2000;35:681–9.

79. Hillege H, Girbes A, De Kam P, et al. Renal function, neurohormonal activation, and survival in patients with chronic heart failure. *Circulation*. 2000;102:203–210.

80. Echemann M, Zannad F, Briançon S, et al. Determinants of angiotensin-converting enzyme inhibitor prescription in severe heart failure with left ventricular systolic dysfunction: the EPICAL study. *Am Heart J*. 2000;39:624–631.

81. Rodeheffer R. Measuring plasma B-type natriuretic peptide in heart failure good to go in 2004? *J Am Coll Cardiol*. 2004;44:740–749.

82. Couvie M, Jourdian P, Maisel A, et al. Clinical applications of B-type natriuretic peptide (BNP) testing. *Eur Heart J*. 2003; 24:1710–1718.

83. Lerman A, Gibbons R, Rodeheffer R, et al. Circulating N-terminal atrial natriuretic peptide as a marker for symptomless left-ventricular dysfunction. *Lancet*. 1993;341:1105–1109.

84. McDonagh T, Robb S, Murdoch D, et al. Biochemical detection of left-ventricular systolic dysfunction. *Lancet*. 1998;351:9–13.

85. Groenning B, Nilsson J, Sondergaard L, et al. Evaluation of impaired left ventricular ejection fraction and increased dimensions by multiple neurohumoral plasma concentrations. *Eur J Heart Fail*. 2001;3:699–708.

86. Luchner A, Burnett J, Jougasaki M, et al. Evaluation of brain natriuretic peptide as marker of left ventricular dysfunction and hypertrophy in the population. *J Hypertens*. 2000;18:1121–1128.

87. Clerico A, Del Ry S, Maffei S, et al. The circulating levels of cardiac natriuretic hormones in healthy adults: effects of age and sex. *Clin Chem Lab Med*. 2002;40:371–377.

88. Davis K, Fish L, Elahi D, et al. Atrial natriuretic peptide levels in the prediction of congestive heart failure risk in frail elderly. *JAMA*. 1992;267:2625–2629.

89. Richards A, Nicholls M, Espiner E, et al. B-type natriuretic peptides and ejection fraction for prognosis after myocardial infarction. *Circulation*. 2003;107:2786–2792.

90. Gottlieb S, Kukin M, Ahern D, et al. Prognostic importance of atrial natriuretic peptide in patients with chronic heart failure. *J Am Coll Cardiol*. 1989;13:1534–1539.

91. Selvais P, Donckier J, Robert A, et al. Cardiac natriuretic peptides for diagnosis and risk stratification in heart failure: influences of left ventricular dysfunction and coronary artery disease on cardiac hormonal activation. *Eur J Clin Invest*. 1998;28:636–642.

92. Swedberg K, Eneroth P, Kjekshus J, CONSENSUS Trial Study Group. Hormones regulating cardiovascular function in patients with severe congestive heart failure and their relation to mortality. *Circulation*. 1990;82:1730–1736.

93. Koglin J, Pehlivanli S, Schwaiblmair M, et al. Role of brain natriuretic peptide in risk stratification of patients with congestive heart failure. *J Am Coll Cardiol*. 2001;38:1934–1941.

94. Berger R, Huelsman M, Strecker K, et al. B-type natriuretic peptide predicts sudden death in patients with chronic heart failure. *Circulation*. 2002;105:2392–2397.

95. Vrtovec B, Delgado R, Zewail A, et al. Prolonged QTc interval and high B-type natriuretic peptide levels together predict mortality in patients with advanced heart failure. *Circulation*. 2003;107:1764–1769.

96. Cheng V, Kazanagra R, Garcia A, et al. A rapid bedside test for B-type peptide predicts treatment outcomes in patients admitted for decompensated heart failure: a pilot study. *J Am Coll Cardiol*. 2001;37:386–391.

97. Anand I, Fisher L, Chiang Y, et al. Changes in brain natriuretic peptide and norepinephrine over time and mortality and morbidity in the Valsartan Heart Failure Trial (Val-HeFT). *Circulation*. 2003;107:1278–1283.

98. Cowie M, Jourdain P, Maisel A, et al. Clinical applications of B-type natriuretic peptide (BNP) testing. *Eur Heart J.* 2003;24:1710–1718.

99. Bouvy M, Heerdink E, Leufkens H, et al. Predicting mortality in patients with heart failure: a pragmatic approach. *Heart.* 2003;89:605–609.

100. Ghio S, Gavazzi A, Campana C, et al. Independent and additive prognostic value of right ventricular systolic function and pulmonary artery pressure in patients with chronic heart failure. *J Am Coll Cardiol.* 2001;37:183–188.

101. Polak J, Holman B, Wynne J, et al. Right ventricular ejection fraction: an indicator of increased mortality in patients with congestive heart failure associated with coronary artery disease. *J Am Coll Cardiol.* 1983;2:217–224.

102. Pozzoli M, Traversi E, Cioffi G, et al. Loading manipulations improve the prognostic value of Doppler evaluation of mitral flow in patients with chronic heart failure. *Circulation.* 1997;95:1222–1230.

103. Campana C, Gavazzi A, Berzuini C, et al. Predictors of prognosis in patients awaiting heart transplantation. *Heart Lung Transplant.* 1993;12:756–765.

104. Gheorghiade M, Gattis W, Adams K, et al. Rationale and design of the pilot randomized study of nesiritide versus dobutamine in heart failure (PRESERVD-HF). *Am Heart J.* 2003;145: S55–S57.

105. Weinfeld M, Chertow G, Stevenson L. Aggravated renal dysfunction during intensive therapy for advanced chronic heart failure. *Am Heart J.* 1999;138:285–290.

106. Krumholz H, Chen Y, Vaccarino V, et al. Correlates and impact on outcomes of worsening renal function in patients 65 years of age with heart failure. *Am J Cardiol.* 2000;85:1110–1113.

107. Rich M, Beckham V, Wittenberg C, et al. A multidisciplinary intervention to prevent the readmission of elderly patients with congestive heart failure. *N Engl J Med.* 1995;333:1190–1195.

108. Anavekar N, McMurray J, Velazquez E, et al. Relation between renal dysfunction and cardiovascular outcomes after myocardial infarction. *N Engl J Med.* 2004;351:1285–1295.

109. Gottlieb S, Brater D, Thomas I, et al. BG9719 (CVT-124), an A1 adenosine receptor antagonist, protects against the decline in renal function observed with diuretic therapy. *Circulation.* 2002;105:1348–1353.

110. Felker G, Gattis W, Leimberger J, et al. Usefulness of anemia as a predictor of death and rehospitalization in patients with decompensated heart failure. *Am J Cardiol.* 2003;92: 625–628.

111. Chandler A, O'Connor C, Gattis W, et al. Patients with preserved systolic function hospitalized for decompensated heart failure have 60-day event rates similar to patients with systolic dysfunction: observations from the IMPACT-HF registry. *J Card Fail.* 2003;9:S12.

112. Gheorghiade M, Gattis W, O'Connor C, et al. Effects of tolvaptan, a vasopressin antagonist, in patients hospitalized with worsening heart failure: a randomized controlled trial. *JAMA.* 2004;291:1963–1971.

113. Konstam MA, Gheorghiade M, Burnett JC Jr, et al. Efficacy of Vasopressin Antagonism in Heart Failure Outcome Study with Tolvaptan (EVEREST) Investigators. Effects of oral tolvaptan in patients hospitalized for worsening heart failure: the EVEREST Outcome Trial. *JAMA.* 2007;297(12):1319–1331. Epub 2007 Mar 25.

114. Gheorghiade M, Konstam MA, Burnett JC Jr, et al. Efficacy of Vasopressin Antagonism in Heart Failure Outcome Study With Tolvaptan (EVEREST) Investigators. Short-term clinical effects of tolvaptan, an oral vasopressin antagonist, in patients hospitalized for heart failure: the EVEREST Clinical Status Trials. *JAMA.* 2007;297(12):1332–1343.

CHAPTER 6

Therapeutic Approach to Heart Failure: An Overview

Daniel L. Dries, MD, MPH/Mariell Jessup, MD

► INTRODUCTION

The lifetime risk of developing heart failure (HF) is 20% in both men and women; this risk changes with age and time.[1,2] The *American College of Cardiology/American Heart Association (ACC/AHA) Guidelines for the Evaluation and Management of Chronic Heart Failure in the Adult* has been instrumental in more clearly articulating the early stages of HF, or the preclinical phase of the disease, and the patterns of disease associated with subsequent progression to clinical symptoms (Fig. 6-1).[3] Those risk factors include hypertension, diabetes, hyperlipidemia, coronary artery disease, or any of these factors in combination. (Obviously, there are less readily identifiable risks as well, such as inherited forms of cardiomyopathy that will one day be easily recognized through gene profiling, but are currently unclear and therefore unhelpful to a busy clinician.)

When a clinician encounters a patient with symptomatic HF, the task is to apply the guidelines to the individual patient in a rational and logical manner. The therapeutic goals for the patient with HF are to improve quality of life and to improve survival. A number of studies have clearly documented that patients with HF, especially severe HF, value the absence of discomfort and

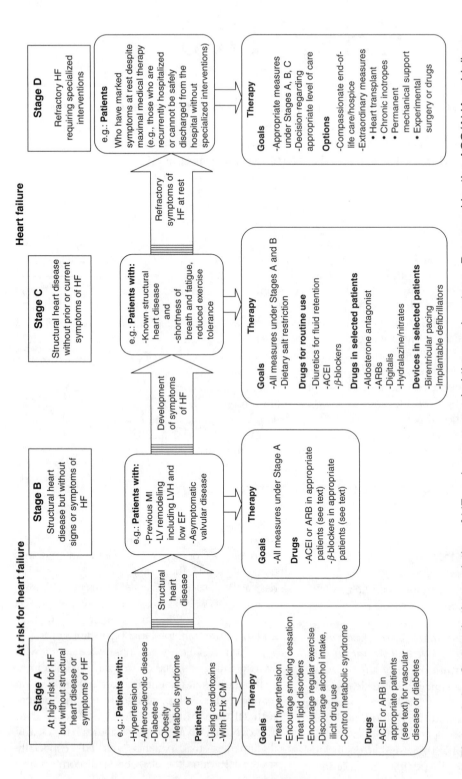

Figure 6-1 Stages in the evolution of HF and recommended therapy by stage. Proposed by the ACC/AHA guidelines for the evaluation and management of chronic HF in adults of 2001. ACC/AHA—American College of Cardiology/American Heart Association; ACEI—angiotensin-converting enzyme inhibitors; ARB—angiotensin receptor blocker; EF—ejection fraction; FHx CM—family history of cardiomyopathy; HF—heart failure; IV—intravenous; LV—left ventricular; MI—myocardial infarction. (Reproduced with permission from Hunt SA, American College of Cardiology, American Heart Association Task Force on Practice Guidelines (Writing Committee to Update the 2001 Guidelines for the Evaluation and Management of Heart Failure). ACC/AHA 2005 guideline update for the diagnosis and management of chronic heart failure in the adult: a report of the American College of Cardiology/American Heart Association Task Force on Practice Guidelines. *J Am Coll Cardiol.* 2005;46(6):E1-E82.)

breathlessness as much or more than the actual duration of their lives.[4] Improvement in the quality of life may mean different things to different patients and may include the absence of hospitalizations, the ability to go shopping with family, or the capacity to continue gainful employment. It is a useful exercise to ask each patient what aspect of his or her illness is most troubling, and then follow the impact of disease management on this perceived disability. Certainly, an improvement of score on a formalized questionnaire used in HF to assess quality of life is an indication of enhanced function. Likewise, an increasing ability to perform during exercise testing is another way to document that this goal is being achieved. Irrespective of the method used to chart functional capacity, clinicians need to periodically assess whether their patients with HF are maintaining or improving quality of life. This is an important goal of therapy and one in which individual patients can be monitored.

There has been a deserved emphasis on the high mortality rate of patients with HF, and as public health advocates, we want to favorably impact survival.[5-7] However, as practicing clinicians, our patients' care can't be dictated by our predictions of their demise. To date, there have been very few reliable methods to accurately calculate an individual's prognosis after HF becomes evident.[8] Rather, clinicians must use those treatments that have been shown in well-designed trials to improve survival, and hope that the broad results are applicable to the single patient at hand. This, then, is the art of medicine. Clinicians must forge ahead with the prescription of drugs that have been shown to be life saving in large studies for an individual patient, who may not resemble the study population.[9,10] The goal of this chapter is to present a general therapeutic approach to the patient with HF, focusing on the patient with HF related to left ventricular systolic function. Many of the specific therapies discussed are addressed in considerably greater detail in dedicated chapters in this book. Our goal is to present a general therapeutic algorithm for the clinician encountering such a patient (Fig. 6-2).

▶ INITIAL THERAPEUTIC APPROACH TO THE PATIENT WITH HEART FAILURE

Differentiate Systolic from Diastolic Heart Failure

The overwhelming numbers of studies performed in an HF population have been in those patients with dilated left ventricles that are poorly contracting, a syndrome often referred to as systolic dysfunction. Although there is a growing recognition that as many as 30–50% of all hospitalized patients with HF have normal cardiac contractility, or a preserved ejection fraction (EF), there remains a paucity of evidence-based recommendations for this group. (This syndrome has been called a variety of names including diastolic HF, or nondilated HF.) Most reviews stress the importance of excluding significant coronary ischemia as an exacerbating cause of HF symptoms, and all agree that meticulous control of hypertension is critical.[11-13] Many of these patients with HF and a normal EF present with atrial arrhythmias, usually atrial fibrillation, and control of heart rate in this situation can be very useful. Obesity, diabetes, arthritis, and renal insufficiency are typical comorbid conditions in this group of patients, so a search for exacerbating drugs used to treat these conditions may be fruitful. Sleep apnea is common, and a screening interview for sleep disturbances is appropriate.[14,15]

Identify Correctable Causes of the Cardiac Dysfunction

If the patient has HF in the setting of a dilated left ventricle and has a low left ventricular EF as determined by an echocardiogram, nuclear ventriculography, or angiography, then the next phase is to pursue, by means of a complete history and physical examination and a few simple diagnostic tests, a search for reversible or correctable causes of the low systolic function. In the United States, the most common cause of dilated cardiomyopathy

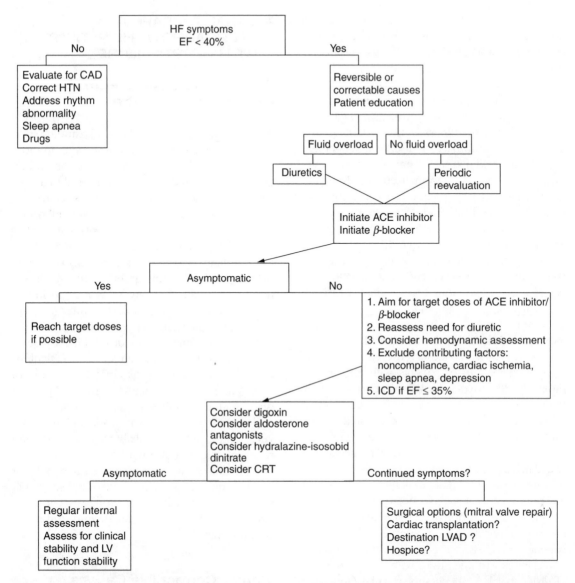

Figure 6-2   A multidrug algorithm for the clinical management of patients with HF symptoms. ACE—angiotensin-converting enzyme; ARB—angiotensin receptor blockers; CAD—coronary artery disease; CRT—cardiac resynchronization therapy; CRT—cardiac resynchronization therapy; EF—ejection fraction; HF—heart failure; HTN—hypertension; ICD—implantable cardiovecterdefibrillator; ICD—implantable cardiac defibrillators; LVAD—Left ventricular assist device; LVEF—left ventricular ejection fraction; MV—mitral valve; VAD—ventricular assist device

is chronic ischemia related to coronary artery obstruction.[16–22] A complete list of potentially correctable etiologies is beyond this chapter, but may include illicit drug use or alcohol abuse, thyroid disorders, or uncontrolled hypertension.

It is important to exclude the role of coronary artery disease as the cause of left ventricular dysfunction. It is estimated that coronary artery disease is the cause of HF in up to two-thirds of patients with left ventricular systolic dysfunction.[23]

It has been demonstrated that coronary revascularization improves symptoms and survival in patients with HF and angina, although patients with markedly impaired ventricular function were not included in these studies.[24] As many as one-third of patients with nonischemic cardiomyopathy may complain of chest pain suggestive of angina, and in these patients noninvasive imaging may demonstrate perfusion defects and segmental wall motion abnormalities. Therefore, it is reasonable to proceed directly to coronary angiography in young patients with HF, angina, and left ventricular systolic dysfunction. It is debated whether or not routine coronary angiography is warranted in all patients, who present with HF and left ventricular dysfunction in the absence of chest pain, because coronary revascularization has not been clearly demonstrated to improve survival in patients without angina.[25] Nonetheless, there are data to suggest that revascularization might improve ventricular function. Therefore, it is a reasonable strategy to exclude coronary artery disease in all patients with newly diagnosed HF and left ventricular systolic dysfunction even in the absence of chest pain.

Recognize and Treat Elevated Cardiac Filling Pressures

The next task when encountering the patient with left ventricular systolic function is to assess the clinical status of the patient. The clinical examination should focus on assessing the volume status of the patient, specifically, the degree of elevation of cardiac filling pressures. Most of the "congestion" that characterizes the HF syndrome is directly related to elevations of left-sided cardiac filling pressure, and provides the largest target for symptomatic improvement. Although the presence of peripheral edema, pulmonary rales, and evidence of pulmonary venous hypertension on chest x-ray are highly specific for elevated cardiac filling pressures, the sensitivity of these signs is low.[26] The clinical examination finding with the highest sensitivity and specificity for elevated left-sided filling pressures is elevation of the jugular venous pressure.

For example, Drazner and colleagues examined the relationship of right- and left-sided filling pressures in 1000 patients with advanced cardiomyopathy, who underwent right heart catheterization.[27] They demonstrated that a right atrial pressure greater than 10 mm Hg correlated with a pulmonary-capillary wedge pressure greater than 22 mm Hg in the large majority (~80%) of patients. The assessment of the jugular venous pressure is a critical skill for the management of patients with HF and can identify the presence of elevated intracardiac filling pressures in the absence of evidence of edema, rales upon auscultation of the lungs, or evidence of pulmonary venous hypertension on chest-x-ray. A "square-wave" systolic blood pressure response to the Valsalva maneuver is also a useful clinical tool to detect elevated left ventricular end-diastolic pressure in patients with dilated cardiomyopathy.[28–30]

When volume overload is identified, the clinician needs to focus attention on a strategy to relieve congestion. Diuretics produce symptomatic benefits more rapidly than any other drug used for HF; they can relieve peripheral or pulmonary edema with hours or days.[31] Diuretics are the only drugs used in the outpatient management of HF that can adequately control fluid retention. Nevertheless, they should never be the sole treatment for patients with Stage C HF, even if the patient becomes asymptomatic after the initiation of a diuresis. Using the skills outlined above, a clinician needs to determine whether a patient has signs or symptoms of fluid retention, and then begin a maintenance diuretic regimen. Although some patients with dilated cardiomyopathy, who have been stabilized on a standard regimen of neurohormonal antagonists may be effectively managed without diuretics, the large majority of patients will need a regular dose of diuretic, usually daily. Diuretic dosage may need to be adjusted as time and other circumstances change. Periodic physical examinations coupled with home weight monitoring and laboratory testing should be done to avoid azotemia or electrolyte imbalances. A key reason for follow-up office visits of the HF patient is to assess the need for diuretic dose adjustment.

Initiate Therapy with Neurohormonal Antagonists

All patients with a low EF (in the absence of aortic outflow obstruction) should be initiated and maintained on both an angiotensin-converting enzyme (ACE) inhibitor and a β-blocker.[3] For historical reasons, clinicians commonly start an ACE inhibitor first and add a β-blocker as a second agent, but recent data suggest that starting a β-blocker as initial therapy has some advantages.[32] Clinicians need to keep in focus that their ultimate task is to maintain patients on both drugs at the highest tolerated dosages. Thus, it is reasonable to start both drugs at very low doses and then uptitrate each drug alternately until target doses are reached or patients become intolerant. If hypotension or azotemia develops, reducing diuretics or staggering the dosing time of the drugs may alleviate symptoms.

Clinicians, in their eagerness, may simultaneously start a patient with newly diagnosed dilated cardiomyopathy and HF on diuretics, ACE inhibitors and β-blockers, all within a 12-hour period. The result is often hypotension, azotemia, or both, and the clinician may wrongly conclude that the patient is intolerant of these life-saving drugs. Once a patient is euvolemic, there is no specific time course that necessitates rushing to get a patient on both drugs. A slow steady approach over several weeks is usually more successful. Many times this can be done without an office visit, but rather through a nurse-administered titration protocol supervised by phone calls.

Unfortunately, not all persons tolerate treatment with an ACE inhibitor. With a 2–10% incidence of a dry cough, potential exacerbation of underlying renal dysfunction and a rare incidence of angioedema, ACE inhibitors have appreciable side effects. In an effort to antagonize the renin-angiotensin system without the side effects of ACE inhibition, direct angiotensin receptor blockers (ARBs) were developed. ARBs bind to angiotensin II receptors, attenuating the diverse effects of this hormone. Now proven effective in treatment of HF, ARBs provide an attractive option in those intolerant of ACE inhibitor therapy.

Determine Need for Implantable Cardiac Defibrillators

The management of patients with systolic HF includes the evaluation for additional nonpharmacologic therapies that have been demonstrated to improve survival. The indications for implantable cardiac defibrillators (ICDs) in the systolic HF population continue to evolve. In patients with cardiac arrest due to ventricular tachycardia (VT) or ventricular fibrillation (VF), or hemodynamically significant sustained VT, an ICD is indicated. The ACC/AHA/NASPE guidelines consider the placement of an ICD a Class IIa indication in patients with ischemic cardiomyopathy with an EF less than 30%, who are at least 1 month postmyocardial infraction or 3 months postcoronary artery revascularization.[33] This recommendation is supported by the results of MADIT II.[34] The release of the results from the Sudden Cardiac Death in Heart Failure Trial (SCD-HeFT) trial suggests that all patients with New York Heart Association (NYHA) Class II HF and an EF less than 35% experience a mortality benefit from an ICD compared to treatment with standard medical therapy, including routine use of β-blockers, or the combination of a β-blocker and amiodarone, in addition to ACE inhibitor therapy. Clinicians encountering patients with HF must, therefore, consider the evaluation for an ICD in conjunction with standard pharmacotherapy. The interpretation and clinical implications of SCD-HeFT will continue to evolve as the data are interpreted by regulatory agencies and additional cost-effectiveness analyses are performed. Strictly interpreted, the data clearly demonstrated that in all patients with symptomatic HF and an EF less than 35%, regardless of etiology, placement of an ICD reduces mortality approximately 23% (hazard ratio 0.77; 95% confidence interval 0.62–0.96; P = 0.007).

Patient and Family Education

Fundamental to our algorithm is the initiation of patient (and family) education.[35] There are some key principals to cover with the patient, including, the potential seriousness of the diagnosis; recommendations about diet, that is, whether the patient needs to restrict fluid or sodium; recommendations about exercise; develop a routine for the patient to self-monitor his or her volume status at home, usually done by daily weights; counsel about alcohol and/or nicotine use; an action plan for the patient, who may develop increasing symptoms; and finally, discuss end-of-life wishes. Although these instructions do take time initially, they will serve both the office staff and the patient well in the future. Moreover, there are an increasing number of electronic educational sites available on the Internet that will reinforce the instructions and teaching done in the office.

Assessment of Response to Therapy

It is important to assess a patient in a routine manner at each visit to accurately determine their symptomatic status. Patients with HF often begin to decrease their attempts at physical activity, usually subconsciously, so that over time their subjective complaints may diminish despite progressive cardiac deterioration. Ask about one or two items that a patient must do on a regular basis, such as making a bed or showering and dressing without stopping, as a routine at each visit. Always ask about social outings or visits with family members, as patients with severe HF or profound fatigue will stop undertaking even pleasurable encounters but may not volunteer this information. Think about incorporating some simple assessment of submaximal exercise into an office visit periodically. This may involve watching the patient walk in place, a measured walk in a hall, or a more formal treadmill test.[36] The amount of information gained, including the possibility of noting marked increases in blood pressure, failure of heart rate to augment, or the aggravation of arrhythmias can often justify the time and expense of the test. There are also some standardized questionnaires that assess quality of life in patients with HF that can be self-administered in the office and maintained in the office

file.[37,38] Additional information that must be acquired and documented at each visit includes any emergency room visits or hospitalizations the patient may have experienced. A review must be made of each medication the patient is taking, including over-the-counter medications that could be exacerbating the HF syndrome. Certain arthritis or pain formulations are common culprits, as are some drugs used for diabetic management.[39–41] Other important historical information includes the possibility of dizziness, syncope, chest pain, or severe sleep disturbances; all of these symptoms may be amenable to treatment or may require intervention.

▶ APPROACH TO THE PATIENT WITH CONTINUED SYMPTOMS

Identify Unrecognized Elevation of Cardiac Filling Pressures

In the patient with continued symptoms, the clinician should continue to assess for evidence of persistent elevation of cardiac filling pressures. These patients often have continued elevation of cardiac filling pressures that is unrecognized. They may benefit from more aggressive diuretic doses, including the combination of a loop agent and a distal agent, although sometimes this approach is limited by cardiorenal limitation, defined by worsening renal function limiting the aggressiveness of diuresis. In these patients, it may be useful to define the underlying hemodynamic profile with a right heart catheterization and using this information to tailor therapy to the individual patient.[42,43] Although not recommended for the routine management of patients with HF, in the refractory patient this approach may reveal a combination of elevated intracardiac filling pressures coupled with elevated systemic vascular resistance, and the judicious use of an intravenous vasodilator coupled with diuretic therapy may be necessary to achieve compensation and transition the patient to a more stable outpatient medical regimen that can sustain the improvements beyond the index hospitalization.[44]

Consider Additional Neurohormonal Antagonists

The clinician might also consider additional pharmacological agents in the patient with persistent HF symptoms despite treatment with adequate doses of a β-blocker and ACE inhibitor. The use of digoxin is a Class I indication for the treatment of symptoms of HF in conjunction with the use of diuretics, an ACE inhibitor, and a β-blocker.[3] There is only one randomized and placebo-controlled clinical trial that evaluated the effect of digoxin therapy on mortality in patients with HF. The Digitalis Investigation Group (DIG) trial randomized 6800 persons with symptomatic HF on ACE inhibitor and diuretic therapy to treatment with digoxin or placebo.[45] Although failing to reach its primary end point, a decrease in all-cause mortality, randomization to digoxin conveyed a significant decrease in risk of death or hospitalization due to worsening HF. Digoxin was well-tolerated and associated with few adverse side effects in this trial. Digoxin dosing should be adjusted for renal dysfunction and concomitant therapy with medications known to increase serum digoxin levels.

The use of an aldosterone antagonist should be considered in patients with recent or current symptoms of HF despite the use of digoxin, diuretics, an ACE inhibitor and a β-blocker. The Randomized Aldactone Evaluation Study (RALES) randomized 1663 persons with NYHA Class III–IV symptoms to treatment with spironolactone or placebo.[46] At baseline, the majority of participants were receiving diuretics, an ACE inhibitor, and digoxin. Spironolactone conferred a significant reduction in the risk of death as well as a reduction in the risk for hospitalization from cardiovascular causes. Favorable side effect and safety profiles were also established as hyperkalemia, renal dysfunction, and hypotension were no different between the spironolactone and placebo groups. Gynecomastia and breast pain were significantly more common in the treatment group, likely due to the steroid activity of spironolactone. Although a single study, the Randomized Aldactone Evaluation Study (RALES) trial established spironolactone as a potent therapeutic agent in advanced HF. The main criticism of this study is the relatively low use of β-blocker therapy in the enrolled subjects. Nonetheless, the current ACC/AHA guidelines recommend use of spironolactone in persons with a history of NYHA Class IIII or IV symptoms, normal renal function, and normal serum potassium levels.[3]

Assess Need for Cardiac Resynchronization Therapy

Data continue to accumulate from randomized controlled clinical trials demonstrating that cardiac resynchronization therapy (CRT) may reduce symptoms, improve functional capacity, and possible improve mortality in select patients with systolic HF.[47,48] Currently, the surface electrocardiogram is used as an indicator to identify patients who may benefit from CRT; patients with a prolonged QRS interval, especially if greater than 140 milliseconds, appear to benefit from CRT. Increasingly, however, there are data to suggest that the surface electrocardiogram lacks sensitivity in identifying patients who have significant mechanical contraction dyssynchrony.[49] The key challenge is to use these techniques to improve our ability to identify patients with the greatest likelihood to benefit from CRT. It is appropriate to consider CRT in patients with refractory symptoms of HF and evidence of either interventricular or intraventricular dyssynchrony.

Evaluate Contribution of Related Comorbidities to Symptoms

In the HF patient with continued symptoms, the clinician should also consider other potential etiologies. Is there evidence of new or exacerbated ischemia that accounts for the patient's symptoms? Perhaps a reevaluation for coronary artery disease should be considered. Is the patient's fatigue and nocturnal restlessness a manifestation of sleep apnea rather than worsening HF with orthopnea? Sleep apnea, both obstructive and central, is common in patients with HF and can be treated.[50,51] Depression is not uncommon in patients with HF and may contribute to increased mortality.[52–54] Highly efficacious therapy is available to treat depression and should be utilized in these patients.

▶ THE PATIENT WITH REFRACTORY HEART FAILURE

Despite great advances in our management strategies for HF, there will always be patients who do not respond to our best efforts or our most efficacious drugs. As our therapeutic approaches improve, the population of patients with advanced cardiomyopathy is increasing. Cardiac transplantation is an option for only a very select few of this group.[55] The results of the Randomized Evaluation of Mechanical Assistance for the Treatment of Congestive Heart Failure (REMATCH) study have revealed that in patients who are not candidates for cardiac transplantation, permanent ventricular assist devices (VAD) may improve survival and quality of life.[56–59] These devices may become technologically improved in the future and may provide a solution for a larger and more meaningful group of patients. Most importantly, a repeat discussion about end-of-life decisions and wishes must be undertaken. Although home inotropic therapy may increase mortality, it may improve quality of life. Recent studies have demonstrated that in many patients with Stage D/refractory HF quality of life is more desired than length of life. Hospice is an appropriate alternative for many patients, as compared to an endless cycle of increasingly longer hospital admissions.[60]

▶ SUMMARY

The clinician evaluating the patient with HF must differentiate systolic from diastolic HF. Diastolic HF is treated with diuretics and pharmacotherapy aimed at controlling heart rate and blood pressure. Randomized clinical trials are lacking in this population. For the patient with systolic HF, reversible causes of systolic dysfunction should be considered. A left heart catheterization to exclude coronary artery disease should be considered. The clinician must then focus upon treatment aimed at improving symptoms and improving survival. Symptom relief depends upon the recognition of elevated cardiac filling pressures and judicious use of diuretic therapy to reduce elevated cardiac filling pressures. Next, pharmacotherapy with an ACE inhibitor and β-blocker therapy is initiated. Frequent follow-up is critical to assess response to therapy as neurohormonal antagonists are uptitrated. Patient education is of paramount importance in achieving and maintaining clinical stability. The clinician must consider a variety of cardiac and noncardiac conditions in the patient with persistent symptoms.

▶ REFERENCES

1. Levy D, Kenchaiah S, Larson MG, et al. Long-term trends in the incidence of and survival with heart failure. *N Engl J Med.* 2002; 347(18):1397–1402.
2. Lloyd-Jones DM, Larson MG, Leip EP, et al. Lifetime risk for developing congestive heart failure: the Framingham Heart Study. *Circulation.* 2002;106(24):3068–3072.
3. Hunt SA, Abraham WT, Chin MH, et al. ACC/AHA 2005 Guideline update for the diognosis and management of chronic heart failure in the adult: summary article. *J Am Call Cardiol.* 2005; 46:1116–1143.
4. Lewis EF, Johnson PA, Johnson W, et al. Preferences for quality of life or survival expressed by patients with heart failure. *J Heart Lung Transplant.* 2001;20(9):1016–1024.
5. Baker DW, Einstadter D, Thomas C, et al. Mortality trends for 23,505 Medicare patients hospitalized with heart failure in Northeast Ohio, 1991 to 1997. *Am Heart J.* 2003;146(2):258–264.
6. Cicoira M, Davos CH, Florea V, et al. Chronic heart failure in the very elderly: clinical status, survival, and prognostic factors in 188 patients more than 70 years old. *Am Heart J.* 2001;142(1): 174–180.
7. Cowie MR, Wood DA, Coats AJ, et al. Survival of patients with a new diagnosis of heart failure:

a population based study. *Heart*. 2000;83(5): 505–510.

8. Cowie MR. Estimating prognosis in heart failure: time for a better approach. [comment.] *Heart*. 2003;89(6):587–588.

9. Khand A, Gemmel I, Clark A, et al. Is the prognosis of heart failure improving? *J Am Coll Cardiol*. 2000;36(7):2284–2286.

10. Konstam MA. Progress in heart failure management: lessons from the real world. *Circulation*. 2000;102(10):1076–1078.

11. Zile MR, Brutsaert DL. New concepts in diastolic dysfunction and diastolic heart failure: part II: causal mechanisms and treatment. *Circulation*. March 26, 2002;105(12):1503–1508.

12. Zile MR, Brutsaert DL. New concepts in diastolic dysfunction and diastolic heart failure: part I: diagnosis, prognosis, and measurements of diastolic function. *Circulation*. March 19, 2002;105(11):1387–1393.

13. Gaasch WH, Zile MR. Left ventricular diastolic dysfunction and diastolic heart failure. *Ann Rev Med*. 2004;55:373–394.

14. Bradley TD, Floras JS. Sleep apnea and heart failure: part I: obstructive sleep apnea. *Circulation*. 2003;107(12):1671–1678.

15. LanFranchi PA, Somers VK. Sleep disordered breathing in heart failure: characteristics and implications. *Resp Physiol Neurobiol*. 2003; 136: 153–165.

16. Adams KF, Jr. New epidemiologic perspectives concerning mild-to-moderate heart failure. *Am J Med*. 2001;110(suppl 7A):S6–S13.

17. Adams KF Jr, Dunlap SH, Sueta CA, et al. Relation between gender, etiology and survival in patients with symptomatic heart failure. *J Am Coll Cardiol*. 1996;28:1781–1788.

18. Cowie MR, Wood DA, Coats AJ, et al. Incidence and aetiology of heart failure: a population-based study. *Eur Heart J*. 1999;20:421–428.

19. Dunlap SH, Sueta CA, Tomasko L, et al. Association of body mass, gender and race with heart failure primarily due to hypertension. *J Am Coll Cardiol*. 1999;34(5):1602–1608.

20. Guertl B, Noehammer C, Hoefler G. Metabolic cardiomyopathies. *Int J Exp Pathol*. 2000;81(6): 349–372.

21. Haas GJ. Etiology, evaluation, and management of acute myocarditis. *Cardiol Rev*. 2001;9(2): 88–95.

22. Mair FS, Crowley TS, Bundred PE. Prevalence, aetiology and management of heart failure in general practice. *Br J Gen Pract*. 1996;46:77–79.

23. Gheorghiade M, Bonow RO. Chronic heart failure in the United States: a manifestation of coronary artery disease. *Circulation*. 1998;97: 282–289.

24. Alderman EL, Fisher LD, Litwin P, et al. Results of coronary artery surgery in patients with poor left ventricular function (CASS). *Circulation*. October 1983;68(4):785–795.

25. Eagle KA, Guyton RA, Davidoff R, et al. ACC/AHA guidelines for coronary artery bypass graft surgery: executive summary and recommendations: a report of the American College of Cardiology/American Heart Association Task Force on Practice Guidelines (committee to revise the 1991 guidelines for coronary artery bypass graft surgery). *Circulation*. 1999;100(13): 1464–1480.

26. Stevenson L, Perloff J. The limited reliability of physical signs for estimating hemodynamics in chronic heart failure. *JAMA*. February 10, 1989;261(6):884–888.

27. Drazner MH, Hamilton MA, Fonarow G, et al. Relationship between right and left-sided filling pressures in 1000 patients with advanced heart failure. *J Heart Lung Transplant*. 1999;18(11): 1126–1132.

28. Sanders GP, Mendes LA, Colucci WS, et al. Noninvasive methods for detecting elevated left-sided cardiac filling pressure. *J Card Fail*. June 2000;6(2):157–164.

29. Schwammenthal E, Popescu BA, Popescu AC, et al. Noninvasive assessment of left ventricular end-diastolic pressure by the response of the transmitral a-wave velocity to a standardized Valsalva maneuver. *Am J Cardiol*. July 15, 2000; 86(2):169–174.

30. Schwengel RH, Hawke MW, Fisher ML, et al. Abnormal Valsalva blood pressure response in dilated cardiomyopathy: association with "pseudonormalization" of echocardiographic Doppler transmitral filling velocity pattern. *Am Heart J*. November 1993;126(5):1182–1186.

31. Haller H. Diuretics in congestive heart failure: new evidence for old problems. *Nephrol Dial Transplant*. 1999;14:1358–1360.

32. Sliwa K, Norton GR, Kone N, et al. Impact of initiating carvedilol before angiotensin-converting enzyme inhibitor therapy on cardiac function in newly diagnosed heart failure. *J Am Coll Cardiol*. November 2, 2004;44(9): 1825–1830.

33. Gregoratos G, Abrams J, Epstein AE, et al. ACC/AHA/NASPE 2002 guideline update for implantation of cardiac pacemakers and antiarrhythmia devices: summary article: a report of

the American College of Cardiology/American Heart Association Task Force on Practice Guidelines (ACC/AHA/NASPE committee to update the 1998 pacemaker guidelines). *J Cardiovasc Electrophysiol*. November 2002; 13(11):1183–1199.

34. Moss AJ, Zareba W, Hall WJ, et al. Prophylactic implantation of a defibrillator in patients with myocardial infarction and reduced ejection fraction. *N Engl J Med*. 2002;346(12):877–883.

35. Colonna P, Sorino M, D'Agostino C, et al. Nonpharmacologic care of heart failure: counseling, dietary restriction, rehabilitation, treatment of sleep apnea, and ultrafiltration. *Am J Cardiol*. 2003;91(9A):F41–F50.

36. Demers C, McKelvie RS, Negassa A, et al. Reliability, validity, and responsiveness of the six-minute walk test in patients with heart failure. *Am Heart J*. 2001;142(4):698–703.

37. Rector T, Cohn J. Assessment of patient outcome with the Minnesota Living with Heart Failure questionnaire: reliability and validity during a randomized, double-blind, placebo-controlled trial of pimobendan. *Am Heart J*. 1992;124:1017.

38. Alla F, Briancon S, Guillemin F, et al. Self-rating of quality of life provides additional prognostic information in heart failure: insights into the EPICAL study. *Eur J Heart Fail*. 2002;4(3): 337–343.

39. Tang WH, Francis GS, Hoogwerf BJ, et al. Fluid retention after initiation of thiazolidinedione therapy in diabetic patients with established chronic heart failure. [see comment.] *J Am Coll Cardiol*. 2003;41(8):1394–1398.

40. Page J, Henry D. Consumption of NSAIDs and the development of congestive heart failure in elderly patients: an underrecognized public health problem. *Arch Intern Med*. 2000;160(6): 777–784.

41. Feenstra J, Heerdink ER, Grobbee DE, et al. Association of nonsteroidal anti-inflammatory drugs with first occurrence of heart failure and with relapsing heart failure: the Rotterdam Study. *Arch Intern Med*. 2002;162(3): 265–270.

42. Stevenson LW, Massie BM, Francis GS. Optimizing therapy for complex or refractory heart failure: a management algorithm. *Am Heart J*. 1998;135(6 Pt 2 Su):S293–S309.

43. Stevenson LW. Tailored therapy to hemodynamic goals for advanced heart failure. *Eur J Heart Fail*. 1999;1(3):251–257.

44. Steimle AE, Stevenson LW, Chelimsky-Fallick C, et al. Sustained hemodynamic efficacy of therapy tailored to reduce filling pressures in survivors with advanced heart failure. *Circulation*. 1997;96(4):1165–1172.

45. The Digitalis Investigation Group. The effect of digoxin on mortality and morbidity in patients with heart failure. *N Engl J Med*. February 20, 1997;336(8):525–533.

46. Pitt B, Zannad F, Remme WJ, Randomzed Aldactone Evaluation Study Investigators.. The effect of spironolactone on morbidity and mortality in patients with severe heart failure. *N Engl J Med*. September 2, 1999;341(10):709–717.

47. Abraham WT. Cardiac resynchronization therapy: a review of clinical trials and criteria for identifying the appropriate patient. *Rev Cardiovasc Med*. 2003;4(suppl 2):S30–S37.

48. Abraham WT, Fisher WG, Smith AL, et al. Cardiac resynchronization in chronic heart failure. *N Engl J Med*. 2002;346(24):1845–1853.

49. Kass DA. Predicting cardiac resynchronization response by QRS duration: the long and short of it. *J Am Coll Cardiol*. December 17, 2003;42(12): 2125–2127.

50. Villa M, Lage E, Quintana E, et al. Prevalence of sleep breathing disorders in outpatients on a heart transplant waiting list. *Transplant Proc*. August 2003;35(5):1944–1945.

51. Trupp RJ, Hardesty P, Osborne J, et al. Prevalence of sleep disordered breathing in a heart failure program. *Congest Heart Fail*. September–October 2004;10(5):217–220.

52. Junger J, Schellberg D, Muller-Tasch T, et al. Depression increasingly predicts mortality in the course of congestive heart failure. *Eur J Heart Fail*. March 2, 2005;7(2):261–267.

53. de Denus S, Spinler SA, Jessup M, et al. History of depression as a predictor of adverse outcomes in patients hospitalized for decompensated heart failure. *Pharmacotherapy*. October 2004;24(10):1306–1310.

54. O'Connor CM, Joynt KE. Depression: are we ignoring an important comorbidity in heart failure? *J Am Coll Cardiol*. May 5, 2004;43(9): 1550–1552.

55. Hunt SA. Current status of cardiac transplantation. *J Am Med Assoc*. 1998;280(19):1692–1698.

56. Frazier OH, Rose EA, Oz MC, et al. Multicenter clinical evaluation of the HeartMate vented electric left ventricular assist system in patients awaiting heart transplantation. *J Thorac Cardiovasc Surg*. 2001;122(6):1186–1195.

57. Goldstein D, Oz MC, Rose EA. Implantable left ventricular assist devices. *N Engl J Med*. 1998;339(21):1522–1533.

58. Holman WL, Davies JE, Rayburn BK, et al. Treatment of end-stage heart disease with outpatient ventricular assist devices. *Ann Thorac Surg.* 2002;73(5):1489–1493; [discussion] 1493–1484.

59. Mancini D, Oz M, Beniaminovitz A. Current experience with left ventricular assist devices in patients with congestive heart failure. *Curr Cardiol Rep.* 1999;1(1):33–37.

60. Albert NM, Davis M, Young J. Improving the care of patients dying of heart failure. *Cleve Clin J Med.* April 2002;69(4):321–328.

CHAPTER 7

How to Evaluate Patients with Symptoms Suggestive of Heart Failure

SHARON HUNT, MD

▶ INTRODUCTION

A patient presenting to a physician or to emergency services with the new onset of dyspnea on exertion or with new lower extremity edema represents a challenge, sometimes of major proportions, to the treating physician. While such symptoms are sometimes accompanied by obvious evidence of heart failure, it is often the case that their cause is not clear and other disease entities as primary or contributing factors need to be entertained. In this situation, it is helpful to pursue a standardized, or at least organized, approach to sorting out the issues and arriving at a diagnosis or diagnoses. This chapter will discuss suggested approaches to the various presenting symptoms.

▶ DYSPNEA—THE HISTORY

The sensation of dyspnea, defined as difficult or labored breathing, is a normal sensation in healthy people after strenuous exertion and in deconditioned people after moderate exertion. It is considered abnormal when it occurs with activity previously well-tolerated or at rest. Dyspnea that occurs only at rest and not with exercise is almost always functional. It is a most distressing symptom for most patients, and when they develop dyspnea as a consequence of customary physical exertion many will initially instinctively curtail their physical activity in order to avoid the sensation. In obtaining a history, it is often helpful to inquire about daily activity levels and whether these have decreased in any subtle ways, even predating the patient's awareness of symptoms. A slow onset of progressive symptoms can be compatible with heart failure, and also with primary pulmonary disease (asthma, chronic obstructive pulmonary disease [COPD], pleural disease or effusions, etc.), anxiety, or simple poor physical conditioning or obesity. More abrupt onset or change of symptoms is more suggestive of heart failure, but is also compatible with pneumothorax, pulmonary embolism, or pulmonary infection. Since heart and lung disease often coexist, the determination of which contributes primarily to a patient's symptomatic deterioration can be most difficult.

Further inquiry regarding respiratory symptoms should look for accompanying ones to suggest heart failure; specifically, to elicit (or exclude) the symptoms of orthopnea or paroxysmal nocturnal dyspnea (PND). Orthopnea, defined as difficult breathing except in the upright position, is due to a further increase in an elevated pulmonary capillary hydrostatic pressure in the supine position causing interstitial and alveolar edema and stiffening of the lungs. Many patients with heart failure instinctively sleep with one or more extra pillows to avoid the unpleasant sensation of dyspnea. The symptom of true orthopnea is distinctly uncommon in the absence of elevated pulmonary capillary pressure and its presence is a strong suggestion pointing to the cardiac cause of dyspnea.

PND, the often quite frightening onset of dyspnea, cough, and diaphoresis occurring several hours after the onset of sleep and often recurring during the night, is a second symptom, which is most strongly suggestive of heart failure as a cause of dyspnea. The symptoms are relieved by sitting up or walking around; in true PND, the patient is not able to simply turn over and go back to sleep. Nocturnal dyspnea can be associated with pulmonary disease, but in that situation the symptom is usually relieved by coughing to clear secretions rather than by sitting up.

▶ LOWER EXTREMITY EDEMA—THE HISTORY

Edema in the lower extremities, usually starting in the feet and ascending to the ankles, pretibial area, and ultimately to the presacral area (as anasarca) is a characteristic complaint in heart failure and is generally accompanied by weight gain. Peripheral edema is due to fluid retention consequent to perturbed neurohormonal activation (as described in Chap. 4), which in turn leads to elevated right-sided venous filling pressures and transudation of fluid from the soft tissue capillaries in a gravity-related fashion, starting in the feet in the upright patient. It is felt that a weight gain of 5–10 lb of fluid is necessary to produce edema in the average-sized person.

Edema can, of course, be caused by things other than heart failure. These include venous insufficiency, renal insufficiency, and hypoproteinemia. Asymmetric distribution of edema is more characteristic of venous disease, but prior orthopedic injury or vein harvest with coronary artery bypass graft (CABG) can also be associated with more prominent edema in one extremity than the other. Edema affecting primarily the face and/or arms is rarely attributable to heart failure and should lead to investigation for a cause of venous or lymphatic obstruction at a higher level.

▶ THE PHYSICAL EXAMINATION

The physical examination can provide important clues to the underlying cause of dyspnea as well as edema. Inspection of the thorax can reveal a "barrel-shaped" configuration typical of emphysema or skeletal abnormalities such as severe kyphoscoliosis that can be associated with cor pulmonale. On auscultation of the lungs during exaggerated respiration, crackles (or rales) can be heard in patients with elevated pulmonary venous pressure of any cause and generally occur according to the dictates of gravity over the lower lung fields first and ascend toward the apices as the pressures increase. However, in longstanding heart failure, the ability of the pulmonary lymphatic system to compensate for extra fluid transudation may resolve the existence of rales, and in chronic heart failure their presence has more to do with acuteness of decompensation than with severity of the disease. The same can be said for the wheezing (cardiac asthma) that often accompanies heart failure.

Palpation and auscultation of the heart can provide circumstantial evidence of structural heart disease to account for heart failure and the associated elevation of pulmonary venous pressures.

Murmurs suggestive of stenotic or regurgitant valvular lesions or congenital malformations are particularly important, as are diastolic filling sounds (S_3 or S_4). Such findings in themselves, however, do not necessarily mean that heart failure is the cause of dyspnea.

Inspection of the jugular venous pulse and examination of the abdomen can provide further evidence pointing to a cardiac etiology for edema. The internal jugular vein on the right side lies in a virtually straight line from the right atrium and best transmits pressures and waveforms from the atrium. Estimation of the height of the oscillating top of the column of blood in the internal jugular pulse is a fairly accurate measure of mean right atrial pressure. Elevation of the pressure 4 cm above the sternal angle (equal to central venous pressure of 9 cm) is abnormal. When edema is due to venous disease or hypoproteinemia, this pressure should be normal. If the jugular venous pressure is normal at rest, assessment of the presence of abdominal jugular reflux should be sought by applying pressure to the periumbilical region with the patient breathing quietly. In normal subjects, there can be at most a brief 3 cm increase in the jugular venous pressure. In patients with right or left ventricular failure, the jugular pressure can become markedly elevated and remain so for more than 15 seconds. With chronic and marked elevation of the jugular venous pressure, there can also be enlargement and even pulsatility of the liver as well as evidence of ascites on abdominal examination.

▶ LABORATORY ASSESSMENT

The history and physical examination can point strongly toward or away from the diagnosis of heart failure as the cause of a patient's symptoms, but virtually always need to be supplemented by laboratory assessment. At its most basic, such assessment will include a chest x-ray, a 12-lead electrocardiogram, appropriate hematologic and blood chemistry determinations, and usually an echocardiogram. Abnormalities on any of these

can point toward a diagnosis of heart failure, but no single finding is diagnostic of heart failure. There is increasing recognition that many patients with heart failure, especially the elderly and women, have predominantly diastolic (as opposed to systolic) dysfunction.[1-3] In the past, these patients often had their symptoms attributed to the normal consequence of aging or other coexistent illnesses when their systolic function was shown to be normal on the echocardiogram. However, it is clear that the presence of a normal left ventricular ejection fraction on echocardiography does not exclude the diagnosis of heart failure, nor are indices of diastolic function sufficiently sensitive or reproducible enough to exclude the diagnosis.

Because of the lack of sensitivity of all of these assessment modalities, there have been efforts in recent years to identify alternative means of diagnosing heart failure. Two such tests, measurements of brain natriuretic peptide (BNP) and N-terminal prohormone brain natriuretic peptide (proBNP) have been shown to improve the accuracy of heart failure diagnosis when combined with clinical judgment in an urgent care setting.[4,5] The utility of the measurement of BNP levels in the urgent care setting has led to the assumption that the assay might also be useful in the diagnosis and management of chronic heart failure. However, elevation of these peptides occurs not only with elevation of left ventricular filling pressures, but also with acute myocardial infarction and can occur with acute pulmonary embolism.[6] Levels are less elevated in obese patients with heart failure and in those with heart failure associated with preserved ejection fraction, although a normal BNP in association with a normal echocardiogram in a patient with dyspnea makes the diagnosis of heart failure unlikely.[7,8] Levels are also sensitive to factors such as age, gender, and renal function.[9,10] At the present time, elevated levels of either BNP or N-terminal proBNP certainly lend weight to a clinically suspected diagnosis of heart failure and may lead to consideration of heart failure when the diagnosis is unknown, but should not be used in isolation to confirm or exclude the diagnosis or to guide therapy.[11,12]

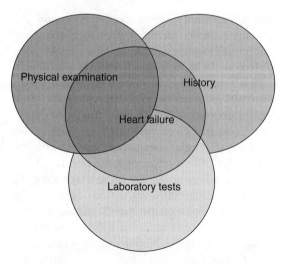

Figure 7-1 Diagnosis of heart failure depends heavily on the clinical skills and judgment of the physician, supplemented by the choice of appropriate testing.

Situations when cardiac and pulmonary diseases most likely coexist present the most challenging diagnostic dilemma. When the contribution of heart failure to the limitation of exercise limitation is an issue, maximal exercise testing with measurement of respiratory gas exchange and/or blood oxygen saturation can be useful to differentiate cardiac versus pulmonary limitations.[13]

▶ **CONCLUSION**

There is no one definitive diagnostic test for heart failure and its diagnosis depends heavily on the clinical skills and judgment of the physician supplemented by the choice of appropriate testing (Fig. 7-1).

▶ **REFERENCES**

1. Senni M, Redfield MM. Heart failure with preserved systolic function: a different natural history? *J Am Coll Cardiol.* 2001;38:1277–1282.
2. Hogg K, Swedberg K, McMurray J. Heart failure with preserved left ventricular systolic function [State of the Art paper]. *J Am Coll Cardiol.* 2004; 43:317–327.
3. Zile MR, Baicu CF, Gaasch WH. Diastolic heart failure: abnormalities in active relaxation and passive stiffness of the left ventricle. *New Engl J Med.* 2004;350:1953–1959.
4. McCullough PA, Nowak RM, McCord J, et al. B-type natriuretic peptide and clinical judgment in emergency diagnosis of heart failure: analysis from Breathing Not Properly (BNP) Multinational Study. *Circulation.* 2002;106:416–422.
5. Maisel AS, Krishnaswamy P, Nowak RM, et al. Rapid measurement of B-type natriuretic peptide in the emergency diagnosis of heart failure. *New Engl J Med.* 2002;347:161–167.
6. Ishii J, Nomura M, Ito M, et al. Plasma concentration of brain natriuretic peptide as a biochemical marker for the evaluation of right ventricular overload and mortality in chronic respiratory disease. *Clin Chim Acta.* 2000;301:19–30.
7. Lubien E, DeMaria A, Krishnaswamy P, et al. Utility of B-natriuretic peptide in detecting diastolic dysfunction: comparison with Doppler velocity recordings. *Circulation.* 2002;105: 595–601.
8. Krishnaswamy P, Lubien E, Clopton P, et al. Utility of B-natriuretic peptide levels in identifying patients witn left ventricular systolic or diastolic dysfunction. *Am J Med.* 2001;111:274.
9. Wang TJ, Larson MG, Levy D, et al. Impact of age and sex on plasma natriuretic peptide levels in healthy adults. *Am J Cardiol.* 2002;90:254–258.
10. Redfield MM, Rodeheffer RJ, Jacobson SJ, et al. Plasma brain natriuretic peptide concentration: impact of age and gender *J Am Coll Cardiol.* 2002;40:976–982.
11. Bozkurt B, Mann DL. Use of biomarkers in the management of heart failure: are we there yet? *Circulation.* 2003;107:1231–1233.
12. Packer M. Should B-type natriuretic peptide be measured routinely to guide the diagnosis and management of chronic heart failure? *Circulation.* 2003;108:2950–2953.
13. Gibbons RJ, Balady GL, Bricker JT, et al. ACC/AHA 2002 guideline update for exercise testing: summary article: a report of the ACC/AHA Task Force on practice guidelines (committee to update the 1997 exercise testing guidelines). *Circulation.* 2002;106:1883–1892.

CHAPTER 8

Nonpharmacologic Treatment of Heart Failure

ANDREW J.S. COATS, MA, DM, DSc, FRACP, FRCP,
FESC, FACC, FAHA, MBA

▶ INTRODUCTION

Chronic heart failure (CHF) is a common condition with a poor prognosis. It generates many debilitating symptoms for the sufferer. Nonpharmacologic treatment modalities play an important role alongside effective modern pharmaceutical, surgical, and device therapies. These treatments include those lifestyle measures that reduce the risk of underlying diseases such as coronary artery disease, diabetes, hypertension, and hyperlipidemia and those lifestyle interventions that benefit either the symptoms or prognosis of established heart failure (HF). The former will have formed a part of the management of the patients prior to the development of HF and should continue. This chapter will review the latter nonpharmacologic treatments that have a role in the management of the patient with HF.

Patient and Care-Giver Education

For patients to get the optimum benefit from their therapy, they and their principal caregivers need to have a good understanding of the nature and causes of CHF. Further information such as awareness of symptoms, diet, salt and fluid restriction, the nature and purpose of their drugs, and how to manage work and other physical activities, lifestyle changes, and measures of self-management of their disease is also important. Nonpharmacologic treatment should include dietary and other lifestyle advice, advice on appropriate levels of physical exercise, and health-care education. The support engendered by learning these aspects with caregivers and other patients and their families can also be of major benefit. These educational programs should form part of a comprehensive multidisciplinary program organized by the treating physician in conjunction with other health-care workers and primary care doctors, nurses, and, especially, the patients and their families. Other specialists including pharmacists dieticians, physiotherapists, psychologists, nurses, and social workers will play important supporting roles.[1]

Rest and Exercise

For many years, patients with HF were routinely advised to avoid all strenuous and even mild exertion. From the late 1980s, reports told, however, of the benefits of carefully constructed exercise training regimens for patients with stable mild to moderate CHF. These benefits have now been confirmed for many grades and stages of HF, and beneficial effects have been shown for symptoms, quality of life (QoL), exercise tolerance, and many surrogate measures of HF severity and complications.

In the first randomized controlled trial (RCT) of exercise training in CHF, we showed that training could increase exercise tolerance and improve the symptoms of dyspnea and fatigue.[2] In 11 patients with CHF secondary to ischemic heart disease (mean [SEM] age 63 [2.3] years; left ventricular ejection fraction (LVEF) 19 [8]%), 8 weeks of home-based bicycle exercise training and 8 weeks of activity restriction were prescribed in random order in a physician-blind, random-order, crossover trial. Training increased exercise duration from 14.2 (1.1) minutes to 16.8 (1.3) minutes and peak oxygen (VO_2) consumption from 14.3 (1.1) mL/min/kg to 16.7 (1.3) mL/min/kg. Heart rates at submaximum workloads and rate-pressure products were significantly reduced by training, and there was also a significant improvement in patient-rated symptom scores. No adverse events occurred during the training phase. This was a home-based physical training program that was shown to be feasible even in severe CHF. Subsequent studies have shown the benefits of exercise training extend to measures of autonomic and neurohormonal balance, muscle structure and function, endothelial and vascular function, ventilatory control, myocardial perfusion, and psychological well-being.

In 1999, Belardinelli and colleagues randomized 99 stable CHF patients (59 ± 14 years of age; 88 men and 11 women) to exercise training at 60% of peak capacity, initially three times a week for 8 weeks, then twice a week for 1 year, or control.[3] Ninety-four patients completed the protocol (48 trained and 46 in control). Both QoL and exercise tolerance were improved and mortality was lower after training (n = 9 vs. n = 20 for those with training vs. those without; relative risk (RR) = 0.37; 95% confidence interval [CI], = 0.17–0.84; P = 0.01). Fewer hospital readmissions for HF were seen in the trained group (5 vs. 14; RR = 0.29; 95% CI, 0.11–0.88; P = 0.02). Although showing a significant reduction in mortality and morbidity, this was not a prospective trial powered and designed to evaluate this effect, so we should not consider that this trial alone proved a mortality-reducing benefit of exercise training in CHF. While we wait for definitive evidence from a well-powered major multicenter trial as to whether training has prognostic as well as symptomatic benefit, the next best thing, an individual patient data meta-analysis, has suggested a significant reduction in both the risk of death and in the number of hospitalizations for HF. We coordinated a collaborative meta-analysis with inclusion criteria of all randomized parallel group-controlled trials of exercise training for at least 8 weeks with individual patient data on survival for at least 3 months.[4] Nine datasets, totaling 801 patients were identified and analyzed; 395 patients received exercise training and 406 were in controls. During a mean (SD) follow-up of 705 (729) days, there were 88 (22%) deaths in the exercise arm and 105 (26%) in the control arm. Exercise training significantly reduced mortality (hazard ratio [HR] 0.65, 95% CI, 0.46–0.92; log rank chi-square = 5.9; P = 0.015). The secondary end point of death or admission to hospital was also reduced (HR 0.72, 95% CI, 0.56–0.93; log rank chi-square = 6.4; P = 0.011). No statistically significant subgroup-specific treatment effect was observed. We can summarize that training in selected CHF patients is beneficial and safe and can reduce mortality and morbidity. It should therefore be recommended for all stable Class I–III CHF patients.

In a second overview approach, we searched the Cochrane Controlled Trials Register (The Cochrane Library Issue 2, 2001), MEDLINE (2000 to March 2001), EMBASE (1998 to March 2001), CINAHL (1984 to March 2001) and reference lists of articles, supplemented by direct enquiry of published experts. We selected all RCTs of exercise-based interventions for adults of all ages with CHF. The comparison group was usual medical care, as defined by the study, or placebo. Only those studies with criteria for diagnosis of HF (based on clinical findings or objective indices) were included. Studies were selected, and data were abstracted, independently by two reviewers supplemented by direct enquiry of authors, where possible, to obtain missing information. Twenty-nine studies were found to meet the inclusion criteria, with 1126 patients randomized. The majority of studies included both patients with primary and secondary HF, New York Heart Association (NYHA) Class II or III. None of the studies specifically examined the effect of exercise training on mortality and morbidity as most were of short duration. Exercise training significantly increased $VO_{2\ max}$ by (weighted mean difference [WMD] random effects model) 2.16 mL/kg/min (95% CI, 2.82–1.49), exercise duration increased by 2.38 minutes (95% CI, 2.85–1.9), work capacity by 15.1 Watts (95% CI, 17.7–12.6), and distance on the 6-minute walk by 40.9 m (95% CI, 64.7–17.1). Improvements in peak oxygen consumption were greater for training programs of greater intensity and duration. Health-Related Quality of Life (HRQoL) improved in the seven of nine trials that measured this outcome. We concluded that exercise training improves exercise capacity and QoL in patients with mild to moderate HF in the short term.[5]

Several questions remain unanswered. We do not know the best and safest training regimens. Although the early trials used almost exclusively an aerobic training regimen (approximately 3 days a week for 20–60 minutes per session), more recent trials have also looked at the efficacy and

safety of exercise including resistance training. One study evaluated the effects of combined endurance/resistance training on NT-proBNP levels in patients with CHF. In this study, of 27 consecutive patients with stable CHF and LVEF <35% were enrolled in a 4-month nonrandomized combined endurance/resistance training program. After 4 months, exercise training caused a significant reduction in circulating concentrations of NT-proBNP (2124 ± 397 pg/mL before, 1635 ± 304 pg/mL after training; P = 0.046, interaction), whereas no changes were observed in an untrained HF control group. This suggests that combined endurance/resistance training significantly reduced circulating levels of NT-proBNP in patients with CHF, arguing against any increase in adverse remodeling.[6] Other recent trials have shown an element of resistance as well as aerobic training to be beneficial, especially for improving muscle strength, bulk, and endurance. Some supervised in-hospital training is necessary, especially at the commencement of a training program, and may well be beneficial for encouraging long-term adherence at regular indefinite intervals. Home-based training can also be recommended in well-evaluated patients to make this a more practical treatment option for larger numbers of patients.

Diet and Nutrition

Obesity is a risk factor for many of the antecedents of HF, including coronary artery disease, diabetes, hypertension, and hyperlipidemia. Adult obesity has been shown to increase the likelihood of later HF. Despite this, in what has been described as the "obesity paradox," once a patient has HF, a higher body mass index (BMI) is actually protective, and weight loss is an ominous sign of worsening HF and a poor prognosis.[7,8] Described as cardiac cachexia, this complication is a dramatic and catastrophic complication of HF in a way that cachexia can complicate other chronic disorders. The challenge of the dietary management of the HF patient is to balance these conflicting needs, aiming for an optimal weight that may mean weight loss early in the natural history and strategies to prevent weight loss later in the clinical course. Data on weight from 7767 patients with stable HF enrolled in the Digitalis Investigation Group (DIG) trial were recently reported. Crude all-cause mortality rates decreased in a near-linear fashion across successively higher BMI groups, from 45% in the underweight group to 28.4% in the obese group (P = 0.001). After multivariable adjustment, overweight and obese patients were at lower risk for death (HR 0.88, 95% CI, 0.80–0.96; and HR 0.81, 95% CI, 0.72–0.92, respectively), compared with patients at a healthy weight. In contrast, underweight patients with stable HF were at increased risk for death (HR 1.21, 95% CI, 0.95–1.53).[9]

Pasini and colleagues have reported that CHF patients have on average a higher total energy expenditure (1700 ± 53 vs. 1950 ± 43 kcal/day; P <0.01), a negative calorie balance (104 ± 35 vs. −186 ± 40 kcal/day; P <0.01), a negative nitrogen balance (2.2 ± 0.5 vs. −1.7 ± 0.4 g/day; P <0.01), and a hypercatabolic hormonal status (cortisol/insulin ratio 32 ± 1.7 vs. 65 ± 5.1; P <0.01). This suggests a relatively inadequate calorie intake for daily activities, with consequent important protein breakdown that causes muscular wasting.[10] In another study, the effects of nutritional supplementation were assessed. A supervised nutritional intervention was shown to improve clinical status and QoL.[11] Sixty-five patients with HF were assigned to one of two groups: the intervention group (IG) (n = 30), received a sodium-restricted diet (2000–2400 mg/day) with restriction of total fluids to 1.5 L/day, and the control group (CG) (n = 35) received traditional medical treatment and general nutritional recommendations. After 6 months, kilocalories, macronutrients, and fluid intakes were significant lower in the IG than in the CG. Urinary excretion of sodium decreased significantly in the IG and increased in the CG (−7.9% vs. 29.4%, P <0.05). IG patients had significantly less-frequent edema (37% vs. 7.4%; P = 0.008) and fatigue (59.3% vs. 25.9%; P = 0.012) at 6 months compared to baseline. Functional class also improved significantly. Physical activity increased 2.5 ± 7.4% in the IG and decreased −3.1 ± 12% in the CG (P <0.05). The IG had a greater increase in total QoL compared with the CG (19.3% vs. 3.2%; P = 0.02).

Kuehneman and colleagues have demonstrated an important role for the dietician in a multidisciplinary HF program. Compared with baseline, QoL scores improved by 6.7 points (P <.003) at 3 months and by 5.9 points (P <.04) at 6 months after dietician intervention, suggesting positive findings in terms of improved nutrition and avoidance of worsening HF due to excessive sodium intake.[12]

Psychological Support

Depression has been recognized as a common and adverse feature of CHF.[13] Gottlieb has shown that in 155 patients with stable NYHA functional Class II, III, and IV HF and an ejection fraction <40%, 48% of the patients could be considered depressed.[14] Depressed patients tended to be younger than nondepressed patients. Women were more likely (64%) to be depressed than men (44%). Depressed patients scored significantly worse than nondepressed patients on all components of both the questionnaires measuring QoL. The authors suggested that pharmacologic or nonpharmacologic treatment of depression might have the capacity to improve the QoL of HF patients, although this presently has not been the subject of an adequately powered randomized clinical trial (RCT).[14]

Sleep Disorders

Many patients with CHF complain of poor sleep. Historically this has been attributed to paroxysmal nocturnal dyspnea, or to depression and anxiety. More recently it has been appreciated that many CHF patients also suffer from sleep-disordered breathing (SDB) due to both obstructive and central sleep apnea with frequent episodes of periodic breathing. One study examined the prevalence of sleep disorders in stable HF patients regardless of ejection fraction. On 3 consecutive days in an HF clinic, all patients were asked to participate in a screening for SDB. This screening involved the placement of an outpatient device (ClearPath, Nexan, Inc., Alpharetta, Georgia), which collects thoracic impedance, oxyhemoglobin saturation, and 2-lead electrocardiogram data. Sixteen patients (42%) had moderate or severe SDB, 22 patients (55%) had mild or no significant SDB. Fourteen of the 16 patients with moderate or severe SDB subsequently received treatment by confirming SDB and continuous positive airway pressure (CPAP) in a sleep laboratory. Forty-two percent of patients with stable HF presenting to an HF clinic screened positive for SDB, despite receiving optimal standard of care.[15] This is now recognized as a common condition and one believed to increase the risk of mortality. Treatment of SDB is considered an important part of the management of CHF.[16] Improvements in SDB have shown a positive effect on cardiac output, neurohormonal activity, and QoL. CPAP has been the traditional method used to treat SDB in patients with CHF, but more recent devices such as a mandibular advancement device have also been shown to be effective.[17] Nocturnal carbon dioxide inhalation by suppressing chemoreflex drive to ventilation (which is excessive in CHF) has been shown to reduce the frequency of central sleep apnea and improve QoL.[18,19] For obstructive sleep apnea, CPAP has been shown to improve cardiac function, sympathetic activity, and QoL.[20] For nocturnal Cheyne-Stokes breathing, nocturnal-assist servoventilation has been shown to improve daytime sleepiness compared with the control. A total of 30 subjects (29 male) (with mean apnea-hypopnea index 19.8 [SD 2.6] and stable symptomatic CHF [NYHA Class II–IV]) were treated with 1 month's therapeutic (n = 15) or subtherapeutic adaptive servoventilation. Daytime sleepiness Oxford SLEep Resistance test (OSLER test) was measured before and after the trial with change in measured sleepiness the primary endpoint. Active treatment reduced excessive daytime sleepiness; the mean Osler change was +7.9 minutes (SEM 2.9), when compared with the control, the change was −1 minute (SEM 1.7), and the difference was 8.9 minutes (95% CI, 1.9–15.9 minutes; P = 0.014, unpaired t-test). Significant falls also occurred in

plasma brain natriuretic peptide and urinary meta-drenaline excretion rates suggesting beneficial neurohormonal effects.[21] There remains, however, little evidence from RCTs to tell us whether it is cost-effective to screen routinely for SDB in CHF clinics and to treat all cases so detected.

Specialist Heart Failure Clinics and Nurses

In recent years, the value of comprehensive hospital and community-based HF management programs has been accepted, and they have become established as the standard of care in many countries. In the Netherlands, for example, 60% of hospitals support an HF management program. Most of the programs are organized as HF outpatient clinics. In all HF programs, cardiologists and nurses are involved. Other health-care providers involved are, amongst others, general practitioners (29%), dieticians (59%), physical therapists (47%), social workers (30%), and psychologists (17%). All programs offer follow-up after discharge from the hospital and in most of the programs patients have increased access to a health-care provider. Behavioral interventions (68%), psychosocial counseling (64%), patient education (88%), and support of the informal caregivers (59%) are important components. In 90% of the programs, physical examination is the responsibility of the HF nurse and in 65% of the programs nurses are involved in optimizing medical treatment.[22]

After hospital discharge, follow-up of CHF patients at a nurse-led HF clinic has been shown to be associated with fewer patients with events (death or admission) after 12 months (29 vs. 40, P = 0.03) and fewer deaths after 12 months (7 vs. 20, P = 0.005) in one study. The IG had fewer admissions (33 vs. 56, P = 0.047) and days in hospital (350 vs. 592, P = 0.045) during the first 3 months. After 12 months, the intervention was associated with a 55% decrease in admissions/patient/month (0.18 vs. 0.40, P = 0.06) and fewer days in hospital/patient/month (1.4 vs. 3.9, P = 0.02). The IG had significantly higher self-care scores at 3 and 12 months compared to the CG (P = 0.02 and P = 0.01).[23]

Intensive home care of middle-aged patients with severe HF has been shown to result in improved QoL and a decrease in hospital readmission rates.[24] A telephone-mediated nurse care management program for HF has also been shown to reduce the rate of rehospitalization for HF, although it has been suggested such programs may be less effective for patients at low risk compared to higher risk patients.[25,26] Other reports of home health intervention programs have, however, reported less convincing benefits.[27] Success has also been reported of incorporating palliative care regimes into the management of end-stage CHF.[28]

The evidence to suggest that such CHF programs involving individualized multidisciplinary postdischarge health care, with a major focus on specialist nurse management are clinically and economically effective in CHF has recently been reviewed.[29] These programs appear to be most effective in "high-risk" patients who typically have recurrent readmissions in high-cost units. Overall, the literature suggests that these programs are able to reduce recurrent hospital stay by 30–50% relative to usual care (even in the presence of optimal treatment) in the short to medium term with comparable cost benefits.

▶ REFERENCES

1. Colonna P, Sorino M, D'Agostino C, et al. Nonpharmacologic care of heart failure: counseling, dietary restriction, rehabilitation, treatment of sleep apnea, and ultrafiltration. *Am J Cardiol.* May 8, 2003;91(9A):F41–F50.
2. Coats AJ, Adamopoulos S, Meyer TE, et al. Effects of physical training in chronic heart failure. *Lancet.* January 13, 1990;335(8681):63–66.
3. Belardinelli R, Georgiou D, Ginzton L, et al. Effects of moderate exercise training on thallium uptake and contractile response to low-dose dobutamine of dysfunctional myocardium in patients with ischemic cardiomyopathy. *Circulation.* February 17, 1998;97(6):553–561.
4. Piepoli MF, Davos C, Francis DP, , ExTraMATCH Collaborative. Exercise training meta-analysis of trials in patients with chronic heart failure (ExTraMATCH). *BMJ.* January 24, 2004; 328 (7433): 189.
5. Rees K, Taylor RS, Singh S, et al. Exercise based rehabilitation for heart failure. *Cochrane Database Syst Rev.* 2004;(3):CD003331.
6. Conraads VM, Beckers P, Vaes J, et al. Combined endurance/resistance training reduces NT-proBNP levels in patients with chronic heart failure. *Eur Heart J.* October, 2004;25(20): 1797–1805.
7. Anker SD, Ponikowski P, Varney S, et al. Wasting as independent risk factor for mortality in chronic heart failure. *Lancet.* April 12, 1997;349(9058):1050–1053.
8. Anker SD, Negassa A, Coats AJ, et al. Prognostic importance of weight loss in chronic heart failure and the effect of treatment with angiotensin-converting-enzyme inhibitors: an observational study. *Lancet.* March 29, 2003;361(9363):1077–1083.
9. Curtis JP, Selter JG, Wang Y, et al. Body mass index and outcomes in patients with heart failure. *Arch Intern Med.* 2005;165:55–61.
10. Pasini E, Opasich C, Pastoris O, et al. Inadequate nutritional intake for daily life activity of clinically stable patients with chronic heart failure. *Am J Cardiol.* April 22, 2004;93(8A):A41–A43.
11. Colin Ramirez E, Castillo Martinez L, Orea Tejeda A, et al. Effects of a nutritional intervention on body composition, clinical status, and quality of life in patients with heart failure. *Nutrition.* October 2004;20(10):890–895.
12. Kuehneman T, Saulsbury D, Splett P, et al. Demonstrating the impact of nutrition intervention in a heart failure program. *J Am Diet Assoc.* December 2002;102(12):1790–1794.
13. Faris R, Purcell H, Henein MY, et al. Clinical depression is common and significantly associated with reduced survival in patients with non-ischaemic heart failure. *Eur J Heart Fail.* August 2002;4(4):541–551.
14. Gottlieb SS, Khatta M, Friedmann E, et al. The influence of age, gender, and race on the prevalence of depression in heart failure patients. *J Am Coll Cardiol.* May 5, 2004;43(9): 1542–1549.
15. Trupp RJ, Hardesty P, Osborne J, et al. Prevalence of sleep disordered breathing in a heart failure program. *Congest Heart Fail.* September–October 2004;10(5):217–220.

16. Eskafi M. Sleep apnoea in patients with stable congestive heart failure an intervention study with a mandibular advancement device. *Swed Dent J Suppl*. 2004;(168):1–56.

17. Eskafi M, Ekberg E, Cline C, et al. Use of a mandibular advancement device in patients with congestive heart failure and sleep apnoea. *Gerodontology*. June 2004;21(2):100–107.

18. Chua TP, Clark AL, Amadi AA, et al. Relation between chemosensitivity and the ventilatory response to exercise in chronic heart failure. *J Am Coll Cardiol*. March 1, 1996;27(3):650–657.

19. Szollosi I, Jones M, Morrell MJ, et al. Effect of CO_2 inhalation on central sleep apnea and arousals from sleep. *Respiration*. September–October 2004;71(5):493–498.

20. Mansfield DR, Gollogly NC, Kaye DM, et al. Controlled trial of continuous positive airway pressure in obstructive sleep apnea and heart failure. *Am J Respir Crit Care Med*. February 1, 2004;169(3):361–366.

21. Pepperell JC, Maskell NA, Jones DR, et al. A randomized controlled trial of adaptive ventilation for Cheyne-Stokes breathing in heart failure. *Am J Respir Crit Care Med*. November 1, 2003;168(9):1109–1114.

22. Jaarsma T, Tan B, Bos RJ, et al. Heart failure clinics in the Netherlands in 2003. *Eur J Cardiovasc Nurs*. December 2004;3(4):271–274.

23. Stromberg A, Martensson J, Fridlund B, et al. Nurse-led heart failure clinics improve survival and self-care behaviour in patients with heart failure: results from a prospective, randomised trial. *Eur Heart J*. June 2003;24(11):1014–1023.

24. Vavouranakis I, Lambrogiannakis E, Markakis G, et al. Effect of home-based intervention on hospital readmission and quality of life in middle-aged patients with severe congestive heart failure: a 12-month follow up study. *Eur J Cardiovasc Nurs*. July 2003;2(2):105–11.

25. Berg GD, Wadhwa S, Johnson AE. A matched-cohort study of health services utilization and financial outcomes for a heart failure disease-management program in elderly patients. *J Am Geriatr Soc*. October 2004;52(10):1655–1661.

26. DeBusk RF, Miller NH, Parker KM, et al. Care management for low-risk patients with heart failure: a randomized, controlled trial. *Ann Intern Med*. October 19, 2004;141(8):606–613.

27. Feldman PH, Peng TR, Murtaugh CM, et al. A randomized intervention to improve heart failure outcomes in community-based home health care. *Home Health Care Serv Q*. 2004;23(1):1–23.

28. Davidson PM, Paull G, Introna K, et al. Integrated, collaborative palliative care in heart failure: the St. George Heart Failure Service experience 1999-2002. *J Cardiovasc Nurs*. January–February 2004;19(1):68–75.

29. Stewart S, Horowitz JD. Specialist nurse management programmes: economic benefits in the management of heart failure. *Pharmacoeconomics*. 2003;21(4):225–240.

CHAPTER 9

How to Use Diuretics in Heart Failure Patients

ROBERT W. SCHRIER, MD

▶ INTRODUCTION

Renal sodium and water retention is a hallmark of congestive heart failure (CHF).[1,2] Thus, the use of diuretics is a standard component of the therapy for patients with CHF. Since there are approximately 5 million heart failure patients in this country and 500,000 newly diagnosed patients every year, expertise in the use of diuretics in CHF is extremely important.[3] This expertise will be an ever-increasing need by physicians as the age of Americans and the prevalence of CHF continues to increase. The present chapter will discuss the pathophysiology of sodium and water retention in CHF, the various diuretics used in CHF including their mechanisms of action and side effects, and the potential effect of diuretics on renal function in patients with CHF.

▶ PATHOPHYSIOLOGY OF SODIUM AND WATER RETENTION IN CONGESTIVE HEART FAILURE

The renal retention of sodium and water in the patient with CHF presents several dilemmas, which have been difficult to understand. Early proposals suggested that a decrease in total blood volume was the initiator of sodium and water retention by the kidney in patients with heart failure. In fact, based on this belief, sodium chloride administration was even recommended for treatment of cardiac failure. However, when the methodology to accurately measure total blood volume in patients with heart failure became available, blood volumes were found to be increased.[4] Thus, the undefined and enigmatic term "effective blood volume" was proposed to be decreased in heart failure with resultant triggering of the intact kidney to retain sodium and water. Extrarenal reflexes are incriminated in CHF since the kidney no longer retains sodium and water after a successful heart transplant.

Search for the effective blood volume led to the proposal that a decrease in cardiac output provided the afferent stimulus for renal sodium and water retention in heart failure. However, there were other circumstances in which the normal kidney retains excess amounts of sodium and water in the presence of an increase in cardiac output. Foremost is high-output cardiac failure, which may occur with beriberi, thyrotoxicosis, and cirrhosis, and lead to renal sodium and water retention.

On this background, we proposed that body fluid volume was regulated by the normal kidney in response to the absolute or relative filling of the arterial vascular tree.[5,6] There are estimates that total blood volume is distributed 85% on the venous side and 15% on the arterial side of the circulation. In this context, total blood volume could be increased if the expansion was predominantly on the venous side of the circulation, yet the kidney could be retaining sodium and water primarily due to underfilling of the arterial circulation. Based on this, we proposed that the arterial circulation could be underfilled either in an absolute manner by a decrease in cardiac output or relatively underfilled by arterial vasodilation, or a combination thereof.[5,6]

There are several baroreceptors capable of sensing an underfilling of the arterial circulation, due to either a decrease in cardiac output or arterial vasodilation. The baroreceptors in the carotid sinus and aortic arch respond to stretch. Under normal arterial filling, there is a tonic inhibition of adrenergic outflow from the central nervous system, which is mediated via the vagus and glossopharyngeal nerves from these arterial baroreceptors. There are also receptors in the afferent arterioles of the glomerulus, which respond to stretch as well as β-adrenergic stimulation.[7] Thus, patients with severe autonomic insufficiency could still respond to arterial underfilling via the renal receptors. The ventricular receptors have been less well studied, but may be important in elderly cardiac failure patients with diastolic dysfunction but normal left ventricular ejection fractions. In this regard, it has been estimated that as many as 50% of elderly patients with heart failure are due to diastolic, rather than systolic dysfunction. There are also studies showing that impaired baroreceptor sensitivity occurs in patients with cardiac failure, and, therefore, could also be a factor in the increase in sympathetic tone associated with CHF.[8] The mortality in CHF correlates directly with plasma norepinephrine, and the sympathetic nervous system (SNS) is a known potent stimulator of the renin-angiotensin-aldosterone system (RAAS).[9,10]

In addition to the arterial baroreceptors, there are receptors on the low pressure side of the circulation. Specifically, in normal subjects, an increase in atrial pressure is known to (1) decrease arginine vasopressin (AVP) concentrations and cause a solute-free water diuresis, (2) increase atrial natriuretic peptide (ANP) and cause a natriuresis, and (3) decrease renal sympathetic tone.[11-13] In contrast, in subjects with CHF the increase in atrial pressure is associated with sodium and water retention and renal vasoconstriction. These observations suggest that the low-pressure receptors are either impaired in cardiac failure patients or are overridden by arterial baroreceptor-mediated increased activity of the SNS and RAAS and the nonosmotic release of AVP.

Our body fluid volume hypothesis is depicted in Fig. 9-1 for arterial underfilling secondary to a decrease in cardiac output and in Fig. 9-2 for arterial vasodilation. While this hypothesis provides a potential sequence of events whereby normal kidneys retain excess sodium and water in association with cardiac failure, several dilemmas exist with respect to the efferent arm of this body fluid volume regulation.[14] With renal vasoconstriction, a fall in glomerular filtration rate (GFR) could contribute to the sodium and water retention in cardiac failure, but it is well established that sodium retention occurs in CHF prior to a decrease in GFR. Thus, enhanced tubular reabsorption must be involved in the sodium retention with cardiac failure. The role of increased aldosterone in this increased tubular reabsorption therefore emerged as a potential factor. However, several problems arose. Specifically, all patients with cardiac failure do not have elevated plasma aldosterone concentrations and large exogenous doses of aldosterone to normal individuals do not cause edema. This is because of the so-called aldosterone escape phenomenon from the hormone's sodium-retaining effect, in which urinary sodium excretion returns to intake levels in spite of continued aldosterone administration. Moreover, patients with CHF do not demonstrate

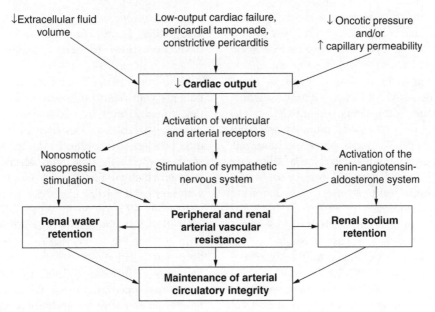

Figure 9-1 Sequence of neurohumoral and hemodynamic responses to arterial underfilling secondary to decrease in cardiac output, which maintain arterial circulatory integrity. (Published with permission from Schrier RW. Body fluid volume regulation in health and disease: a unifying hypothesis. *Ann Intern Med.* 1990;113:155–159.)

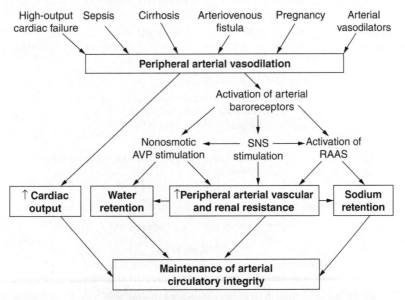

Figure 9-2 Sequence of neurohumoral and hemodynamic responses to arterial underfilling secondary to an arterial vasodilation, which maintain arterial circulatory integrity. AVP—arginine vasopressin; RAAS—renin-angiotensin-aldosterone system; SNS—sympathetic nervous system. (Published with permission from Schrier RW. Body fluid volume regulation in health and disease: a unifying hypothesis. *Ann Intern Med.* 1990;113:155–159.)

the aldosterone escape phenomenon. Patients with cardiac failure have also been shown to be resistant to the natriuretic response to increasing doses of ANP.[15] There is evidence that the effects of increased angiotensin II and adrenergic activity to increase proximal tubule sodium reabsorption in cardiac failure limits sodium delivery to the collecting duct sites of aldosterone and ANP action (Fig. 9-3). We have proposed that this diminished distal sodium delivery is a major factor in the failure of the CHF patient to escape from the sodium-retaining effect of aldosterone and to respond normally to ANP.[16]

Experimental results indicate that aldosterone not only increases Na-K-ATPase activity as well as the expression and membrane trafficking of the collecting duct epithelial sodium channel (ENaC) but may also increase the NaCl cotransporter (thiazide sensitive cotransporter) in the distal convoluted and connecting tubules. There is also evidence that angiotensin II, independent of aldosterone, is an important factor in ENaC activity. There is substantial evidence that aldosterone increases cardiac fibrosis and angiotensin II as a major factor in cardiac remodeling.[17,18] Thus, angiotensin-converting enzyme (ACE) inhibitors and angiotensin receptor blockers (ARBs) as well

as non-natriuretic doses of mineralocorticoid antagonists (spironolactone and eplerenone) have been shown to increase survival in cardiac patients (*vide infra*).

The renal sodium and water retention in patients with heart failure may have substantial deleterious effects in addition to causing pulmonary congestion. The resultant increased cardiac preload is associated with myocardial wall stress, cardiac dilatation, and ventricular hypertrophy, which are factors known to be associated with increased cardiac morbidity and mortality in CHF. Thus, in addition to ACE inhibition, ARBs, and low-dose mineralocorticoid antagonists, diuretics need to be considered in the therapeutic armamentarium in cardiac failure patients. Figure 9-4 shows a deleterious vicious cycle, which may occur in cardiac failure patients and where several proven and unproven interventions, including diuretics, may intervene.[19]

Use of Loop Diuretics in Congestive Heart Failure

The loop diuretics available in the United States include furosemide, bumetanide, ethacrynic acid,

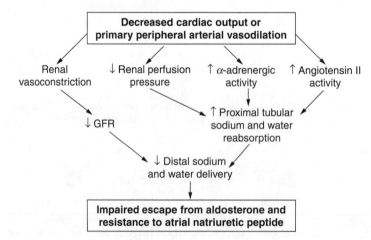

Figure 9-3 Pathways whereby arterial underfilling due to a decrease in cardiac output or arterial vasodilation lead to a decrease in sodium and water delivery to the collecting duct site of action of aldosterone and atrial natriuretic peptide. GFR—glomerular filtration rate.

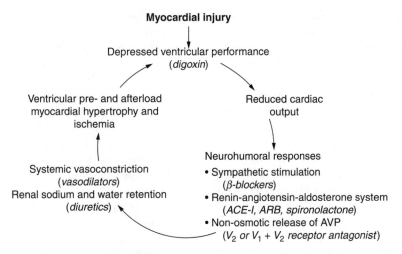

Myocardial injury

Depressed ventricular performance
(*digoxin*)

Ventricular pre- and afterload
myocardial hypertrophy and
ischemia

Reduced cardiac
output

Systemic vasoconstriction
(*vasodilators*)
Renal sodium and water retention
(*diuretics*)

Neurohumoral responses
• Sympathetic stimulation
   (*β-blockers*)
• Renin-angiotensin-aldosterone system
   (*ACE-I, ARB, spironolactone*)
• Non-osmotic release of AVP
   (*V₂ or V₁ + V₂ receptor antagonist*)

Figure 9-4 Vicious cycle for worsening of ventricular function in chronic congestive heart failure with potential interventions in parenthesis. ACE—angiotensin-converting enzyme; ARB—angiotensin receptor blocker; AVP—arginine vasopressin (Published with permission from Schrier RW, Abdallah JC, Weinberger HH, et al. Therapy of heart failure. *Kidney Int.* 2000;57:1418–1425.)

and torsemide.[20] The half-lives of these agents are short and range from 1 hour with bumetanide to 3–4 hours for torsemide. After oral administration of loop diuretics, the peak serum concentration occurs within 0.5–2 hours, with furosemide being somewhat slower than bumetanide and torsemide. The predominant effect of loop diuretics is to inhibit the electroneutral Na-K-2Cl cotransporter at the apical surface of the thick ascending limb cells whereby up to 25% of filtered Na and Cl can be excreted.[21] The transepithelial voltage of the thick ascending limb is oriented normally with lumen positive and this accounts for absorption of Na, Ca, and Mg via the paracellular pathway.[22] In fact, this paracellular pathway accounts for approximately 50% of Na transport by the thick ascending limb. Loop diuretics inhibit both the transcellular and paracellular pathways in the thick ascending limb for Na transport, and increase Ca and Mg excretion primarily by inhibiting the paracellular pathway secondary to abolishing the lumen positive transepithelial voltage.

Furosemide has been shown to stimulate prostaglandin E_2 production from thick ascending limb cells.[23] Loop diuretics reduce renal vascular

resistance and increase renal blood, an effect that depends at least in part on prostaglandins. Inhibition of prostaglandin synthesis with nonsteroidal anti-inflammatory drugs (NSAIDs) has been shown to decrease the diuretic potency of loop diuretics.[24] Prostaglandins may also be the primary mediator of the venodilatory effect of loop diuretics.[25] This venodilatory effect and the resultant increased splanchnic compliance no doubt accounts for the effect of loop diuretics to decrease cardiac preload and pulmonary edema prior to any effect on urinary electrolyte excretion.[26]

In patients with chronic CHF, however, loop diuretic administration may acutely increase cardiac afterload, left ventricular end-diastolic pressure, and worsen pulmonary edema.[27] This response is probably due to the effect of loop diuretics to stimulate the renin-angiotensin system and secondarily the SNS system. Macula densa cells are in the cortical thick ascending limb and mediate renin secretion and tubuloglomerular feedback (TGF). An increase in NaCl transport across the apical membrane of the macula densa cells via the Na-K-2Cl cotransporter activates TGF and increases renin secretion in association with constriction of the glomerular afferent arteriole and a resultant decrease in GFR. Loop diuretics block this NaCl transport in the macula densa cells and therefore inhibit TGF.[28] This may be the reason that GFR is maintained during loop diuretic administration even in the presence of a decrease in extracellular fluid volume (ECFV). The effect of loop diuretics to increase prostaglandin E_2 and nitric oxide (neuronal nitric oxide synthase [NOS] is highly expressed in the macula densa) has been proposed to account for adenosine 3'5' cyclic monophosphate (cyclic AMP)-mediated renin secretion.[29] In this regard, inhibition of prostaglandins with NSAIDs has been shown to block the effect of loop diuretics to increase renin secretion.[30] In contrast, any effect of nitric oxide to induce renin secretion appears only to be permissive, since loop diuretics still increase renin secretion in experimental knockout models of NOS.[31] The effect of loop diuretics to stimulate the RAAS theoretically can have adverse effects on cardiac function (Fig. 9-5).

The potential beneficial effects of loop diuretics in CHF patients are shown in Fig. 9-6. The resultant negative sodium and water balance will

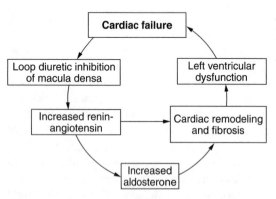

Figure 9-5 Mechanisms whereby loop diuretics may worsen cardiac failure. On this background, it can be theoretically argued that loop diuretics should always be accompanied by treatment with angiotensin-converting enzyme inhibitor or angiotensin receptor blockade in heart failure patients.

not only improve pulmonary congestion, but the associated decrease in ventricular filling pressure can diminish ventricular dilatation. Myocardial function then may improve secondary to a decrease in mitral insufficiency and endomyocardial ischemia as cardiac dilatation is ameliorated. In this setting of improved myocardial function, renal function may actually improve during loop diuretic therapy. Excess diuresis in CHF, however, may further decrease cardiac output and worsen renal function. This particularly occurs in the presence of ACE inhibitor or ARB therapy, which predisposes to a fall in glomerular filtration pressure, and thus decreased GFR, by blocking the vasoconstrictor effect of angiotensin II on the glomerular efferent arteriole.[32] Nevertheless, since angiotensin II and aldosterone are known to mediate cardiac remodeling and fibrosis respectively, and ACE inhibitors and ARBs have been shown to decrease mortality in CHF patients, their use is indispensable, even if some decrease in renal function occurs.[17,18] Decreasing the loop diuretic dose and lessening the degree of sodium restriction should be considered if blood urea nitrogen (BUN) and serum creatinine concentration are rising during diuretic therapy in a CHF patient.

As discussed above, loop diuretics activate the RAAS by blocking the Na-K-2Cl cotransporter in the macula densa independent of any effect on ECFV. Moreover, this effect on RAAS can be accentuated by ECFV depletion if the diuretic-inducing renal excretion rate exceeds the estimated 12–14 mL/min mobilization of interstitial fluid into the circulation in CHF patients.[33] Ultrafiltration has been used in CHF, particularly in the setting of diuretic resistance. It has several potential advantages over loop therapy.[34] The RAAS activation in CHF need not be accentuated with ultrafiltration if the rate of fluid removal does not exceed the rate of interstitial fluid mobilization. Also, for the same volume of negative fluid balance, more sodium is removed with ultrafiltration than diuretic-induced fluid loss. This is because the diuresis with loop diuretics is always hypotonic, in contrast to the isotonic fluid removal with ultrafiltration. In this regard, it is the amount of sodium removal that

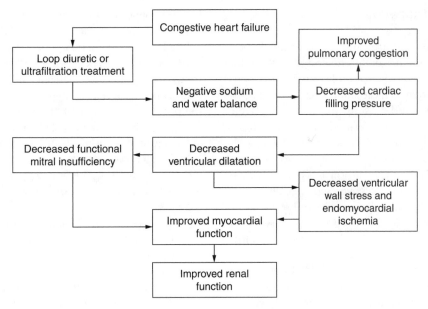

Figure 9-6 Mechanisms in congestive heart failure whereby negative sodium and water balance by loop diuretics or ultrafiltration therapy may improve myocardial and renal function.

determines the effect on ECFV. Ultrafiltration is invasive and more expensive than diuretic therapy. However, with newer ultrafiltration instrumentation and the use of peripheral access, the potential for diminished hospitalization may make this approach cost-effective.

In addition to overzealous use and activation of the RAAS, there are other potential adverse effects of loop diuretic use. Urinary potassium and magnesium losses can lead to deleterious effects on cardiac function secondary to hypokalemia and hypomagnesemia. In addition to the inhibition of Na-K-2Cl cotransporter, the effect of loop diuretics to increase potassium delivery to the collecting duct site of aldosterone-mediated potassium secretion is also involved. Hypokalemia also contributes to loop diuretic-related metabolic alkalosis by stimulating ammonium production.[35] Loop diuretics can also cause excess urinary calcium losses, which can potentially decrease plasma-ionized Ca and worsen cardiac function in a patient with CHF. Loop diuretics may cause hyponatremia, however this is less

frequent than with distal convoluted tubule (DCT) diuretics.[36] This may be because loop, but not DCT, diuretics impair urinary concentration. Ototoxicity, sometimes irreversible, may also occur with loop diuretic therapy. This complication has occurred with the rapid infusion of high doses of a loop diuretic in patients with impaired renal function.[37] Thus, it is recommended not to infuse loop diuretics faster than 4 mg/min. With metabolic alkalosis secondary to loop diuretics, the usual method of saline infusion to decrease proximal tubule bicarbonate reabsorption and correct metabolic alkalosis obviously cannot be used in patients with CHF. In this setting, a carbonic anhydrase inhibitor, such as acetazolamide, can be used to increase urinary bicarbonate excretion and correct metabolic alkalosis in CHF when saline infusion is not indicated.[38] An increase in urinary pH >7 indicates bicarbonaturia is present. It is important to remember that bicarbonaturia increases urinary potassium loss and thus can worsen hypokalemia if potassium replacement is not instituted.

Thiazide Diuretics

Thiazide diuretics are benzothiadiazide derivatives.[39] Other structurally related diuretics are quinazolinones (e.g., metolazone) and benzophenone (e.g., chlorthalidone). These diuretics inhibit Na and Cl transport along the DCT and thus have been termed "DCT diuretics." Acute administration of these diuretics is associated with inhibition of carbonic anhydrase with increased Na, K, Cl, bicarbonate (HCO_3), phosphate, and urate. However, chronically these DCT diuretics primarily increase urinary Na, Cl, and K excretion. In fact, as ECFV decreases with DCT diuretic use, increased uric acid reabsorption may lead to hyperuricemia and precipitate gout in predisposed patients. DCT diuretics also decrease calcium excretion and thus are used to treat nephrolithiasis. Increased urinary Mg excretion and hypomagnesemia may also occur with DCT diuretics.

The molecular site of action of the DCT diuretics has been identified as a transport protein entitled thiazide-sensitive cotransporter (TSC) or sodium chloride cotransporter (NCC).[40] This transport protein has been identified in all mammalian species that have been examined.[41]

Since there is less NaCl reabsorption in the DCT than the thick ascending limb of Henle's loop, these DCT diuretics are less potent than loop diuretics in patients with CHF. However, the addition of a DCT diuretic to a CHF patient receiving a loop diuretic may dramatically increase NaCl excretion. Similar to loop diuretics, DCT diuretics are highly protein bound in the circulation and thus reach the tubular lumen primarily by the organic anion secretory pathway in the proximal tubule rather than by glomerular filtration.[42] In contrast to loop diuretics, the TGF mechanism is not blocked by DCT diuretics since their nephron site of action is beyond the macula densa.[43]

Therapy with DCT diuretics is associated with more hyponatremia and hypokalemia than loop diuretics.[44] With respect to the hyponatremia, the DCT diuretics impair solute-free water excretion

but, in contrast to loop diuretics, which impair urinary concentration, DCT diuretics do not impair solute-free water reabsorption. Because of the effect of loop diuretics to impair the countercurrent concentrating mechanism, these agents can lead to the excretion of hypotonic urine even in the presence of antidiuretic hormone (i.e., AVP).[45] There is also evidence that furosemide may attenuate the action of AVP at the nephron level.[46] Since patients with CHF exhibit a nonosmotic stimulation of AVP and are generally receiving loop diuretics, the addition of a DCT diuretic may increase the occurrence of hyponatremia.[47]

There are reasons why DCT diuretics may be associated with more hypokalemia than loop diuretics. First of all, DCT diuretics have a longer duration of action than loop diuretics and this is particularly true of chlorthalidone and metolazone.[48] Both DCT and loop diuretics increase tubule flow rate in the connecting tubule and collecting duct, the main sites of potassium secretion. Thus, in the presence of hyperaldosteronism associated with CHF, both diuretics will increase urinary potassium excretion. Thus, resultant hypokalemia is a particularly adverse side effect when a DCT diuretic is added to loop diuretic therapy in a patient with cardiac failure. There is also evidence that high luminal concentrations of calcium, which occur with loop diuretics but not with DCT diuretics, inhibit the functional activity of ENaC and thus decrease potassium excretion.[49] Hypomagnesemia, which occurs with both DCT and loop diuretics, has also been shown to increase urinary K excretion, and magnesium replacement may diminish K losses.[50] Taken together, diuretic-related hypokalemia and hypomagnesemia may predispose to cardiac arrhythmias, particularly in patients with CHF receiving cardiac glycosides, for example, digoxin. Potassium replacement may also obviate the hyperglycemic effect of DCT by normalizing pancreatic insulin release.[51] In the Antihypertensive and Lipid-Lowering Treatment to Prevent Heart Attack Trial (ALLHAT) the effect of the DCT diuretic chlorthalidone on total cholesterol versus placebo was only an increase of 2.2 mg/dL.[52]

Cortical Collecting and Connecting Tubule Diuretics

Diuretics whose action is localized in the cortical collecting and/or connecting tubule have been referred to as potassium-sparing diuretics.[53] Filtered potassium is mostly reabsorbed in the proximal portions of the nephron so that the rate of urinary potassium excretion is primarily determined by potassium secretion in the connecting tubule and cortical collecting duct.[54] These are the sites where the potassium-sparing diuretics inhibit potassium secretion. The apical membrane of connecting tubule and principal cells of the collecting tubule express Na and K channels.[55] The mechanism for sodium reabsorption in these sites is through conductive ENaC. The basolateral Na-K-ATPase by extruding cellular sodium creates a low intracellular sodium reabsorption, which provides an electrochemical gradient for sodium entry through the sodium channels.[56] Thus, sodium entry into the cell creates a lumen-negative transepithelial potential difference, which provides the electrochemical driving force, along with the Na-K-ATPase-generated high intracellular potassium, for potassium secretion. Amiloride and triamterene decrease potassium secretion by blocking these sodium conductance channels, thereby decreasing the electrochemical gradient for potassium excretion.[57] This effect of these two diuretics occurs independent of aldosterone action. The sodium channel is comprised of three homologous subunits (α, β, γ-ENaC), which in the mouse are expressed in the apical membrane during a sodium-retaining state.[58] In mammals, aldosterone has been shown to increase the abundance of the α-subunit of ENaC and to redistribute all three subunits to the apical region of the principal cells in the collecting duct.[59] The mechanism of action of mineralocorticoid receptor blockers, namely spironolactone, is by blocking the nuclear localization of the mineralocorticoid receptors.[60] The natriuretic effect of spironolactone is modest, 1–2% of filtered sodium, and is dependent on the presence of aldosterone.[61] Spironolactone is, therefore, ineffective in adrenalectomized animals and patients with Addison's disease. The peak response of spironolactone may occur as late as 48 hours and the effect wanes over a period of 48–72 hours after stopping the diuretic.[62] Eplerenone is another competitive aldosterone antagonist, which appears to be 50–70% as potent as spironolactone, but does not have the estrogenic side effects of spironolactone (e.g., gynecomastia, breast tenderness, menstrual irregularities, decreased libido, and impotence).[63]

The use of the potassium-sparing diuretics as an adjunct to loop diuretics, so as to prevent hypokalemia, is quite effective. These potassium-sparing diuretics should, however, *not* be used in conjunction with potassium supplements, since this agent's main side effect is hyperkalemia. The hyperkalemia of mineralocorticoid receptor antagonists is most likely to occur in elderly patients, patients with diabetes, and patients with reduced kidney function, all of which can occur in association with CHF.[64] Since CHF patients are receiving ACE inhibitors, ARBs, and β-blockers, all of which have been shown to improve survival, but also predispose to potassium retention, the use of potassium-sparing diuretics must be monitored carefully in this setting. The potassium-losing effect of loop diuretics may, however, attenuate this potential adverse side effect of hyperkalemia during use of potassium-sparing diuretics in the CHF patients. By blocking hydrogen ion secretion, as well as potassium secretion, amiloride, triamterene, and mineralocorticoid, antagonists may predispose to, or worsen, hyperchloremic metabolic acidosis.[65]

Spironolactone has been shown to improve mortality in CHF (Randomized Aldactone Evaluation Study [RALES]), and eplerenone has been shown to improve mortality in patients with left ventricular dysfunction following myocardial infarction.[66,67] These effects are observed at non-natriuretic doses of these mineralocorticoid receptor antagonists; however, these agents may also be useful in treating sodium retention in CHF, albeit with higher doses.[68] Diuretic resistance to loop diuretics

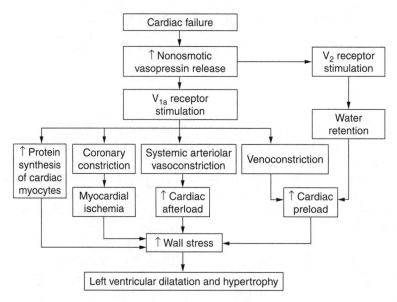

Figure 9-7   Pathways whereby vasopressin stimulation of V_2 and V_{1a} receptors can contribute to events that worsen cardiac function.

involves secondary hyperaldosteronism and upregulation of NCC and ENaC effects, which can be reversed by mineralocorticoid antagonists.[69] In fact, in cirrhosis, another edematous disorder with secondary hyperaldosteronism, spironolactone has been shown to be the diuretic of choice.[70]

Agents that increase solute-free water excretion, so-called aquaretics, are under study by several pharmaceutical companies in phase II and III of clinical trials.[71] These agents cause a water diuresis by blocking the V_2 vasopressin receptor on the basolateral membrane of the collecting duct and have been shown to correct hyponatremia in cardiac failure patients.[72,73] There is little effect with these agents on the hormonal status of CHF patients, since two-thirds of the solute-free water excretion is removed from the intracellular space and only one-third from the extracellular fluid (ECF) compartment. There are also AVP antagonists, which block both the V_2 and V_1 vascular receptors. The potential benefits of these combined V_1 and V_2 antagonists are shown in Fig. 9-7. The effect of these antagonists on morbidity and mortality in CHF patients has yet to be demonstrated. Pretreatment hyponatremia is a dire prognostic risk factor for mortality in CHF patients, but this most likely relates to the severity of the cardiac disease.[74] Similarly, the hyponatremic patient with advanced cardiac failure appears to be at increased risk for cardiac arrhythmias. A primary deleterious effect of hyponatremia on cardiac function remains to be demonstrated. In vitro studies in vascular smooth muscle, however, have shown that hypo-osmolality is associated with an increase in cytosolic calcium concentration and enhanced contractile response to vasoconstrictor agents.[75]

The author would like to acknowledge the excellent editorial assistance of Jan Darling.

▶ REFERENCES

1.   Schrier RW. Pathogenesis of sodium and water retention in high-output and low-output cardiac failure, nephrotic syndrome, cirrhosis, and pregnancy. Part I. *N Engl J Med.* 1988;319: 1065–1072.

2. Schrier RW. Pathogenesis of sodium and water retention in high-output and low-output cardiac failure, nephrotic syndrome, cirrhosis, and pregnancy. Part II. *N Engl J Med*. 1988;319:1127–1134.

3. Ghali JK, Cooper R, Ford E. Trends in hospitalization rates for heart failure in the United States, 1973-1987: evidence for increasing population prevalence. *Arch Intern Med*. 1990;150:769–773.

4. Schrier RW, Ecder T. Unifying hypothesis of body fluid volume regulation: implications for cardiac failure and cirrhosis. *Mt Sinai J of Med*. 2001;68:350–361.

5. Schrier RW. Body fluid volume regulation in health and disease: a unifying hypothesis. *Ann Intern Med*. 1990;113:155–159.

6. Schrier RW, Abraham WT. Hormones and hemodynamics in heart failure. *N Engl J Med*. 1999;341:577–585.

7. Henrich WL, Berl T, McDonald KM, et al. Angiotensin II, renal nerves, and prostaglandins in renal hemodynamics during hemorrhage. *Am J Physiol*. 1978;235:F46–F51.

8. Ferguson DW, Berg WJ, Roach PJ, et al. Effects of heart failure on baroreflex control of sympathetic neural activity. *Am J Cardiol*. 1992;69:523–531.

9. Cohn JN, Levine TB, Olivari MT, et al. Plasma norepinephrine as a guide to prognosis in patients with chronic congestive heart failure. *N Engl J Med*. 1984;311:819–823.

10. Brooks VL. Interactions between angiotensin II and the sympathetic nervous system in the long term control of arterial pressure. *Clin Exp Pharmacol Physiol*. 1997;24:83–90.

11. Henry JP, Gauer OH, Reeves JS. Evidence of atrial location of receptors in influencing urine flow. *Circ Res*. 1956;4:85–90.

12. Mulrow PJ, Schrier RW. *Atrial Hormones and Other Natriuretic Factors*. Clinical Physiology Series. Bethesda, MD: American Physiological Society; 1987.

13. Linden RJ, Kappagoda CT. *Atrial Receptors*. Cambridge, England: Cambridge University Press; 1982.

14. Schrier RW. An odyssey into the milieu intéreur: pondering the enigmas. *J Am Soc Nephrol*. 1992;2:1549–1559.

15. Cody RJ, Covit AB, Schaer GL. Sodium and water balance in chronic heart failure. *J Clin Invest*. 1986;77:144–52.

16. Schrier RW, Better OS. Peripheral arterial vasodilation hypothesis: implications for impaired aldosterone escape. *Eur J Gstroenterol Hepatol*. 1991;3:721–729.

17. Weber K. Mechanisms of disease: aldosterone in chronic heart failure. *N Engl J Med*. 2001;345:1689–1697.

18. Hirsch AT, Pinto YM, Schunkert H, et al. Potential role of the tissue renin-angiotensin system in the pathophysiology of congestive heart failure. *Am J Cardiol*. 1990;66:D22–D30.

19. Schrier RW, Abdallah JG, Weinberger H, et al. Therapy of heart failure. *Kidney Int*. 2002;57:1418–1425.

20. Ellison DH, Okusa MD, Schrier RW. Mechanisms of diuretic action. In: Schrier RW, ed. *Diseases of the Kidney and Urinary Tract*. 8th ed. Philadelphia, PA: Lippincott Williams and Wilkins; 2007.

21. Gamba G. Molecular physiology and pathophysiology of electroneutral cation-chloride cotransporters. *Physiol Rev*. 2005;85:423–493.

22. Hebert SC, Reeves WB, Molony DA, et al. The medullary thick limb: function and modulation of the single-effect multiplier. *Kidney Int*. 1987;31:580–588.

23. Miyanoshita A, Terada M, Endou H. Furosemide directly stimulates prostaglandin E2 production in the thick ascending limb of Henle's loop. *J Pharmacol Exp Ther*. 1989; 251:1155–1159.

24. Kirchner KA. Prostaglandin inhibitors alter loop segment chloride uptake during furosemide diuresis. *Am J Physiol*. 1985;248:F698–F704.

25. Dikshit K, Vyden JK, Forrester JS, et al. Renal and extrarenal hemodynamic effects of furosemide in congestive heart failure after acute myocardial infarction. *N Engl J Med*. 1973;288:1087–1090.

26. Bourland WA, Day KD, Williamson HE. The role of the kidney in the early natriuretic action of furosemide to reduce elevated left atrial pressure in the hypervolemic dog. *J Pharmacol Exp Ther*. 1977;202:221–229.

27. Francis GS, Siegel RM, Goldsmith SR, et al. Acute vasoconstrictor response to intravenous furosemide in patients with chronic congestive heart failure. *Ann Intern Med*. 1985;103: 1–6.

28. Wright FS, Schnermann J. Interference with feedback control of glomerular filtration rate by furosemide, triflocin, and cyanide. *J Clin Invest* 1974;53:1695–1708.

29. Schricker K, Hamann M, Kurtz A. Nitric oxide and prostaglandins are involved in the macular densa control of renin system. *Am J Physiol* 1995;269:F825–F830.

30. Frölich JC, Hollifield JW, Dormois JC, et al. Suppression of plasma renin activity by indomethacin in man. *Circ Res.* 1976; 39:447–452.

31. Sun D, Samuelson LC, Yang T, et al. Mediation of tubuloglomerular feedback by adenosine: evidence from mice lacking adenosine 2 receptors. *Proc Natl Acad Sci USA.* 2001;98:9983–9988.

32. Packer M, Lee WH, Medina N, et al. Functional renal insufficiency during long-term therapy with captopril and enalapril in severe congestive heart failure. *Ann Intern Med.* 1987;106:346–354.

33. McCurley J, Hanlon S, Shao-kui W, et al. Furosemide and the progression of left ventricular dysfunction in experimental heart failure. *J Am Coll Cardiol* 2004;44:1301–1307.

34. Agostoni P, Marenzi G, Lauri G. Sustained improvement in functional capacity after removal of body fluid with isolated ultrafiltration in chronic cardiac insufficiency: failure of furosemide to provide the same result. *Am J Med.* 1994;96:191–199.

35. Tannen RL. The effect of uncomplicated potassium depletion on urine acidification. *J Clin Invest.* 1970;49:813–827.

36. Schrier RW, Gurevich AK, Abraham WT. Renal sodium excretion, edematous disorders, and diuretic use. In: Schrier RW, ed. *Renal and Electrolyte Disorders.* 6th ed. Philadelphia, PA: Lippincott Williams and Wilkins; 2003:64–114.

37. Wigand ME, Heidland A. Ototoxic side effects of high doses of furosemide in patients with uremia. *Postgrad Med J.* 1971;47:54–56.

38. Preisig PA, Toto RD, Alpern RJ. Carbonic anhydrase inhibitors. *Renal Physiol.* 1987;10:136–159.

39. Eknoyan G, Suki WN, Martinez-Maldonado M. Effect of diuretics on urinary excretion of phosphate, calcium, and magnesium in thyroparathyroidectomized dogs. *J Lab Clin Med.* 1970;76:257–266.

40. Miyanoshita A, Gamba G, Lytton J, et al. Primary structure and functional expression of the rat renal thiazide-sensitive NA+:Cl− cotransporter. In *Proceedings of the 12th International Congress of Nephrology.* 1993;110.

41. Bostanjoglo M, Reeves WB, Reilly RF, et al. 11b-hydroxysteroid dehydrogenase, mineralocorti-coid receptor and thiazide-sensitive Na-Cl cotransporter expression by distal tubules. *J Am Soc Nephrol.* 1998;9:1347–1358.

42. Brater DC. Diuretic pharmacokinetics and pharmacodynamics. In: Seldin DW, Giebisch G, eds. *Diuretic Agents: Clinical Physiology and Pharmacology.* San Diego, CA: Academic Press; 1997:189–208.

43. Okusa MD, Erik A, Persson G, et al. Chlorothiazide effect on feedback-mediated control of glomerular filtration rate. *Am J Physiol.* 1989;257:F137–F144.

44. Ashraf N, Locksley R, Arieff A. Thiazide-induced hyponatremia associated with death or neurologic damage in outpatients. *Am J Med.* 1981;70:1163–1168.

45. Hartman D, Rossier B, Kohlman R, et al. Rapid correction of hyponatremia in the syndrome of inappropriate secretion of antidiuretic hormone. *Ann Intern Med.* 1973;78:870–875.

46. Szatalowicz VL, Miller PD, Lacher JW, et al. Comparative effect of diuretics on renal water excretion in hyponatremic, edematous disorders. *Clin Sci.* 1982;62:235–238.

47. Szatalowicz VL, Arnold PE, Chaimovitz C, et al. Radioimmunoassay of plasma arginine vasopressin in hyponatremic patients with congestive heart failure. *N Engl J Med.* 1981;305: 263–266.

48. Ram CV, Garrett BN, Kaplan, NM. Moderate sodium restriction and various diuretics in the treatment of hypertension. *Arch Intern Med.* 1981;141:1015–1019.

49. Okusa MD, Velazquez H, Ellison DH, et al. Luminal calcium regulates potassium transport by the renal distal tubule. *Am J Physiol.* 1990;258:F423–F428.

50. Rude RK. Physiology of magnesium metabolism and the important role of magnesium in potassium deficiency. *Am J Cardiol.* 1989; 63:G31–G34.

51. Helderman JH, Elahi D, Andersen DK, et al. Prevention of the glucose intolerance of thiazide diuretics by maintenance of body potassium. *Diabetes.* 1983;32:106–111.

52. The Antihypertensive and Lipid-Lowering Treatment to Prevent Heart Attack Trial (ALL-HAT) Study Group. Major outcomes in high-risk hypertensive patients randomized to angiotensin-converting enzyme inhibitor or calcium channel blocker vs diuretic. *JAMA.* 2002;288:2981–2997.

53. Baer J, Jones C, Spitzer S, et al. The potassium sparing and natriuretic activity of N-amidino-3,4- diamino-6-chloropyrazinecarboxamide hydrochloride dihydrate (amiloride hydr). *J Pharmacol Exp Ther.* 1967;157:472–485.

54. Peterson LN, Levi M. Disorders of potassium metabolism. In: Schrier RW, ed. *Renal and Electrolyte Disorders.* 6th ed. Philadelphia, PA: Lippincott Williams and Wilkins; 2003:171–215.

55. Meneton P, Loffing J, Warnock DG. Sodium and potassium handling by the aldosterone-sensitive distal nephron: the pivotal role of the distal and connecting tubule. *Am J Physiol Renal Physiol.* 2004;287:F593–F601.

56. Garty H, Palmer LG. Epithelial sodium channels: function, structure, and regulation. *Physiol Rev.* 1997;77:359–396.

57. Bull MB, Laragh JH. Amiloride: A potassium-sparing natriuretic agent. *Circulation.* 1968;37:45–53.

58. Loffing J, Pietri L, Aregger F, et al. Differential subcellular localization of EnaC subunits in mouse kidney in response to high-and low-sodium diets. *Am J Physiol Renal Physiol.* 2000;279:F252–F258.

59. Masilamani S, Kim GH, Mitchell C, et al. Aldosterone-mediated regulation of ENaC α, β and γ subunits. *J Clin Invest.* 1999;104:R19–R23.

60. Couette B, Lombes M, Baulier EE, et al. Aldosterone antagonists destabilize the mineralocorticoid receptor. *Biochem J.* 1992;282:697–702.

61. Coppage WS, Liddle GW. Mode of action and clinical usefulness of aldosterone antagonists. *Ann NY Acad Sci.* 1960;88:815–821.

62. Sungaila I, Bartle WR, Walker SE, et al. Spironolactone pharmacokinetics and pharmacodynamics in patients with cirrhotic ascites. *Gastroenterology.* 1992;102:1680–1685.

63. Rose LI, Underwood RH, Newmark SR, et al. Pathophysiology of spironolactone-induced gynecomastia. *Ann Intern Med.* 1977;87:398–403.

64. Tamirisa KP, Aaronson KD, Koelling TM. Spironolactone-induced renal insufficiency and hyperkalemia in patients with heart failure. *Am Heart J.* 2004;148:971–978.

65. Gabow PA, Moore S, Schrier RW. Spironolactone-induced hyperchloremic acidosis in cirrhosis. *Ann Intern Med.* 1979;90:338–340.

66. Effectiveness of spironolactone added to an angiotensin-converting enzyme inhibitor and a loop diuretic for severe chronic congestive heart failure (The randomized aldactone evaluation study [RALES]). *Am J Cardiol.* 1996;78:902–907.

67. Pitt B, Williams G, Remme W, Eplerenone Post-AMI Heart Failure Efficacy and Survival Study. The EPHESUS trial: eplerenone in patients with heart failure due to systolic dysfunction complicating acute myocardial infarction. *Cardiovasc Drugs Ther.* 2001;15:79–87.

68. Hensen J, Abraham WT, Durr JA, et al. Aldosterone in congestive heart failure: analysis of determinants and role in sodium retention. *Am J Nephrol.* 1991;11:441–446.

69. Abdallah JG, Schrier RW, Edelstein C, et al. Loop diuretic infusion increases thiazide-sensitive Na^+-Cl^- cotransporter abundance: role of aldosterone. *J Am Soc Nephrol.* 2001;12:1335–1341.

70. Perez-Ayuso RM, Arroyo V, Planas R, et al. Randomized comparative study of efficacy of furosemide versus spironolactone in nonazotemic cirrhosis with ascites: relationship between the diuretic response and the activity of the renin-aldosterone system. *Gastroenterology.* 1983;84:961–968.

71. Schrier RW, Chen YC, Cadnapaphornchai MA. From finch to fish to man: role of aquaporins in body fluid and brain water regulation. *Neuroscience.* 2004;129:897–9904.

72. Abraham WT, Shamshirsaz AA, McFann K, et al. Aquaretic effect of lixivaptan, an oral non-peptide selective V2 receptor vasopressin antagonist, in the NYHA Class II and III chronic heart failure patients. *J Am Coll Cardiol.* In revision.

73. Gheorghiade M, Gattis WA, O'Connor CM, et al. Effects of tolvaptan, a vasopressin antagonist, in patients hospitalized with worsening heart failure: a randomized controlled trial. *JAMA.* 2004;291:1963–1971.

74. Lee WH, Packer M. Prognostic importance of serum sodium concentration and its modification by converting-enzyme inhibition in patients with severe chronic heart failure. *Circulation.* 1986;73:257–267.

75. Okada K, Ishikawa S, Caramelo C, et al. Enhancement of vascular action of arginine vasopressin by diminished extracellular sodium concentration. *Kidney Int.* 1993;44:755–763.

CHAPTER 10

How to Use Neurohormonal Antagonists in Heart Failure

ALEXANDER E. FRALEY, MD/BARRY H. GREENBERG, MD

▶ OVERVIEW

The development of clinical heart failure (HF) is a progressive process that can be initiated by a variety of conditions that alter cardiac performance either by directly injuring the myocardium or imposing an increase in loading conditions. When this occurs, neurohormonal systems are activated in an attempt to augment cardiac output and tissue perfusion. Although activation of the renin-angiotensin-aldosterone and sympathetic nervous system (SNS) may help to maintain circulatory homeostasis over the short run, it is clear that their sustained effects have adverse consequences on cardiac structure and function that ultimately result in progression of disease and clinical deterioration.

One of the fundamental strategies of HF management is to interrupt maladaptive neurohormonal activation by blocking production of effector peptides or preventing the action of these molecules with their target receptor. There is now convincing evidence that this strategy results not only in symptomatic improvement, but also significant reduction in morbidity and mortality.

The present chapter describes the use of neurohormonal blocking agents in the treatment of HF with particular focus on practical aspects related to their initiation, uptitration, and long-term maintenance. The classes of drugs that will be discussed are the angiotensin-converting enzyme (ACE) inhibitors, angiotensin receptor blockers (ARBs), β-blockers, and aldosterone antagonists.

▶ INHIBITORS OF THE RENIN-ANGIOTENSIN SYSTEM

Initial activation of the renin-angiotensin system (RAS) involves secretion of renin by the kidney in response to hypoperfusion resulting from intravascular volume depletion or low cardiac output. The fact that renin secretion is enhanced by adrenergic stimulation of the kidney highlights the interaction and synergism between various neurohormonal systems. Renin cleaves angiotensinogen, initiating a cascade that concludes in the generation of angiotensin II (AngII), the main effector molecule of the RAS. The effects of AngII are mediated by its interaction with its Type I (AT_1), and Type II (AT_2) receptors. Of these, the AT_1 mediates most known physiologic effects of AngII. AngII-AT_1-receptor effects result in sodium (Na^+) retention, vasoconstriction, norepinephrine (NE) secretion, and aldosterone release. AT_1-receptor activation also has direct trophic effects on cardiac myocytes and stimulates fibroblasts to increase extracellular matrix production. These latter effects, in particular, contribute to the adverse remodeling that results in progressive left ventricular (LV) dysfunction. In experimental animal models, blocking AngII-AT_1-receptor interactions attenuates this maladaptive process. Pharmacologically, this is accomplished by inhibiting ACE from cleaving AngI to AngII or by direct antagonism of the AT_1 receptor. The application of ACE inhibitors and AT_1-receptor blockers has been shown in human HF trials to inhibit remodeling, ameliorate symptoms, improve hemodynamics, reduce hospitalizations, and prolong survival.

Angiotensin-Converting Enzyme Inhibitors in Chronic Heart Failure

Clinical Evidence

ACE inhibitors were the first class of neurohormonal blocking agents that were shown to have a mortality benefit in patients with chronic HF and left ventricular dysfunction (LVD). The randomized, placebo-controlled trial (RCT), Cooperative North Scandinavian Enalapril Survival Study (CONSENSUS), was a seminal study, which established the concept that ACE inhibitors have favorable effects on the clinical course of HF.[1] In this study, after 6 months of treatment, enalapril reduced mortality in patients with advanced HF by 40% relative to placebo. Improved survival, reduced hospitalization, and other clinical benefits have also been reported in the Studies Of Left Ventricular Dysfunction (SOLVD) trials and other studies encompassing a broader spectrum of HF patients and using a variety of different ACE inhibitors (see Table 10-1).[2,3] The Assessment of Treatment with Lisinopril and Survival (ATLAS) trial demonstrated that the effects of ACE inhibitors appear to be dose dependent, at least for a combined morbidity/mortality endpoint.

How to Use Angiotensin-Converting Enzymes Inhibitors in Chronic Heart Failure

Inhibition of the RAS is a cornerstone of neurohormonal treatment of HF and it is now widely accepted that all patients with LV dysfunction should receive an ACE inhibitor titrated to the target dose, unless such treatment is contraindicated (see Table 10-2). Treatment with ACE inhibitors is usually initiated at a low dose that can then be rapidly uptitrated. When patients are being treated in-hospital, this is usually completed within a matter of days, while in outpatients a more gradual approach is taken. The major limiting factors for the initiation and uptitration of ACE inhibitors are hypotension, impaired renal function, and elevated serum potassium (K^+) levels. In general, advised practice is to initiate and uptitrate ACE inhibitors in patients with systolic pressures

▶ Table 10-1 Angiotensin-converting enzyme inhibitors heart failure trials

Trial (n)	Agent	Target dose	NYHA class enrolled	Follow-up	All-cause mortality	Other
CONSENSUS (n = 253)	Enalapril	20 mg bid	• NYHA Class IV	6 months, 12 months	• 40% RRR at 6 months (P = 0.02) • 31% RRR at 12 months (P = 0.001)	• 50% RRR progressive HF(P = 0.001)
SOLVD Treatment (n = 2569)	Enalapril	10 mg bid	• NYHA Class II–III	41.4 months	• 16% RR (95% CI 5–26%; P = 0.0072)	• 22% RRR death secondary to progressive HF (P <0.009)
SOLVD Prevention (n = 4228)	Enalapril	10 mg bid	• NYHA Class I–II	37.4 months	• Nonsignificant mortality trend favoring enalapril	• 20% RRR death or hospitalization for HF (P <0.001)
ATLAS (n = 3164)	Lisinopril	Low (2.5–5 mg) vs. high dose (32.5–35 mg)	• NYHA III–IV or Class II with HF exacerbation in prior 6 months	45.7 months	• Nonsignificant trend showing 8% mortality reduction in high dose lisinopril group	• 12% RRR for all-cause mortality + hospitalization (P = 0.002) • 24% RRR of hospitalization for HF (P = 0.002)

CONSENSUS—Cooperative North Scandinavian Enalapril Survival Study; SOLVD—Studies Of Left Ventricular Dysfunction trial; ATLAS—Assessment of Treatment with Lisinopril and Survival trial; NYHA—New York Heart Association; RRR—relative risk reduction; CI—confidence interval; HF—heart failure
Source: The CONSENSUS Trial Study Group. Effects of enalapril on mortality in severe congestive heart failure. Results of the Cooperative North Scandinavian Enalapril Survival Study (CONSENSUS). *N Engl J Med.* 1987;316(23):1429–1435.
The SOLVD Investigators. Effect of enalapril on survival in patients with reduced left ventricular ejection fractions and congestive heart failure. *N Engl J Med.* 1991;325(5):293–302.
Packer M, ATLAS Study Group, et al. Comparative effects of low and high doses of the angiotensin-converting enzyme inhibitor, lisinopril, on morbidity and mortality in chronic heart failure. *Circulation.* 1999;100(23):2312–2318.

▶ **Table 10-2** Angiotensin-converting enzyme inhibitors target doses

Agent	Initial dose	Target dose
Captopril	12.5 mg tid	50 mg tid
Ramipril	2.5 mg bid	5 mg bid
Trandolapril	1 mg qd	4 mg qd
Enalapril	2.5 mg bid	20 mg bid
Fosinopril	10 mg qd	40 mg qd
Lisinopril	5 mg qd	40 mg qd
Quinapril	5 mg bid	20 mg bid

≥80 mm Hg, limiting uptitration only by the development of symptomatic hypotension rather than by a level of blood pressure, per se. Patients at greatest risk for developing symptoms for low blood pressure include those (1) with borderline pressure to begin with, (2) who have recently undergone extensive diuresis, (3) with New York Heart Association (NYHA) functional Class IV symptoms, and/or (4) who have low levels of serum Na+. If symptomatic hypotension occurs, initial management includes a reduction of other vasodilators and diuretics (see Patient Monitoring and Management later in the chapter). The basic chemistry panel should be drawn within a few days following ACE inhibitor initiation to assess renal function and serum K+. These measurements should be repeated periodically thereafter with the frequency determined by the stability of the patient and the initial levels of creatinine and K+. If serum K+ levels >4.5 mEq/L, amount of potassium replacement should be reduced. When this proves insufficient, addressing sources of potassium in the diet and discontinuing supplemental K+ may be necessary. When the K+ levels >5.5 mEq/L despite these measures, halving (or greater) of the ACE inhibitor dose is usually recommended. In some patients, ACE inhibitors cannot be continued because of persistent hyperkalemia.

A change in creatinine can be anticipated in the elderly and those patients with limited renal reserve. Increases in creatinine of <30% are generally considered acceptable if there is no clinical evidence of progressive fluid overload or associated hyperkalemia. "Dry" patients who develop renal insufficiency can be treated by cautiously decreasing the diuretic dose by 25–50%. The strict use of a daily weight log to detect changes in volume status can also be of value in adjusting the diuretic dose during this period in order to maintain euvolemia in HF patients. When hyperkalemia occurs it is critical to review the patients' medications and to eliminate or reduce contributing medications, such as nonsteroidal anti-inflammatory drugs (NSAIDs), K+ sparing diuretics, or K+ replacement.

Angiotensin-Converting Enzyme Inhibitors Postmyocardial Infarction

Clinical Evidence
Based on the results of studies in experimental animal models, their efficacy in chronic HF and the results of initial studies demonstrating a favorable impact on post-myocardial infarction (post-MI) cardiac remodeling, the effects of ACE inhibitors on the clinical course of post-MI patients were evaluated in a series of large well-designed RCTs. These trials, Survival and Ventricular Enlargement (SAVE), Acute Infarction Ramipril Efficacy (AIRE) and Trandolapril Cardiac Evaluation (TRACE), Survival of Myocardial Infarction Long-term Evaluation (SMILE), included patients with evidence of LV dysfunction and/or HF following an MI (summarized in Table 10-3) and demonstrated significant reductions in all-cause mortality, hospitalization, progressive HF, and other relevant cardiovascular (CV) endpoints.[4–6] As a result, the use of ACE inhibitors has emerged as a cornerstone of long-term medical therapy for patients with post-MI LV dysfunction.

How to Use ACE Inhibitors in the Post-Acute Myocardial Infarction Patient
Following an acute myocardial infarction (AMI), all patients should undergo assessment of LV function. Those patients with an ejection fraction (EF) <40% or symptoms of HF should be started

▶ **Table 10-3** Angiotensin-converting enzyme inhibitors post-acute myocardial infarction trials

Trial (n)	Agent	Target dose	NYHA class enrolled	Follow-up	All-cause mortality	Other
SAVE (n = 2231)	Captopril	50 mg tid	• Asymptomatic patients • 3 days post-AMI with LV dysfunction	42 months	• 19% RRR (95% CI 3–32%; P = 0.019)	• 22% RRR in HF hospitalization (P = 0.019) • 37% RRR in open-labeled ACEI for progressive HF (P <0.001) • 24% RRR death CV cause, CHF, or AMI (P < 0.001)
AIRE (n = 1986)	Ramipril	5 mg bid Initiation of ACEI 3–10 days post-AMI	• AMI with clinical evidence of HF requiring diuretics or vasodilators • Class IV patients excluded	Average 15 months	• 27% RRR (95% CI 11–40%; P = 0.002)	• 19% RRR death, AMI, progressive HF, CVA (P = 0.008)
TRACE (n = 1749)	Trandolapril	4 mg qd Initiation of ACEI 3–7 days post-AMI	• Randomized 3–7 days post-AMI • LV dysfunction	24–50 months	• 22% RRR (95% CI 9–33%; P = 0.001)	• 29% RRR for progression of HF (P = 0.003)
SMILE (n = 1556)	Zofenopril	Zofenopril 30 mg bid	• Randomized within 24 hours of anterior MI to 6 weeks of therapy	12 months	• 29% RRR (95% CI 6–51%; P = 0.011)	• 46% RRR for severe HF at 6 weeks (P = 0.018)

SAVE—Survival and Ventricular Enlargement; AIRE—Acute Infarction Ramipril Efficacy trial; TRACE—Trandolapril Cardiac Evaluation; SMILE—Survival of Myocardial Infarction Long-Term Evaluation; AMI—acute myocardial infarction; NYHA—New York Heart Association; LV—left ventricular; HF—heart failure; MI—myocardial infarction; RR—relative risk reduction; CVA—coronary vascular accident; CV—cardiovascular

Source: Pfeffer MA, The SAVE Investigators, et al. Effect of captopril on mortality and morbidity in patients with left ventricular dysfunction after myocardial infarction. Results of the survival and ventricular enlargement trial. *N Engl J Med.* 1992;327(10):669–677.

The Acute Infarction Ramipril Efficacy (AIRE) Study Investigators. Effect of ramipril on mortality and morbidity of survivors of acute myocardial infarction with clinical evidence of heart failure. *Lancet.* 1993;342(8875):821–828.

Kober L, et al. A clinical trial of the angiotensin-converting-enzyme inhibitor trandolapril in patients with left ventricular dysfunction after myocardial infarction. *N Engl J Med.* 1995;333(25):1670–1676.

Ambrosioni E, Borghi C, Magnani B, The Survival of Myocardial Infarction Long-Term Evaluation (SMILE) Study Investigators. The effect of the angiotensin-converting-enzyme inhibitor zofenopril on mortality and morbidity after anterior myocardial infarction. *N Engl J Med.* 1995;332(2):80–85.

on an ACE inhibitor (along with other therapies including aspirin, a statin, and β-adrenergic receptor blocker). It is advisable that treatment be initiated prior to hospital discharge both in order to increase the likelihood that this beneficial form of therapy will be used and to provide early protection to the MI survivor. In fact, studies such as GISSI-3 and ISIS-4 indicate that the benefits and early initiation of ACE inhibitors post-MI are substantial.[8,9] While in-hospital, a short acting ACE inhibitor such as captopril is usually initiated at a low dose (e.g., 6.25 mg thrice daily). The dosage is then rapidly increased over a period of days to the target dose of 150 mg daily. Switching to a longer acting ACE inhibitor at the time of discharge can simplify the patients' medical regimen and improve compliance. Careful monitoring of blood pressure, serum creatinine, and potassium levels is mandatory during the initiation and uptitration of ACE inhibitors in post-MI patients.

Angiotensin Receptor Blockers in Chronic Heart Failure

Clinical Evidence

The use of ARBs in chronic HF offers an alternative approach to blocking RAS. The main theoretical advantage would appear to be the ability of the ARBs to block effects of AngII, regardless of whether the peptide is generated by the action of ACE or through alternative pathways that appear to predominate in the tissue-based RAS. Unlike ACE inhibitors, ARBs do not enhance bradykinin (BK) levels by inhibiting ACE-mediated breakdown of this peptide. Whereas this latter effect has been associated with the excess cough seen with the ACE inhibitors, BK accumulation may contribute to the beneficial effects of the ACE inhibitors since it has vasodilating and antigrowth properties.

Although ACE inhibitors are the foundation of contemporary HF therapy, clinical trials (see Table 10-4) have established an important supporting role for ARBs. Evaluation of Losartan in the Elderly (ELITE II) compared the effect of losartan to that of captopril in patients with

chronic HF and LV dysfunction.[10] Although the results failed to demonstrate the superiority of the ARB, it did provide evidence that losartan was better tolerated. The Candesartan in Heart Failure: Assessment of Reduction in Mortality and Morbidity (CHARM)-Alternative study studied the effects of candesartan in ACE inhibitor-intolerant patients with symptomatic HF and LV systolic dysfunction.[11] The results demonstrated a highly favorable effect on the combined endpoint of CV mortality and HF hospitalization. These studies, along with an analysis of patients in Valsartan Heart Failure Trial (Val-HeFT) who were not receiving ACE inhibitors, provide convincing evidence of the efficacy of ARBs in systolic HF and establish their place as an alternative therapy in ACE-intolerant patients.[12] Both Val-HeFT and the CHARM-Added study evaluated the impact of adding an ARB in addition to a therapeutic regimen that already included an ACE inhibitor.[13] In each study, there was a significant reduction in the primary composite endpoint of morbidity and mortality. The CHARM-Added study, in which high doses of candesartan were used, also showed a 15% reduction in CV mortality with the addition of the ARB. While there was suggestion from post-hoc analysis of Val-HeFT that the addition of an ARB to a regimen that already included an ACE inhibitor and β-blocker might have adverse consequences, this possibility was not confirmed in the predesignated analysis of this interaction in the CHARM-Added study.

How to Use Angiotensin Receptor Blockers in Chronic Heart Failure with Left Ventricular Dysfunction

In starting ARB therapy, one follows similar guidelines to those summarized above in regards to the initiation of ACE inhibitors. The ARB is started at a low dose (see Table 10-5). Potassium supplementation is decreased by 25–50% if K$^+$ >4.5 mEq/L. A history of symptomatic hypotension is sought and K$^+$ and renal function are remeasured at 1 week. If systolic blood pressure (SBP) >80 and the patient does not have symptoms of orthostasis, continue to uptitrate the dose. In euvolemic

▶ Table 10-4 Angiotensin receptor blocker chronic heart failure trials

Trial (n)	Comparison	Agent	Patient population	Follow-up	All-cause mortality	Other
ELITE II (n = 3152)	ACEI vs. ARB	Losartan or captopril	• NYHA Class II–IV	Median 18 months	• NS	NS for SCD, hospitalization, composite
Val-HeFT (n = 5010)	ACEI + ARB vs. ACE	Valsartan or placebo	• NYHA Class II–IV	24 months	• NS	• 13% RRR in mortality + morbidity (SCD + HF hospitalization + HF exacerbation) (P = 0.009)
CHARM-Added (n = 2548)	ACEI + ARB vs. ACE	Candesartan	• NYHA Class II + cardiac admission in past 6 months or NYHA Class III–IV	Median 41 months	• NS	• 15% RRR CV death or hospitalization for HF (P = 0.011) • 16% RRR CV death (P = 0.029) • 17% RRR hospitalization for HF (P = 0.014)
CHARM-Alternative (n = 2028)	ARB vs. placebo	Candesartan	• NYHA Class II–IV • Intolerant of ACEI therapy	Median 33.7 months	• NS	• 23% RRR CV death or hospitalization for HF (P = 0.0004) • 32% RRR hospitalization for HF (P <0.0001)

ELITE II—Evaluation of Losartan in the Elderly; Val-HeFT—Valsartan Heart Failure Trial; CHARM—Candesartan in Heart Failure: Assessment of Reduction in Mortality and Morbidity; ACE—angiotensin-converting enzyme; ARB—angiotensin receptor blocker; ACEI—angiotensin-converting enzyme inhibitors; NYHA—New York Heart Association; SCD—sudden cardiac death; RR—relative risk reduction; HF—heart failure; CV—cardiovascular; NS—not significant

Source: Pitt B, et al. Effect of losartan compared with captopril on mortality in patients with symptomatic heart failure: randomised trial—the Losartan Heart Failure Survival Study ELITE II. *Lancet.* 2000;355(9215):1582–1587.

Granger CB, et al. Effects of candesartan in patients with chronic heart failure and reduced left-ventricular systolic function intolerant to angiotensin-converting-enzyme inhibitors: the CHARM-Alternative trial. *Lancet.* 2003;362(9386):772–776.

Cohn JN, Tognoni G. A randomized trial of the angiotensin-receptor blocker valsartan in chronic heart failure. *N Engl J Med.* 2001;345(23):1667–1675.

Granger CB, McMurray JJ, Ostergen J, Swedberg K, et al. Effects of candesartan in patients with chronic heart failure and reduced left-ventricular systolic function taking angiotensin-converting-enzyme inhibitors: the CHARM-Added trial. *Lancet.* 2003;362(9386):767–771.

▶ **Table 10-5** Angiotensin receptor blocker target doses

Agent	Initial dose	Target dose
Losartan	12.5 mg qd	50 mg qd
Valsartan	40 mg bid	160 mg bid
Candesartan	4 mg qd	32 mg qd

patients with symptomatic hypotension, altering the timing of the dosing regimen to separate administration of the ARB from that of other vasoactive drugs or administration as a single dose at bedtime often alleviates the problem. With more refractory orthostasis, consider decreasing diuretics by 25–50% and eliminating other vasodilators wherever possible.

When administering an ARB in addition to an ACE inhibitor, problems related to hypotension, hyperkalemia, and worsening renal function are more likely than with each individual agent. More stringent surveillance of these patients using the management strategies outlined above is clearly warranted.

Angiotensin Receptor Blockers in Acute Myocardial Infarction

Clinical Evidence
The Optimal Trial in Myocardial Infarction with the Angiotensin II Antagonist Losartan (OPTI-MAAL) and Valsartan in Acute Myocardial Infarction (VALIANT) trials have helped to define the role of ARBs in the post-MI patient. OPTI-MAAL was a head-to-head comparison between losartan and captopril in post-MI patients with LV dysfunction.[14,15] For the primary endpoint of all-cause mortality, there was an insignificant trend in favor of the ACE inhibitor, but there was evidence that the ARB was better tolerated with a lower rate of discontinuation (17% vs. 23%, $P < 0.0001$). This study has been criticized, however, based on the low dose and delayed titration schedule for the ARB. VALIANT examined the efficacy of captopril, valsartan, and their combination

therapy in patients with post-MI LV dysfunction. The study demonstrated "noninferiority" of the ARB, valsartan, to ACE inhibitor therapy. Treatment with the combination of valsartan and captopril provided no additional morbidity or mortality benefit and resulted in an increased incidence of adverse events. These trials established ARBs as an alternative agent in the ACE inhibitor-intolerant patient with post-MI LV dysfunction.

How to Use Angiotensin Receptor Blockers in the Post-Acute Myocardial Infarction Patient
When selecting an ARB (or replacing an ACE inhibitor) for treatment of post-MI LV dysfunction, the drug should be started in conjunction with other treatments including a β-adrenergic receptor blocker, aspirin, and a statin. In patients with elevation of creatinine due to the effects of the contrast load delivered during emergency angiography, initiation of therapy should be delayed until creatinine stabilizes. Treatment is usually initiated in a monitored environment, prior to hospital discharge, but this degree of caution is not necessary since serious immediate side effects are rare. When the drug is started in the in-patient setting, rapid titration to target can be accomplished with minimal risk. Management of hypotension and other issues (with the exception of cough and angioneurotic edema) are similar as with ACE inhibitors and are managed in a similar manner.

Patient Monitoring and Management of Adverse Effects During Chronic Therapy with Angiotensin-Converting Enzymes Inhibitors and/or Angiotensin Receptor Blockers

Hypotension
Initially, one should confirm that new symptoms of dizziness and fatigue correspond to a reduction in SBP (usually to <80 mm Hg) or that orthostatic hypotension (a decrease in SBP or diastolic blood pressure [DBP] of 20 or 10 mm Hg, respectively, within 3 minutes after standing) is present.[16]

Although hypotension is a well-recognized side effect of ACE inhibitors and ARBs, symptoms may be due to other agents as shown in the SOLVD prevention study where the incidence of hypotension was reported as 57% in ACE inhibitor-treated patients and 50% in the placebo group.[3] Combination therapy with an ACE inhibitor and ARB is more likely to cause hypotension than a single drug. In VALIANT, hypotension was reported in 18.2% of patients on combination RAS blockade compared to 15.1% and 11.9% in the groups randomized to valsartan or captopril, respectively.[15] Overall, the discontinuation rate was low with 1.9%, 1.4%, and 0.8% of patients in the valsartan-captopril, valsartan, and captopril groups, respectively. In patients with symptomatic hypotension, it is essential to assess volume status (by assessing weight, estimating jugular venous pressure [JVP], measuring serum bicarbonate, blood urea nitrogen [BUN], and creatinine levels). If the patient is volume depleted, decrease the diuretic dose by 25–50%. If the patient is euvolemic and receiving other vasodilators, reduce or eliminate these medications wherever possible. Hypervolemic and hypotensive patients may require hospitalization for decompensated congestive heart failure (CHF). If hypotension persists in the ambulatory patient, decrease the RAS blocker dose and attempt to titrate back to target in 2–3 weeks.

Progressive Renal Dysfunction

ACE inhibitors and ARBs decrease intraglomerular pressure, an effect that results in decreased filtration of renal plasma flow through the glomeruli (GFR). In patients who develop increases in creatinine while receiving an ACE inhibitor or ARB, it is important to consider reversible etiologies of azotemia including volume depletion, medications (NSAIDs, antibiotics), and post-renal outflow obstruction. If no reversible etiology is identified and a >30% increase occurs, reduce the dose of the ACE inhibitor or ARB by 50%.

Hyperkalemia

Patients receiving either an ACE inhibitor, an ARB, or, particularly, the combination are at increased risk for hyperkalemia. The groups receiving low- and high-dose lisinopril from the ATLAS trial reported a 4% and 6% incidence of hyperkalemia, respectively. However, only 0.2% and 0.4% of these patients required eventual ACE inhibitor discontinuation. If K^+ rises to >5.5 mEq/L, discontinue concurrent K^+ supplements or K^+ sparing diuretics, such as spironolactone or eplerenone. Patients receiving dual therapy with an ARB and ACE inhibitor should discontinue one of these agents. If these measures are ineffective, decrease the ACE inhibitor dose by 50% and repeat serum chemistries in 1 week.

Cough

ACE inhibitor-associated cough is estimated to occur in 5–10% of treated patients and may require discontinuation of therapy. Before considering a medication change, confirm that the cough is not a result of progressive HF, exacerbation of reactive airway disease, chronic obstructive pulmonary disease (COPD), or upper respiratory infection. In ATLAS, the low- and high-dose lisinopril group reported an incidence of cough of 13% and 11%, respectively, suggesting that cough is not dose related. In our experience, there is usually not a benefit in switching from one ACE inhibitor to another. If no other cause is identified and the patient cannot tolerate the cough, we recommend changing to an ARB.

Angioneurotic Edema

Angioneurotic edema is a rare adverse event occurring in 0.1–0.5% of patients treated with an ACE inhibitor.[14,15,17] The incidence appears to occur more frequently in African Americans.[18] Angioneurotic edema is very unlikely with ARBs but it does occur. When this characteristic interstitial fluid accumulation occurs in patients receiving an ACE inhibitor, our usual practice is to stop the ACE inhibitor and replace it with an ARB unless the syndrome included airway obstruction. In that case, we exclude both classes of drug from the patients' regimen and seek alternative therapies such as the combination of nitrates and hydralazine.

Contraindication in Pregnancy

Numerous case reports of RAS inhibition suggest the potential for organodysplasia and fetal renal dysfunction in both human and animal models.[19] These risks are greatest in the second and third trimester of pregnancy and once pregnancy is recognized it is imperative to discontinue ACE inhibitor or ARB therapy. These medications should be used with caution in women of reproductive age not using birth control.

ACE Inhibitor and Aspirin Therapy

The question of whether or not there is an interaction between aspirin and RAS inhibition in HF has not been prospectively studied. Analyses of HF patients from SOLVD suggest that concurrent use of aspirin diminished the mortality benefit of ACE inhibitors. It is proposed that aspirin attenuated ACE inhibitor-mediated vasodilatation.[20] These findings were not reproduced in a meta-analysis, including data from SOLVD, and the authors concluded that ACE inhibitor treatment reduced mortality in HF patients regardless of whether concurrent aspirin therapy was administered.[21] It is our practice to continue low-dose, aspirin therapy in patients receiving an ACE inhibitor or ARB, particularly if there is a history of coronary disease or the patient is post-MI.

The Use of Angiotensin-Converting Enzyme Inhibitors and Angiotensin Receptor Blockers in Special Populations

Diabetes Mellitus

Diabetes is an independent risk factor for death from HF and it contributes to vascular inflammation, endothelial dysfunction, and to an increase in "oxidative stress."[22] In diabetic hypertensives, ACE inhibitors and ARBs have been shown to reduce progression of renal dysfunction.[23–25] The Heart Outcomes Prevention Evaluation (HOPE) and Microalbuminuria Cardiovascular and Renal Outcomes-HOPE (MICRO-HOPE) trials enrolled diabetic patients with a prior CV event or a single CV risk factor and randomized them to ramipril or placebo.[26,27] Treatment with ramipril resulted in a 24% and 37% relative reduction in all-cause mortality and CV death, respectively. HOPE excluded patients with HF, but treatment with ramipril reduced the relative risk of HF in the diabetic population by 20%. TRACE, a similarly designed study that included HF patients, concluded that ACE inhibitor treatment reduced mortality and progressive HF to a greater extent in diabetic than their nondiabetics counterparts.[28] Overall, it appears that whereas all patients with HF and LVD benefit from treatment with an RAS blocker, this benefit is more pronounced in diabetic patients.

Heart Failure with Preserved Left Ventricular Function

The optimal treatment for patients with HF and preserved LV systolic function remains poorly defined. The CHARM-Preserved trial was designed to address this question and enrolled NYHA functional Class III–IV, or Class II patients with recent hospitalization and an LVEF >40%.[29] Patients were randomized to candesartan or placebo in addition to background therapy with ACE inhibitor (20%), β-blocker (55%), and spironolactone (11%). There was a nonsignificant trend toward a reduction in the combined endpoint of CV mortality and hospitalization for HF. Hospitalizations for HF were significantly reduced by the ARB. This modest trend came at a significant increase in the risk of hypotension, renal insufficiency, and hyperkalemia. Thus, at this time the value of RAS blockade in HF with preserved LV function is uncertain. The ongoing irbesartan in HF with preserved systolic function (I-PRESERVE) trial should help resolve this issue.[30]

Race

Many of the trials investigating the impact of RAS blockers were performed in Northern Europe and enrolled only a small numbers of black or African American patients. Data from the Val-HeFT II comparing the effects of enalapril to the combination of hydralazine and isosorbide dinitrate (ISDN) suggested a diminished effect of enalapril on blood pressure and mortality in

African Americans versus the Caucasian subgroup, or alternatively an enhanced response to hydralazine-ISDN not present in Caucasians.[31] A retrospective analysis of the data collected from the SOLVD trial (conducted mostly in the United States) suggests that African Americans with impaired LV function are at greater risk of death and progressive HF than their Caucasian counterparts.[32] This data set, however, also concluded that African American patients experienced an equivalent risk reduction when treated with enalapril. Despite contradictory and incomplete data, we recommend the use of ACE inhibitors and ARBs in the African American population for the same indications and in the same way as in other patients.

Sympathetic Nervous System Blockade

The SNS primarily functions during stress or exercise to maintain or elevate blood pressure and tissue perfusion through a cascade of selective α- and β-stimulation that increases heart rate and myocyte contractility and helps regulate peripheral vascular resistance. SNS action is potent and rapid in onset. Its short-term role in maintaining circulatory homeostasis is complemented by the intermediate and long-term effect of the RAS and aldosterone system. A reduction

in cardiac function disturbs this balanced system and results in persistent sympathetic activation and elevation of serum catecholamines. The pathologic milieu of excess catecholamines results in an increase in afterload as well as a variety of direct effects on the heart including β-receptor downregulation, alteration of myocyte phenotype and compromised cell viability. If this sympathetic activation is unopposed, cardiac remodeling is enhanced and HF progresses. Chronic β-receptor stimulation contributes to increased mortality from pump failure as well as sudden death from arrhythmia. The consequences of chronic SNS activation, however, can be ameliorated by β-adrenergic receptor blockade.

Adrenergic receptor antagonists are a diverse class and can be classified by their variable selectivity on α_1 and α_2, and β_1 and β_2 receptor subtypes and other ancillary properties (see Table 10-6). Given the diversity in pharmacology between adrenergic blocking agents, it is not warranted to describe the beneficial effects of a single agent as being due to a "class effect" as is done with ACE inhibitors. For the latter, the bulk of evidence would suggest that the effects of the ACE inhibitor can be generalized to all drugs within the class and it is our practice to use the ACE inhibitors interchangeably. For β-blockers, however, we recommend using only specific β-receptor antagonists proven to reduce morbidity and mortality in RCTs in HF or post-MI.

▶ **Table 10-6** β-Blocker target doses

Agent	Generation (action)	Initial dose	Target dose
Bisoprolol	Second (β_1R)	1.25 mg qd (dose unavailable in United States)	10 mg qd
Carvedilol	Third (β_1R,β_2R,α_1R)	3.125 mg bid in HF 6.25 mg bid in post-MI LVD	25 mg bid (50 mg bid when weight greater than 85 kg)
Metoprolol succinate	Second (β_1R)	25 mg qd or 12.5 mg qd in NYHA Class III or IV HF	200 mg qd

HF—heart failure; LVD—left ventricular dysfunction; MI—myocardial infarction; NYHA—New York Heart Association

β-Receptor Blockers in Chronic Heart Failure

Clinical Evidence

Initial trials, which randomized HF patients to β-receptor blockers demonstrated improvements in exercise capacity, LVEF, and HF symptoms. These trials were not adequately powered to evaluate the impact on mortality. The U.S. Carvedilol Heart Failure Study group evaluated the safety and efficacy of β-receptor blockers in patients with symptomatic HF and a reduced LVEF ≤35% on stable therapy with an ACE inhibitor and diuretic. Although not specifically powered for assessing these endpoints, the results showed that carvedilol was associated with a significant reduction in morbidity and mortality as well as reduced progression of disease.[32] Cardiac Insufficiency Bisoprolol Study II (CIBIS-II)[34] and Metoprolol Controlled-Release Randomized Intervention Trial in Heart Failure (MERIT-HF)[35] were designed to assess the effects of bisoprolol and metoprolol succinate, respectively, on mortality as the primary endpoint and definitively demonstrated evidence of improved survival with these drugs (Table 10-7). However, these studies included patients with mostly NYHA functional Class II–III symptoms and their

▶ **Table 10-7** β-Blockers in chronic heart failure

Trial (n)	Agent	Patient population	Follow-up	All-cause mortality	Other
U.S. Carvedilol (n = 1094)	Carvedilol	• NYHA Class II–IV	Mean 6.5 months	• 65% RRR (95% CI 39–80%; P <0.001)	• Hospitalization for CV cause 27% reduction in risk of hospitalization (P = 0.036)
CIBIS II (n = 2647)	Bisoprolol	• NYHA Class III–IV	Mean 16 months	• 34% RRR (95% CI 19–46%; P <0.0001)	• SCD 44% RRR (P = 0.0011) • Progressive HF 36% RRR (P = 0.0001)
MERIT-HF (n = 3991)	Metoprolol succinate	• NYHA Class II–IV	Mean 12 months	• 34% RRR (95% CI 19–47%; P = 0.00009)	• SCD 41% RRR (P = 0.0002)
COPERNICUS (n = 2289)	Carvedilol	• NYHA Class IV	Mean 10.4 months	• 35% RRR (95% CI 19–48%; P = 0.0014)	• Composite of death or hospitalization 24% RRR (P <0.001)

CIBIS II— Cardiac Insufficiency Bisoprolol Study II; MERIT-HF— Metoprolol Controlled-Release Randomized Intervention Trial in Heart Failure; COPERNICUS— Carvedilol Prospective Randomized Cumulative Survival; NYHA—New York Heart Association; RR—relative risk reduction; CI—confidence interval; CV—cardiovascular; HF—heart failure

Source: Packer M, et al. The effect of carvedilol on morbidity and mortality in patients with chronic heart failure. *N Engl J Med.* 1996;334(21):1349–1355.

The Cardiac Insufficiency Bisoprolol Study II (CIBIS-II): a randomised trial. *Lancet.* 1999;353(9146):9–13.

Effect of metoprolol CR/XL in chronic heart failure: Metoprolol CR/XL Randomised Intervention Trial in Congestive Heart Failure (MERIT-HF). *Lancet.* 1999;353(9169):2001–2007.

Packer M, et al. Effect of carvedilol on survival in severe chronic heart failure. *N Engl J Med.* 2001;344(22):1651–1658.

results did not provide convincing evidence that β-blockade could either be tolerated or were beneficial in patients with more advanced HF and with more severe symptoms. In fact, the concept that patients with more advanced HF had progressed to a state of "sympathetic dependence" and would be unable to tolerate β-receptor blockade without hemodynamic decompensation was considered to be a real possibility. Results from the Carvedilol Prospective Randomized Cumulative Survival (COPERNICUS) trial, however, established that carvedilol, a nonselective antagonist of the β_1, β_2, and α_1 receptors with additional antioxidant activity, was well tolerated and that it significantly reduced mortality in patients with EF <25% and Class IIIb–IV HF symptoms (see Table 10-7).[36] The increased severity of HF in patients studied in COPERNICUS compared to other trials is apparent from the substantially higher rate of placebo mortality in this study compared to mortality seen in the placebo groups of the CIBIS-II and MERIT-HF trials. Thus, the conclusion reached from the results of this robust database is that there is incontrovertible evidence that when β-blockers are added to an ACE inhibitor, outcomes including mortality and hospitalizations are markedly improved. Moreover, these beneficial effects are present over a wide spectrum of HF patients including those with advanced disease.

How to Use β-Antagonists in Chronic Heart Failure

Despite the fact that clinical evidence clearly demonstrates that select β-blockers reduce morbidity and mortality in patients with HF, registry data indicate that these drugs remain underutilized in the population at risk. The Initiation Management Predischarge process for Assessment of Carvedilol Therapy for Heart Failure (IMPACT-HF) trial confirmed that β-receptor antagonists can be safely initiated in patients hospitalized for HF prior to discharge.[37] Predischarge initiation significantly increased β-blocker utilization when compared to initiation in the ambulatory setting. The criteria for

introduction of a β-blocker are the same as in the outpatient setting. Thus, the drugs can and should be started in all patients with symptomatic HF due to systolic dysfunction as soon as they reach (or are approaching) the euvolemic state in the absence of contraindications such as symptomatic hypotension or bradycardia, active bronchospastic disease, or conduction disease greater then first-degree atrioventricular (AV) block.

Before initiating therapy, we recommend documenting the patients' euvolemic or "dry weight." Patients who do not tolerate the initial dose (see Table 10-6) due to increasing fluid retention, bradycardia (<60 beats/min) or symptomatic hypotension, or SBP <80 mm Hg, can be challenged with half of the initial dose. The dose should be uptitrated approximately every 2 weeks, but some patients will require a longer titration period. It is not uncommon for patients with severe HF to become somewhat more symptomatic before improving. A period of 3–6 months to achieve maximal tolerated or target dose is not uncommon in these severely ill patients. Most patients, however, are easily titrated up to target dose and surprisingly few experience even transient symptoms of worsening HF as catecholamine stimulation of the heart is progressively blocked.

In patients who develop evidence of decompensation secondary to fluid retention, we usually reduce the dose of β-blocker by half and double their diuretic dose for 3 days with careful monitoring of body weight, creatinine, and electrolytes. We then resume uptitration of the β-blocker over the next 2–3 weeks. In rare cases, patients will develop hypotension, fluid retention, and rapid progression of HF during the initiation/uptitration phase. These individuals usually require hospitalization for acute HF exacerbation (see below).

In patients with symptomatic hypotension, it is our practice to treat this side effect using one or more of the following approaches: (1) eliminate other nonessential vasodilators (e.g., calcium channel blockers); (2) alternate the dosing of RAS blockers in the morning with β-receptor blockers in the evening (when once daily formulations of these agents are being used) or, when both drugs are given on a bid regimen, separate the dosing of the agents by 1–2 hours; (3) administer the β-blocker with meals when its absorption (e.g., carvedilol) can be delayed by this approach; (4) consider reducing the diuretic dose if the patient is euvolemic; and (5) temporarily reduce the dose of RAS blockers. Since blood pressure often improves over time with β-blockers, the RAS blockers can often be increased to target dose at a later date. Patients who develop bradycardia should be queried for a history of syncope or presyncope. Asymptomatic patients without AV block and exertional HR >55 require no further intervention. Patients with severe HF and symptomatic bradycardia, or evidence of AV block that limits initiation and/or uptitration of a β-blocker can be considered for a permanent pacemaker.[38]

How to Select a β-Receptor Blocker in Heart Failure

The discordant results of BEST, which showed no benefit of bucindolol therapy, and COPERNICUS that demonstrated a mortality reduction in NYHA Class IIIb–IV patients, support the concept that the benefits of β-blockade should not be considered a class effect.[39] COMET tested this hypothesis in patients with mainly NYHA Functional Class II and III HF.[40] Patients were randomized and titrated to a target dose of 25 mg bid of carvedilol or 50 mg of metoprolol tartrate bid. Treatment with carvedilol conferred a 17% reduction in all-cause death relative to metoprolol tartrate. These data emphasize the importance of selecting only specific agents proven to reduce morbidity and mortality in RCTs. Unlike the results of clinical trials with ACE inhibitors, which indicated that the beneficial effects of these drugs could be considered a "class effect," only three β-receptor antagonists have been shown to reduce mortality in HF patients: carvedilol, metoprolol succinate (e.g., Toprol XL, a longer acting formulation of metoprolol), and bisoprolol. Thus, only these three β-receptor blocking agents should be used in the treatment of patients with symptomatic HF due to LV systolic dysfunction.

ACE Inhibitor or β-Receptor Blocker; Which One to Start First in Heart Failure Patients?

Historically, ACE inhibitors have been the initial neurohormonal agent added to the treatment regimen of HF patients based both on the fact that they were the first approved for clinical practice and that they can acutely improve cardiac function by providing afterload reduction. The latter property being of particular benefit in patients presenting with decompensated HF. In contrast, data supporting the use of β-receptor blockers in stable HF patients are relatively more recent and therefore, in practice, these agents are commonly instituted after the ACE inhibitor. However, clinical trial data indicate that the overall impact of β-blockers on the clinical course may be of greater magnitude than that of the RAS blockers and there is evidence from a small recent study that NYHA Functional Class II–III HF patients with idiopathic dilated cardiomyopathy may actually have better outcomes when initially treated with a β-blocker. In this study, patients receiving digoxin and diuretics were randomized to initial therapy of either carvedilol or perindopril, an ACE inhibitor. After 6 months, the carvedilol group was additionally treated with an ACE inhibitor and the perindopril group was started on carvedilol. A functional assessment at 6 and 12 months favored the group initially receiving carvedilol as these patients tolerated a higher dose of the β-blocker and required a lower dose of diuretic, and experienced significant symptomatic improvement and lower plasma NT-BNP.[40] Although, this small study, in a nonischemic HF population, suggests that initial therapy with a β-receptor blocker might be preferable, this possibility needs to be further evaluated in a larger, more diverse population including patients with an ischemic etiology of their HF.

β-Receptor Blockers in Heart Failure and Post-Acute Myocardial Infarction

Clinical Evidence

Although the long term use of β-receptor antagonists in the post-MI patient has been demonstrated in RCTs to reduce mortality, sudden cardiac death, and reinfarction rate, registry data suggest that these agents are markedly underutilized in this population.[42] This situation appears to be most pronounced in high risk patients with LV dysfunction.[43] This is, at least in part, a consequence of the fact that high risk post-MI patients and/or those with evidence of LVD were generally excluded from the earlier post-MI β-blocker trials. The CAPRICORN trial, however, evaluated the use of β-receptor blockers in patients, with documented LV dysfunction, 3–21 days following AMI.[44] In this study, all-cause mortality was reduced by 23% in patients who were randomized to the carvedilol-treated group. Of note is the fact that this improvement in outcome in the primary endpoint of the trial was seen in the context of contemporary therapy that included aspirin, statins, anticoagulants, revascularization (where deemed appropriate), and ACE inhibitors.

How to Use β-Antagonists in Post-AMI Patient with LV Dysfunction

In the post-MI period, all patients require imaging to evaluate LV function. Patients with reduced LV function should be considered for angiography and revascularization. All patients with depressed LVEF in this setting should receive a β-blocker regardless of the presence or absence of clinical HF. At the time of initiation of therapy, patients should be euvolemic, maintained on a stable dose of oral diuretics, and receiving an RAS blocker. If the initial dose is not tolerated (see Table 10-6) start the drug at half dose. Patients require ambulatory follow-up 7–10 days after hospital discharge and every 2 weeks thereafter as the β-blocker is uptitrated. This is accomplished by doubling the dose unless limited by symptoms of orthostasis, SBP <80, HR <60 or progressive HF.

In the case of bradycardia, discontinue other elective SA and/or AV nodal blocking agents, such as calcium channel blockers (CCB). If the patient is asymptomatic, HR >55 with effort and no evidence of AV nodal disease continue at the current dose and reevaluate in 2–3 weeks. Patients with AV nodal disease and symptomatic

bradycardia should be considered for placement of a permanent pacemaker. In the case of hypotension, confirm adequate peripheral perfusion, evaluate for evidence of excess diuretics, and then consider withdrawing other vasodilators, adjust the timing of ACE inhibitor administration and β-blocker dosing and/or reduce the diuretic dose. If patients remain symptomatic, decrease the β-blocker dose by 50% and reevaluate shortly thereafter. Patients, who experience functional LV recovery, should continue on target therapy or maximal tolerated dose indefinitely.

Treatment of Special Population

Diabetes Mellitus

Diabetic patients are at increased risk of developing HF and, when HF is present, they have an increased risk of death when compared to nondiabetics. An analysis of the diabetic subgroups from CIBIS, COPERNICUS, and MERIT-HF trials demonstrate that β-blocker treatment results in a mortality reduction in both diabetic and nondiabetic patients.[45] Though the relative mortality reduction appeared greater in HF patients without diabetes, given that diabetics have a greater overall risk of death it seems reasonable to conclude that diabetics also receive a substantial benefit from β-blocker therapy.

There have been concerns that β-blockers exacerbate hyperglycemia and worsen other CV risk factors in diabetics. The GEMINI investigators explored the impact of a selective β_1-receptor antagonist, metoprolol versus carvedilol, a nonselective agent with α_1-receptor action and additional antioxidant activity, in high-risk hypertensive diabetic patients without HF.[46] These patients received concurrent treatment with a RAS blocker. The agents were titrated to achieve good hypertensive control and after 5 months of treatment this had been achieved in over two-thirds of patients in both arms of the trial. At this time, however, the HbA_{1c} in the metoprolol group had increased with no significant change in the carvedilol group. Though both agents were well-tolerated, carvedilol was shown at equal antihypertensive doses to have more favorable effects on metabolic parameters such as HbA_{1c}, insulin sensitivity, and microalbuminuria compared to metoprolol.

Reactive Airway Disease

HF patients with comorbid airway disease may have restrictive or obstructive disease or components of both. In our experience, patients who carry a diagnosis of COPD often have little or no reactive airway component so that initiation/uptitration of β-blockers can be carried out without difficulty. Patients with reactive airway disease or who are being acutely treated with steroids should not be initiated on β-receptor antagonist therapy. However, because of the reduction in mortality associated with β-blockers, patients with RAD in whom bronchospasm is well-controlled can be considered for treatment using a selective β_1-receptor antagonist. Given its nonselective activity that includes blockade of the β_2-receptor, we generally avoid the use of carvedilol in the relatively small percentage of HF patients with well-documented RAD. Metoprolol succinate has selective action on the β_1-receptor and is preferred in those patients with stable RAD. Patients with all but the most severe RAD tolerate treatment well and minor exacerbations can be managed in most cases with inhaled β_2-receptor agonists.

Race-Based Therapeutics

The natural history of HF in the African American population is more likely to be a sequela of hypertensive heart disease than in the non-African American population. These patients are also more likely to have comorbid diabetes and LVH. Whether related to this or to other factors this subpopulation has been shown to have worse outcomes. Retrospective analysis of the African American cohort from the U.S. Carvedilol Heart Failure study group did not detect an impact of race on the benefits of therapy.[47] Therefore, β-blockers are recommended as first-line treatment of all HF patients regardless of their race.

Application in Acute Decompensated HF

Patients with acutely decompensated HF already on β-blockers who are maintaining adequate peripheral and organ profusion can be continued on their current regimen or the dose can be reduced transiently to half of their outpatient regimen. This approach, however, does not apply to patients who require inotropes for support due to evidence of hypoperfusion. It is our usual practice to halve or discontinue the β-blocker dose while inotropic agents are being given. When an inotrope is given, we usually use milrinone as opposed to dobutamine since the effects of the latter are more likely to be influenced by the presence of β-blockade. β-blocker naïve patients should not be started on therapy acutely, but should receive their first dose prior to hospital discharge at the time when their clinical course has stabilized and they have achieved or are approaching the euvolemic state.

Aldosterone Blockade in Heart Failure and Post-Acute Myocardial Infarction

Aldosterone secretion, once thought to be solely under the regulation of AngII (via the AT_1-receptor), is now known to be influenced by norepinephrine, adrenocorticotropic hormone, nitric oxide, serum potassium levels, and BK. This RAS-independent secretion is the likely cause of the phenomena of "aldosterone escape," which occurs after reduction of serum ATII levels by RAS inhibition or after interactions between AngII and its receptor have been blocked by an ARB.[48] Aldosterone is secreted not only by the adrenal gland, but also from vascular endothelium, vascular smooth muscle, and other tissue. Aldosterone acts both systemically, on the widely distributed mineralocorticoid receptor and is synthesized locally, acting in a paracrine fashion in the brain, blood vessels, and heart.

Aldosterone acts on the distal nephron in the kidney to promote retention of Na^+ and, simultaneously, secretion of K^+. These effects contribute to fluid overload and also K^+ depletion. The latter is of particular importance in the HF population and/or post-MI population who are already at increased risk of sudden cardiac death and who are often being treated with loop or thiazide diuretics that potentiate K^+ loss. Local aldosterone production, within the heart, is believed to contribute to cardiac myocyte hypertrophy and interstitial fibrosis. An increase in the quantity of fibrous tissue in the heart decreases ventricular compliance and also, by disturbing the homogeneity of electrical conduction, creates a substrate for arrhythmias. In the vasculature, aldosterone contributes to endothelial dysfunction by impairing acetylcholine and NO-mediated vasodilatation. It also increases vascular inflammation by recruiting macrophages and promoting monocyte infiltration of vessel walls. The discovery of "aldosterone escape" following treatment with RAS blockers raised the possibility that direct aldosterone blockade might provide incremental benefits and protection for the HF population.[48]

Aldosterone Blockade in Chronic Heart Failure Patients with LV Dysfunction

The RALES trial evaluated the effects of spironolactone on all-cause mortality in patients with advanced HF symptoms and evidence of systolic dysfunction who were already receiving an ACE inhibitor as background treatment.[49] Patients received spironolactone 25–50 mg qd, or placebo, in addition to contemporary therapy with diuretics (100%), digoxin (~75%), and an ACE inhibitor (~95%). However, β-blockers were used in only ~10% of patients. The trial was terminated early after a 30% relative mortality reduction was reported in patients randomized to spironolactone. There was a 29% relative reduction in sudden cardiac death and 36% reduction in death due to progressive HF. The risk of severe hyperkalemia was low, at 2%, in this carefully monitored group. RALES proved that spironolactone, when added to contemporary therapy in a carefully controlled setting with well-defined follow-up monitoring of renal function and electrolytes, is well-tolerated and provides substantial clinical benefit.

Aldosterone Blockade in Post-Acute Myocardial Infarction Patients with LV Dysfunction

The Eplerenone in Patients with Heart Failure Due to Systolic Dysfunction Complicating Acute Myocardial Infarction (EPHESUS) trial assessed the effects of aldosterone blockade following AMI in patients with LV dysfunction and HF.[50] Patients with symptomatic HF were randomized 3–14 days after the index event to eplerenone, a selective mineralocorticoid receptor blocker, or placebo. Diabetics, a group at high risk for CV events, were enrolled after the index MI with or without symptoms of HF. Eplerenone was added to standard therapy that included diuretics (60%), ACE inhibitor (86%), and β-blocker (75%). Many of these patients were also receiving aspirin (88%) and a statin (47%). Despite the already comprehensive therapy that was being administered to these patients, treatment with eplerenone resulted in significant 15% all-cause and 17% CV mortality reductions. These findings indicate that following AMI, patients with impaired LV function and DM or HF should receive eplerenone to reduce their risk of death and hospitalization for HF. Moreover, the results of EPHESUS indicate that this approach is of incremental benefit even in the setting of background treatment with other neurohormonal blocking agents.

How to Use Aldosterone Blockers in Heart Failure and Post-Acute Myocardial Infarction Patients with LV Dysfunction

The use of aldosterone blockade in patients with HF requires careful monitoring of serum K^+ and renal function. It should only be added once patients are on a stable dose of a diuretic, RAS blocker, and β-receptor blocker. Supplemental K^+ should be reduced or discontinued unless serum K^+ levels fall below the lower limit of the normal range followed up at 1 and 4 weeks following initiation dose of 25 mg. The dose should be cut in half if $K^+ > 5$ mEq/L and discontinued if > 5.5 mEq/L. At 4 weeks, if the eplerenone 25 mg/day is well-tolerated, increase the dose to 50 mg/day.

Adverse Events and Patient Monitoring

Monitoring for Hyperkalemia

In both the RALES and EPHESUS trials, there was a significant increase in the incidence of hyperkalemia in those patients treated with spironolactone or eplerenone compared with patients receiving placebo (2% vs. 1% and 5.5 vs. 3.9%, respectively). Notably, patients receiving placebo in the EPHESUS study were more likely to develop hypokalemia, an equally life-threatening electrolyte imbalance and this risk was significantly ameliorated by treatment with eplerenone. Following the publication of RALES, two groups documented a greater incidence of hyperkalemia and inadequate patient selection in both the community and an academic setting.[51,52] Treating HF with aldosterone blockade has a narrow therapeutic index, requires strict monitoring, and is indicated only in high-risk patients or those with HF, post-MI with depressed LVEF, and/or diabetes. In patients with less severely symptomatic HF or in those whom some time has passed since an MI that resulted in reduced EF, the benefits of aldosterone antagonists is uncertain. In these settings, the potential benefits of treatment should be carefully weighed against the known risks.

Aldosterone antagonists should only be initiated in patients with serum Cr $\leq$2.5 mg/dL or K^+ $\leq$5 mEq/L and on a stable regimen of an ACE inhibitor, β-receptor blocker, and loop diuretic. If the patient is currently receiving K^+ supplementation, cut the dose by one-half. The risk for severe hyperkalemia can be mitigated by close monitoring of serum creatinine and potassium levels. For this purpose we use the "rule of ones" that is, measurement of renal function and serum electrolytes is carried out 1 day prior to and 1 week and 1 month after drug treatment is begun. In monitored patients who later develop Cr >4 mg/dL or K^+ >5.5 mEq/L, stop the medication. The medication should also be stopped during periods of acute illness causing dehydration or renal dysfunction. In more mild cases of hyperkalemia, K^+ 5–5.5 mEq/L, decrease the dose by half or if only tolerating 12.5 mg, change to qd dosing.

Gynecomastia

Spironolactone has activity at the androgen and estrogen receptor, which can result in gynecomastia. In RALES, 9% of male patients were affected by this condition compared to a 1% incidence in the placebo group. Patients who develop gynecomastia on spironolactone should be switched to eplerenone, which has substantially lower affinity for the androgen, progesterone, and estrogen receptors and, which does not increase the likelihood of gynecomastia above that seen with placebo.[50]

▶ REFERENCES

1. The CONSENSUS Trial Study Group. Effects of enalapril on mortality in severe congestive heart failure. Results of the Cooperative North Scandinavian Enalapril Survival Study (CONSENSUS). *N Engl J Med.* 1987;316(23): 1429–1435.

2. The SOLVD Investigators. Effect of enalapril on survival in patients with reduced left ventricular ejection fractions and congestive heart failure. *N Engl J Med.* 1991;325(5): 293–302.

3. The SOLVD Investigators. Effect of enalapril on mortality and the development of heart failure in asymptomatic patients with reduced left ventricular ejection fractions. *N Engl J Med.* 1992;327(10):685–691.

4. Pfeffer MA, The SAVE Investigators, et al. Effect of captopril on mortality and morbidity in patients with left ventricular dysfunction after myocardial infarction. Results of the survival and ventricular enlargement trial. *N Engl J Med.* 1992;327(10):669–677.

5. The Acute Infarction Ramipril Efficacy (AIRE) Study Investigators. Effect of ramipril on mortality and morbidity of survivors of acute myocardial infarction with clinical evidence of heart failure. *Lancet.* 1993;342(8875):821–828.

6. Kober L, et al. A clinical trial of the angiotensin-converting-enzyme inhibitor trandolapril in patients with left ventricular dysfunction after

myocardial infarction. *N Engl J Med.* 1995; 333(25):1670–1676.

7. Ambrosioni E, Borghi C, Magnani B, The Survival of Myocardial Infarction Long-Term Evaluation (SMILE) Study Investigators. The effect of the angiotensin-converting-enzyme inhibitor zofenopril on mortality and morbidity after anterior myocardial infarction. *N Engl J Med.* 1995;332(2):80–85.

8. GISSI-3: effects of lisinopril and transdermal glyceryl trinitrate singly and together on 6-week mortality and ventricular function after acute myocardial infarction. Gruppo Italiano per lo Studio della Sopravvivenza nell'infarto Miocardico. *Lancet.* 1994;343(8906):1115–1122.

9. ISIS-4 (Fourth International Study of Infarct Survival) Collaborative Group. ISIS-4: a randomised factorial trial assessing early oral captopril, oral mononitrate, and intravenous magnesium sulphate in 58,050 patients with suspected acute myocardial infarction. *Lancet.* 1995;345(8951):669–685.

10. Pitt B, et al. Effect of losartan compared with captopril on mortality in patients with symptomatic heart failure: randomised trial—the Losartan Heart Failure Survival Study ELITE II. *Lancet.* 2000;355(9215):1582–1587.

11. Granger CB, et al. Effects of candesartan in patients with chronic heart failure and reduced left-ventricular systolic function intolerant to angiotensin-converting-enzyme inhibitors: the CHARM-Alternative trial. *Lancet.* 2003; 362(9386):772–776.

12. Cohn JN, Tognoni G. A randomized trial of the angiotensin-receptor blocker valsartan in chronic heart failure. *N Engl J Med.* 2001; 345(23):1667–1675.

13. McMurray JJ, Ostergren J, Swedberg K, et al. Effects of candesartan in patients with chronic heart failure and reduced left-ventricular systolic function taking angiotensin-converting-enzyme inhibitors: the CHARM-Added trial. *Lancet.* 2003;362(9386):767–771.

14. Dickstein K, Kjekshus J. Effects of losartan and captopril on mortality and morbidity in high-risk patients after acute myocardial infarction: the OPTI-MAAL randomised trial. Optimal Trial in Myocardial Infarction with Angiotensin II Antagonist Losartan. *Lancet.* 2002;360(9335):752–760.

15. Pfeffer MA, et al. Valsartan, captopril, or both in myocardial infarction complicated by heart failure, left ventricular dysfunction, or both. *N Engl J Med.* 2003;349(20):1893–1906.

16. The Consensus Committee of the American Autonomic Society and the American Academy of Neurology. *Consensus statement on the definition of orthostatic hypotension, pure autonomic failure, and multiple system atrophy. Neurology.* 1996;46(5):1470.

17. Israili ZH, Hall WD. Cough and angioneurotic edema associated with angiotensin-converting enzyme inhibitor therapy: a review of the literature and pathophysiology. *Ann Intern Med.* 1992;117(3):234–242.

18. Sondhi D, Lippman M, Murali G. Airway compromise due to angiotensin-converting enzyme inhibitor-induced angioedema: clinical experience at a large community teaching hospital. *Chest.* 2004;126(2):400–404.

19. Shotan A, Widerhorn J, Hurst A, et al. Risks of angiotensin-converting enzyme inhibition during pregnancy: experimental and clinical evidence, potential mechanisms, and recommendations for use. *Am J Med.* 1994;96(5):451–456.

20. Al-Khadra AS, et al. Antiplatelet agents and survival: a cohort analysis from the Studies of Left Ventricular Dysfunction (SOLVD) trial. *J Am Coll Cardiol.* 1998;31(2):419–425.

21. Teo KK, et al. Effects of long-term treatment with angiotensin-converting-enzyme inhibitors in the presence or absence of aspirin: a systematic review. *Lancet.* 2002;360(9339):1037–1043.

22. Smooke S, Horwich TB, Fonarow GC. Insulin-treated diabetes is associated with a marked increase in mortality in patients with advanced heart failure. *Am Heart J.* 2005;149(1):168–174.

23. Lewis EJ, The Collaborative Study Group. The effect of angiotensin-converting-enzyme inhibition on diabetic nephropathy. *N Engl J Med.* 1993;329(20):1456–1462.

24. Brenner BM, et al. Effects of losartan on renal and cardiovascular outcomes in patients with type 2 diabetes and nephropathy. *N Engl J Med.* 2001;345(12):861–869.

25. Lewis EJ, Hunsicker LG, Rodby RA. A clinical trial in type 2 diabetic nephropathy. *Am J Kidney Dis.* 2001;38(4 Suppl 1):S191–S194.

26. Yusuf S, The Heart Outcomes Prevention Evaluation Study Investigators. Effects of an angiotensin-converting-enzyme inhibitor, ramipril, on cardiovascular events in high-risk patients. *N Engl J Med.* 2000;342(3):145–153.

27. Prevention Evaluation Study Investigators. Effects of ramipril on cardiovascular and microvas-cular outcomes in people with diabetes mellitus: results of the HOPE study and MICRO-HOPE substudy. Heart Outcomes. *Lancet.* 2000; 355(9200):253–259.

28. Gustafsson I, et al. Effect of the angiotensin-converting enzyme inhibitor trandolapril on mortality and morbidity in diabetic patients with left ventricular dysfunction after acute myocardial infarction. *J Am Coll Cardiol.* 1999;34(1):83–89.

29. Yusuf S, et al. Effects of candesartan in patients with chronic heart failure and preserved left-ventricular ejection fraction: the CHARM-Preserved Trial. *Lancet.* 2003;362(9386):777–781.

30. Carson P, Massie BM, Mekelvie R, et al. The irbesartan in heart failure with preserved systolic function (I-PRESERVE) trial: ratinale and design *J Cald Fail.* 2005;11;576–585.

31. Cohn J, et al. A comparison of enalapril with hydralazine-isosorbide dinitrate in the treatment of chronic congestive heart failure. *N Engl J Med.* 1991;325(5):303–310.

32. Dries DL, et al. Efficacy of angiotensin-converting enzyme inhibition in reducing progression from asymptomatic left ventricular dysfunction to symptomatic heart failure in black and white patients. *J Am Coll Cardiol.* 2002;40(2):311–317.

33. Packer M, et al. The effect of carvedilol on morbidity and mortality in patients with chronic heart failure. *N Engl J Med.* 1996;334(21): 1349–1355.

34. The Cardiac Insufficiency Bisoprolol Study II (CIBIS-II): a randomised trial. *Lancet.* 1999; 353(9146):9–13.

35. Effect of metoprolol CR/XL in chronic heart failure: Metoprolol CR/XL Randomised Intervention Trial in Congestive Heart Failure (MERIT-HF). *Lancet.* 1999;353(9169):2001–2007.

36. Packer M, et al. Effect of carvedilol on survival in severe chronic heart failure. *N Engl J Med.* 2001;344(22):1651–1658.

37. Gattis WA, et al. Predischarge initiation of carvedilol in patients hospitalized for decompensated heart failure: results of the Initiation Management Predischarge: Process for Assessment of Carvedilol Therapy in Heart Failure (IMPACT-HF) trial. *J Am Coll Cardiol.* 2004;43(9): 1534–1541.

38. Gregoratos G, et al. ACC/AHA/NASPE 2002 guideline update for implantation of cardiac pacemakers and antiarrhythmia devices: summary article: a report of the American College of Cardiology/American Heart Association Task Force on Practice Guidelines (ACC/ AHA/NASPE Committee to Update the 1998 Pacemaker Guidelines). *Circulation.* 2002;106(16): 2145–2161.

39. A trial of the beta-blocker bucindolol in patients with advanced chronic heart failure. *N Engl J Med.* 2001;344(22):1659–1667.

40. Poole-Wilson PA, et al. Comparison of carvedilol and metoprolol on clinical outcomes in patients with chronic heart failure in the Carvedilol Or Metoprolol European Trial (COMET): randomised controlled trial. *Lancet.* 2003;362(9377):7–13.

41. Sliwa K, et al. Impact of initiating carvedilol before angiotensin-converting enzyme inhibitor therapy on cardiac function in newly diagnosed heart failure. *J Am Coll Cardiol.* 2004;44(9):1825–1830.

42. Antman EM, et al. ACC/AHA guidelines for the management of patients with ST-elevation myocardial infarction: a report of the American College of Cardiology/American Heart Association Task Force on practice guidelines (committee to revise the 1999 guidelines for the management of patients with acute myocardial infarction). *J Am Coll Cardiol.* 2004;44(3):E1–E211.

43. Gottlieb SS, McCarter RJ, Vogel RA. Effect of beta-blockade on mortality among high-risk and low-risk patients after myocardial infarction. *N Engl J Med.* 1998;339(8):489–497.

44. Dargie HJ. Effect of carvedilol on outcome after myocardial infarction in patients with left-ventricular dysfunction: the CAPRICORN randomised trial. *Lancet.* 2001;357(9266):1385–1390.

45. Shekelle PG, et al. Efficacy of angiotensin-converting enzyme inhibitors and beta-blockers in the management of left ventricular systolic dysfunction according to race, gender, and diabetic status: a meta-analysis of major clinical trials. *J Am Coll Cardiol.* 2003;41(9):1529–1538.

46. Bakris GL, et al. Metabolic effects of carvedilol vs metoprolol in patients with type 2 diabetes mellitus and hypertension: a randomized controlled trial. *JAMA.* 2004;292(18):2227–2236.

47. Yancy CW, et al. Race and the response to adrenergic blockade with carvedilol in patients with chronic heart failure. *N Engl J Med.* 2001; 344(18):1358–1365.

48. McKelvie RS, The RESOLVD Pilot Study Investigators, et al. Comparison of candesartan, enalapril, and their combination in congestive

heart failure: Randomized Evaluation of Strategies for Left Ventricular Dysfunction (RESOLVD) Pilot Study. *Circulation*. 1999; 100(10):1056–1064.

49. Pitt B, et al. The effect of spironolactone on morbidity and mortality in patients with severe heart failure. *N Engl J Med*. 1999;341(10):709–717.

50. Pitt B, et al. Eplerenone, a selective aldosterone blocker, in patients with left ventricular dysfunction after myocardial infarction. *N Engl J Med*. 2003;348(14):1309–1321.

51. Bozkurt B, Agoston I, Knowlton AA. Complications of inappropriate use of spironolactone in heart failure: when an old medicine spirals out of new guidelines. *J Am Coll Cardiol*. 2003;41(2):211–214.

52. Juurlink DN, et al. Rates of Hyperkalemia after Publication of the Randomized Aldactone Evaluation Study. *N Engl J Med*. 2004;351(6): 543–551.

CHAPTER 11

Is There Still a Role for Digitalis in Heart Failure?

JOSEPH S. ROSSI, MD/MIHAI GHEORGHIADE, MD

▶ INTRODUCTION

Digitalis preparations have been a common remedy in the treatment of heart disease for centuries. Oral digoxin first became available in the twentieth century, and a large amount of data from clinical trials has demonstrated it to be both safe and effective in the treatment of symptomatic heart failure (HF) with or without atrial fibrillation. Due to its wide availability and lack of patent protection, it did not have extensive support from the pharmaceutical industry, but modern clinical trial data led to its approval by the U.S. Food and Drug Administration in 1999 for use in chronic HF, and recommendations for its use by the American College of Cardiology and American Heart Association (ACC/AHA) as well as the Heart Failure Society of America (HFSA) followed soon after.[1,2] However, the role of digoxin therapy has recently been challenged after its use was associated with increased mortality in women.[3] In addition, its worth has not been studied in the presence of modern therapy with β-blockers and aldosterone antagonists. Accordingly, the new ACC/AHA guidelines no longer recommend digoxin as routine therapy for patients with chronic HF and systolic dysfunction who are in sinus rhythm.[4]

▶ BACKGROUND

The beneficial effects of digitalis preparations have been recognized for centuries, however, they were not formally introduced to the allopathic community until 1785 when first described by Sir William Withering, an English botanist and physician, in his textbook describing the medical uses of foxglove.[5] Withering described the ability of digitalis to cause diuresis and slow the heart rate of patients with irregular pulse. Beginning in the twentieth century, many studies in animals and humans demonstrated positive inotropic properties of digitalis in normal as well as failing myocardium.

In the late 1970s, the use of digoxin was challenged when several nonrandomized studies in patients with HF in normal sinus rhythm (many of which did not assess left ventricular [LV] function) failed to show clinical benefit. In addition, there was a high incidence of digoxin intoxication that was associated with a mortality as high as 40%.[6] These findings led to a decreased emphasis on its use, and newer therapies that included potent diuretics, vasodilators, and new inotropic agents were developed that provided clinicians with important alternative therapies in a growing population of HF patients.

In the 1990s, interest was renewed when (1) newer inotropic agents were found to worsen survival, (2) randomized studies demonstrated clinical benefits of digoxin in combination with diuretics and ACE inhibitors, and (3) lower incidences of digoxin toxicity were demonstrated due to increased recognition of drug interactions, lower dosing, and the monitoring of serum digoxin concentration (SDC). The safety and clinical benefits of digoxin gained widespread acceptance after the publication of the Digitalis Investigation Group (DIG) trial in 1996, when digoxin was shown to significantly decrease hospitalizations and improve symptoms in patients with congestive heart failure (CHF). These results led to strong recommendations for its use by both the ACC/AHA in 2001 and the HFSA in 1999 (Table 11-1).

In the last decade, several landmark studies demonstrating significant mortality benefits of β-blockers and aldosterone antagonists in patients with chronic heart failure have been published. The interest in digoxin faded when these new treatments became widely available. However, background digoxin therapy ranged from 51% to 90% in these clinical trials, leading to speculation about the usefulness of these drugs in the absence of digoxin therapy.[7-10] Digoxin was further challenged by a post-hoc analysis of the DIG trial that reported an increased mortality in women, a finding that has been recently disputed.[3]

Mechanisms of Action

For decades, physicians have debated the exact mechanism by which digitalis increases cardiac

▶ **Table 11-1** Effects of digitalis in systolic heart failure at therapeutic concentrations

Hemodynamic effects:
Increases CO and decreases PCWP and systemic vascular resistance
   At rest
   During exercise
   Alone or in combination with ACE inhibitors or systemic vasodilators
   During chronic therapy
Increases left ventricular ejection fraction

Neurohormonal effects:
Vagomimetic action
Improves baroreceptor sensitivity
Decreases norepinephrine serum concentration
Decreases activation of renin-angiotensin system
May directly increase aldosterone release
Directs sympathoinhibitory effect
At high doses, increases sympathetic CNS outflow
Decreases cytokine concentrations
Increases release ANP and BNP

Electrophysiologic effects:
SA node: decreases automaticity, severe sinoatrial block in patients with sinus node disease
Atrium: no effect or decreases refractory period
AV node: decreases conduction velocity; increases effective refractory period; advanced heart block
   in patients with AV node disease; increases antegrade conduction in accessory AV pathways
Ventricle: no effect; at higher doses or during ischemia

Cholinergic and antiadrenergic effects.
CO—cardiac output; PCWP—pulmonary capillary wedge pressure; ACE—angiotensin-converting enzyme; CNS—central
   nervous system; ANP—atrial natriuretic polypeptide; BNP—brain natriuretic peptide; SA—sinoatrial; AV—atrioventricular.
Source: Adapted from Eichhorn EJ, Gheorghiade M. Digoxin. *Prog in Card Dis.* 2002; 44:251–256, with permission from
   Elsevier.

performance. Basic science studies have demonstrated a clear affinity of the digitalis molecule for the potassium (K^+) receptor of the sodium-potassium adenosine triphosphatase (ATPase). It is through this action that digitalis inhibits the enzyme, resulting in increased levels of intracellular Na. This results in increased transmembrane sodium-calcium (Na-Ca) exchange, increasing intracellular Ca levels, and improving myocardial contractility.[11] This mechanism is also thought to account (at least in part) for the neurohormonal effects of digitalis by increasing baroreceptor sensitivity.[12]

Neuroendocrine Effects

HF causes neurohormonal activation, many phases of which are countered by digitalis and may explain its long-term beneficial effect in this population. These include the following: (1) Baroreceptor function: In patients with CHF, the failure of the carotid sinus to respond properly may lead to stimulation of the sympathetic nervous system, which will increase the production of plasma renin and vasopressin. In low-output HF models, this decrease in baroreceptor function improves with digoxin administration.[12] (2) Vagomimetic effect: At therapeutic doses, digitalis increases vagal tone, resulting in decreased sinoatrial (SA) and atrioventricular (AV) conduction.[13] (3) Direct sympathoinhibitory effect: It is mediated by direct inhibition of sympathetic nerve discharge.[14] This effect is, if independent of the increase in cardiac performance, produced by digoxin, and is not seen in the administration of other medications that increase cardiac output (e.g., dobutamine).

(4) Effect on circulating neurohormones: Therapeutic doses of digoxin decrease plasma renin activity and circulating norepinephrine levels.[15] In the Dutch Ibopamine Multicenter Trial (DIMT), digoxin therapy was associated with a decreased concentration of plasma norepinephrine over a 6-month period. (5) Antifibrotic effects: Aldosterone stimulation of the sodium pump may lead to perivascular fibrosis, which is inhibited experimentally by digoxin.[16]

Electrophysiological Effects

Administration of nontoxic doses of digoxin slows sinus rate by its parasympathomimetic action. This effect prolongs the refractory period of the AV node. Toxic doses predispose atrial fibers to automatic impulse initiation that does not depend on the autonomic nervous system, high-grade AV block that is mediated by cholinergic mechanisms, and an increase in the rate of spontaneous diastolic depolarization leading to the occurrence of rapid spontaneous rhythms of Purkinje fibers. Although it is clear that digitalis intoxication may produce lethal ventricular arrhythmias, therapeutic doses of digoxin do not appear to increase arrhythmias in the absence of ischemia.[17]

Hemodynamic Effects

Digitalis administration does not alter cardiac output in normal subjects, although it does cause significant increase in contractility. This lack of effect on cardiac output is likely due to an increase in systemic vascular resistance produced by digitalis that prevents the increase in contractility from translating into increased forward flow. In patients with reduced systolic function and abnormal central hemodynamics who are in sinus rhythm, digoxin improves LV performance and reduces pulmonary capillary wedge pressure while increasing cardiac output both at rest and during exercise.[18] These beneficial hemodynamic effects are potentiated in the presence of ACE inhibitors and other afterload-reducing agents. In HF, when hemodynamics are normalized first with diuretics and vasodilators, no further improvement in wedge pressure or cardiac output is achieved after acute administration of digoxin.[19] The improvement in hemodynamics persists during chronic therapy due to lack of downregulation of the Na-K-ATPase sites (putative digoxin receptor).

▶ METABOLISM

Digoxin has excellent oral bioavailability, with approximately 80% of the dose being absorbed within 3 hours after ingestion from the distal small bowel and colon. It can be partially inactivated by colonic bacteria, and therefore antibiotic use that depletes enteric flora may increase the amount of active drug that enters the circulation. More than 80% of the active drug is excreted unchanged in the urine. The combination of limited metabolism and relatively large volume of distribution results in a relatively prolonged half-life of 36–48 hours. Steady state serum concentrations therefore generally occur within 7 days after initiation of oral therapy. Digitalis is not removed by dialysis or exchange transfusion.

▶ DRUG INTERACTIONS

Of commonly prescribed medications used to treat cardiovascular illness, it is likely that only warfarin surpasses digoxin in concern regarding dosing and drug interactions (Table 11-2). In particular, many common medications used to treat cardiovascular disease complicate digoxin dosing. Propafenone and verapamil cause decreased renal reabsorption and therefore increase SDC.[20,21] Quinidine therapy decreases nonrenal clearance of digoxin.[22] Amiodarone, spironolactone, and flecainide all have been shown to increase SDC by unknown mechanisms.[23–25] Non-potassium-sparing diuretics could be a major contributing factor to digoxin toxicity by causing hypokalemia.

▶ **Table 11-2** Drug interactions with digoxin

Drug	Mechanism of action	Effects
Non-potassium-sparing diuretics	Hypokalemia, hypomagnesemia, promotes sodium pump inhibition	Increase in the risk of arrhythmias
Intravenous calcium	Increases myocyte calcium	Increase in the risk of arrhythmias
Quinidine, verapamil, amiodarone, propafenone, itraconazole, alprazolam, spironolactone	Reduction in digoxin clearance and decrease in volume of distribution	Increase in serum digoxin concentration
Erythromycin, clarithromycin, tetracycline	Increase digoxin absorption by inactivating intestinal bacterial metabolism	Increase in serum digoxin concentration
Propantheline, diphenoxylate	Increase digoxin absorption by decreasing gut motility	Increase in serum digoxin concentration
Antiacids, anticancer drugs, bran, cholestyramine, kaolin-pectin, metoclopramide, neomyocin, sulfasalazine	Decrease digoxin absorption	Decrease serum digoxin concentration
Rifampin	Increases nonrenal clearance of digoxin	Decreases serum digoxin concentration
Thyroid medications	Increase metabolic state	Decrease serum digoxin concentration
Sympathomimetics	Increase automaticity	Increase the risk of arrhythmias
Succinylcholine	Extrusion of potassium from cells	Increases the risk of arrhythmias
β-adrenergic blockers, nondihydropyridines, calcium channel blockers, flecainide, disopyramide, bepridil	Decrease sinoatrial or atrioventricular node conduction	Increase the risk of sinoatrial and atrioventricular block
ACE inhibitors	May decrease renal function	Increase serum digoxin concentratio
Nonsteroidal anti-inflammatory agents	Decrease renal function	Increase serum digoxin concentration

ACE—angiotensin-converting enzyme
Source: Adapted from Eichhorn EJ, Gheorghiade M. Digoxin. *Prog in Card Dis.* 2002; 44:254–256, with permission from Elsevier.

▶ **ELECTROLYTES**

Electrolyte disorders commonly accompany and/or potentiate the toxic effects of digitalis. Serum potassium levels should be monitored periodically, as most of the effects of digitalis are through its interaction with the K$^+$ site on the Na-K-ATPase enzyme. Decreased serum K$^+$ levels result in the potentiation of the effects of digitalis, potentially leading to ventricular tachycardia or ventricular fibrillation. Similar effects have been observed with hypomagnesemia. In the presence of hyperkalemia, the autonomic effects of digitalis predominate, resulting in decreased AV nodal and SA conduction, leading to heart block or significant bradycardia. Digitalis toxicity itself can also worsen hyperkalemia and lead to ventricular fibrillation. Hypercalcemia or administration of intravenous calcium may lead to life-threatening arrhythmias or other manifestations of digoxin toxicity even in the setting of normal SDC.

▶ DIGOXIN INTOXICATION

Increased serum digitalis concentrations can lead to intoxication, a clinical diagnosis, which can cause a multitude of symptoms, the most concerning of which are the electrophysiological effects, which can lead to life-threatening arrhythmias by mechanisms described previously. The overall incidence of digoxin toxicity is <1% per patient-year, down from 35% in 1971.[6] The commonly described "digitalis effect" on 12-lead electrocardiogram (ECG) should be distinguished from true intoxication. It is commonly manifested by sagging of the ST segments, can occur at normal SDC, and requires no treatment. *Digitalis excess* is defined as the presence of significant ECG changes such as heart block and/or mild clinical symptoms such as nausea or fatigue. Proper treatment includes holding digoxin therapy with close monitoring of electrolytes. True "digitalis intoxication" is a relatively rare occurrence manifested by life-threatening arrhythmias and severe gastrointestinal and neurological symptoms (Table 11-3). It is best treated with antidigoxin antibodies.[26] The results of prospective trials with adults and children have established the effectiveness and safety of antidigoxin antigen binding fragments (Fab) in treating cases of life-threatening digoxin intoxication, including cases of massive ingestion of the drug with suicidal intent (*digoxin overdose*). Although hemodialysis does not remove digoxin from the body, it can often be useful in cases where hyperkalemia is also present.

▶ DIGOXIN IN HEART FAILURE WITH REDUCED SYSTOLIC FUNCTION

In several studies, digoxin withdrawal in patients with systolic dysfunction and sinus rhythm was associated with a decrease in left ventricular (LV) ejection fraction (EF) and exercise tolerance and an increase in resting heart rate, diastolic pressure, body weight, and/or cardiac size on chest x-ray. The majority of double-blind trials examining the effect of digoxin in patients with HF and systolic dysfunction have noted an improvement in clinical status. Although there has been little evidence that digoxin therapy improves survival, the majority of published data consistently describe a variety of clinical benefits.

The body of clinical research establishing the role of digoxin therapy in HF took place in three distinct phases. Initially, observational studies of digoxin withdrawal were performed in patients with chronic heart failure in normal sinus rhythm. Subsequently, placebo-controlled trials were conducted examining withdrawal of digoxin therapy in patients receiving stable background therapy of diuretics with and without ACE inhibitors. Some of these studies also compared the effects of digoxin withdrawal in patients receiving other oral inotropic agents. Data from the Prospective Randomized Study of Ventricular Failure and the Efficacy of Digitalis (PROVED) and the Randomized Assessment of Digitalis on Inhibitors of the Angiotensin Converting Enzyme (RADIANCE) study provided solid evidence that digoxin therapy improved symptoms and decreased hospitalizations in patients with chronic heart failure.[27,28] None, however, addressed the issue of mortality or survival, nor the effects of de novo digoxin therapy in HF. This was the rationale for conducting the DIG trial, a large randomized clinical trial designed to assess the mortality benefit of digoxin therapy for HF patients in normal sinus rhythm who were already receiving angiotensin-converting enzyme (ACE) inhibitors and diuretics (Table 11-4).[29]

Early Randomized Studies

In a multicenter, double-blind, placebo-controlled study conducted by the Captopril-Digoxin Multicenter Research Group, digoxin was compared to captopril and placebo in a population

▶ **Table 11-3** Manifestations of digoxin intoxication

- Cardiac disturbances
- Arrhythmias due to increased automaticity
  - Premature ventricular depolarization
  - Accelerated junctional (nodal) rhythm
  - Unifocal or multifocal ventricular bigeminy
  - Ventricular tachycardia
  - Ventricular fibrillation
  - Bidirectional ventricular tachycardia
- Arrhythmias due to decreased conduction velocity and ERP
  - Asystole
  - Sinoatrial block
  - First or second (Wenckebach) AV block, advanced or complete heart block
  - Acceleration or conduction via accessory pathway in WPW
  - Multifocal or paroxysmal atrial tachycardia with block
  - Idioventricular rhythm; AV dissociation
- Gastrointestinal symptoms
  - Anorexia
  - Nausea
  - Vomiting
  - Diarrhea
  - Abdominal pain
  - Intestinal ischemia/infarction
- Central nervous system
  - Visual disturbances (blurred or yellow vision)
  - Headache
  - Weakness
  - Dizziness
  - Apathy
  - Contusion
  - Mental disturbances (anxiety, depression, delirium, hallucination)
- Other
  - Gynecomastia (especially with spironolactone)
  - Thrombocytopenia
  - Severe hyperkalemia

ERP—effective refractory period; WPW—Wolfe–Parkinson-White syndrome; AV—atrioventricular
Source: Adapted from Eichhorn EJ, Gheorghiade M. Digoxin. *Prog in Card Dis.* 2002; 44:251–256, with permission from Elsevier.

of 300 patients with mild to moderate HF.[30] Patients were randomized to captopril (target dose 50 mg tid), digoxin (target serum level 0.9–3.2 nmol/L), or placebo for 6 months. In the prerandomization phase of the study, only patients who did not deteriorate when digoxin was discontinued were randomized. Despite this initial bias against digoxin, the results for the digoxin group show fewer hospitalizations and emergency room visits for HF, a better EF, and a decrease in diuretic requirements compared to patients randomized to placebo. Except for the changes in EF, similar benefits were also noted in the patients treated with captopril.

▶ Table 11-4 Randomized placebo-controlled studies of digoxin in heart failure

Reference	Study design	Duration (weeks)	No. of patients	FC (NYHA)	EF (%)	Digoxin concentration (ng/mL)	Concomitant therapy (%)		ExT↑	Worsening of HF (%)		Mortality (%)	
							D	V		Dig	P	Dig	P
Dobbs et al., 1977	CO	6	46	NA	NA	1.3	60	0	NA	0	34*	0	0
Lee et al., 1982	CO	9	35	II–III	29	1.15	88	24	NA	24	56*	0	0
Fleg et al., 1982	CO	12	40	II–III	23(FS)	1.4	77	17	NS	10	10	0	0
Taggart et al., 1983	CO	12	22	I–II	NA	0.8	96	36	NA	10	18	0	5
Captopril-Digoxin, 1988	PA	24	196	II–III	25	0.7	86	0	No	15	29*	7	6
Guyatt et al., 1988	CO	7	28	II–III	19(FS)	1.37	90	55	Yes†	0	35*	0	0
German/Austrian Xamoterol, 1988	PA	12	213	I–III	NA	0.9	25	10	No	4	6	0	1
Haerer et al., 1988	PA	3	28	I–III	25(FS)	1.8	0	0	Yes*	14	36	0	0
Milrinone Multicenter Trial, 1989	PA	12	111	II–III	25	1.2	100	48	Yes	15	47*	5	6
Pugh et al., 1989	CO	8	44	NA	27(FS)	1.4	75	9	NA	7	25*	0	0
Fleg et al., 1991	CO	4	10	II–III	33	1.4	100	50	NS	0	0	0	0
Drexler et al., 1992	PA	104	133	II–III	50	NA	9	8	Yes†	9	9	2	2.5
DIMT, 1993	PA	26	108	II–III	26	0.94	0	56	Yes*	0	4	4	6
PROVED, 1993	PA	12	88	II–III	27	1.2	100	0	Yes*	19	39*	2	4
RADIANCE, 1993	PA	12	178	II–III	26	1.2	100	100§	Yes*	7	25*	3.5	1
DIG Trial, 1997	PA	148	6800	I–IV	29	0.9	82	95§	NA	25	34‡	35	35

*P<0.05
†Trend
‡Hospitalization for heart failure
§Angiotensin-converting enzyme inhibitors

EF—ejection fraction; ExT—exercise tolerance; FC—functional class; FS—fractional shortening on echocardiogram; P—placebo; Dig—digoxin; HF—heart failure; NYHA—New York Heart Association; CO—crossover; V—vasodilator; PA—parallel; NA—not available; NS—not significant

Source: Adapted from Eichhorn EJ, Gheorghiade M. Digoxin. *Prog in Card Dis.* 2002; 44:251–256, with permission from Elsevier.

However, digoxin had no effect on the New York Heart Association (NYHA) class or exercise capacity. This study was not powered to assess a mortality difference between groups but demonstrated the effectiveness of digoxin therapy in treating the signs and symptoms of HF in patients receiving optimal doses of diuretic therapy.

As intravenous and oral inotropic agents began to emerge as possible therapies for HF, investigators sought to compare these new therapies to digoxin, the only established oral inotropic therapy available at the time. In a 12-week study randomizing patients to milrinone, digoxin, combination therapy, or placebo, a combination of milrinone and digoxin was found to be equivalent to digoxin alone for improvement in exercise tolerance. Digoxin was superior to placebo and milrinone alone in improvement of exercise tolerance.[31] Patients randomized to digoxin required fewer cointerventions, defined as additional therapy to control symptoms of HF, than those taking placebo. A trial of oral ibopamine, another oral inotropic therapy, likewise failed to demonstrate an advantage over oral digoxin therapy.[32] Both studies confirmed earlier data that digoxin therapy significantly improved exercise tolerance and decreased the frequency of worsening HF compared to placebo.

Prospective Randomized Study of Ventricular Failure and the Efficacy of Digitalis (PROVED) and Randomized Assessment of Digitalis on Inhibitors of the Angiotensin Converting Enzyme (RADIANCE)

The PROVED investigators conducted a randomized, placebo-controlled trial of digoxin withdrawal after a 12-week stabilization period in which all patients received digoxin. Patients received background therapy of diuretics only. A total of 88 patients were randomized. Patients withdrawn from digoxin therapy after 12 weeks of stabilization showed worsened maximal exercise capacity (median change in exercise

time -96 s) compared to those who continued therapy. Patients who received digoxin had a lower body weight and heart rate compared to those who received placebo. There was a two-fold increase in the incidence of worsening HF in patients taking placebo.[27]

Designed as a companion trial to PROVED, RADIANCE was a similarly designed digoxin withdrawal study on the background of ACE inhibitor (captopril or enalapril) and diuretic therapy. All patients had clinical evidence NYHA Class II–III HF, an EF <35%, and LV end-diastolic dimension >60 mm by echocardiography. Exercise testing was performed at baseline and at follow-up intervals and was measured with simple treadmill walk time, and 178 patients were randomized after the stabilization period. Despite the fact that all patients received background ACE inhibitor and diuretics, the investigators found a six-fold increase in worsening HF in the withdrawal group (after a stabilization period as in PROVED) and significant decrease in cardiac performance as measured by decrease in EF and increased heart rate. In addition, body weight was significantly reduced in the digoxin group. Most striking were the data indicating significantly improved quality of life scores in patients who were maintained on digoxin therapy.

Several post-hoc analyses of the PROVED and RADIANCE data have been published. Triple therapy with ACE inhibitors, diuretics, and digoxin was associated with the best outcomes and patients with mild symptoms (NYHA Class II) also benefited from therapy (Fig. 11-1, Table 11-5). The clinical deterioration rate was 5% in patients receiving triple therapy, compared to 30% in patients receiving diuretics alone.[33] In a cost-benefit analysis, one study concluded that digitalis therapy has a 90% likelihood of saving the health-care system between $106 million to $822 million annually.[34] These figures were based on combined data of the two trials, and had the patients in the PROVED study been taking ACE inhibitor therapy, the figures may have been even more robust.

By the time PROVED and RADIANCE were published, ACE inhibitor therapy had become

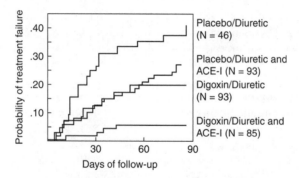

Figure 11-1   Probability of treatment failure in PROVED and RADIANCE: improved outcomes with "triple therapy." ACE-I—angiotensin-converting enzyme inhibitor. (Adapted from Young J, Gheorghiade M, Uretsky B, et al. Superiority of "triple" drug therapy in heart failure: insights from PROVED and RADIANCE trials. *J Am Coll Cardiol.* 1998;3:686–92.)

the standard of care for patients with chronic systolic HF, and it was time for a large randomized study examining the use of digoxin with background ACE inhibitor therapy. Because PROVED and RADIANCE were designed to study digoxin withdrawal, they did not address the impact of de novo digoxin therapy in patients with HF, and they did not include patients with normal systolic function. In addition, these studies were underpowered to study any mortality difference between the groups. The DIG trial was designed to answer these important questions.

▶ **Table 11-5**   PROVED and RADIANCE primary and secondary endpoints

Variable	PROVED study digoxin effects	RADIANCE study digoxin effects
Primary endpoints		
Treadmill time	Improve	Improve
6-minute walk	No change	Improve
Incidence of treatment failure	Improve	Improve
Time to treatment failure	Improve	Improve
Secondary endpoints		
Change in signs and symptoms of CHF	No change	Improve
Quality of life (Minnesota Living with Heart Failure Questionnaire)	No change	Improve
CHF score	No change	Improve
Global evaluation of progress	No change	Improve
LVEF	Improve	Improve
HR and BP	Improve	Improve
Body weight	Improve	Improve

CHF—congestive heart failure; LVEF—left ventricular ejection fraction; HR—heart rate; BP—blood pressure
Source: Adapted from Eichhorn EJ, Gheorghiade M. Digoxin. *Prog in Card Dis.* 2002;44:251–256, with permission from Elsevier.

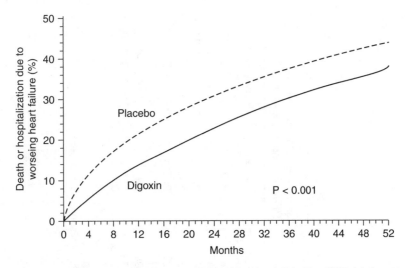

Figure 11-2   Cumulative incidence of the combined endpoint in the DIG trial. (Adapted with permission from the Digitalis Investigation Group (DIG) Trial. The effect of digitalis on mortality and morbidity in patients with heart failure. *N Engl J Med.* 1997;336:525–533.)

The Digitalis Investigation Group Trial

In the largest placebo-controlled trial of digoxin therapy ever conducted, 7788 patients with EF <45% received 0.25 mg of digitalis or placebo. The trial was specifically designed to assess mortality differences between the two groups and the effect of de novo digoxin therapy. Investigators also sought to validate an existing formula for the estimation of SDC. Other important questions were the effect of LVEF, NHYA functional class, and cardiothoracic ratio on clinical outcomes of digoxin therapy. All patients were maintained on background CHF therapy of ACE inhibitors and diuretics as needed. Approximately one-half of patients entering the trial were already taking digitalis prior to randomization.

At 37 months' mean follow-up, there was no difference in mortality between digitalis and placebo. The overall cardiovascular mortality was approximately 30%. However, there was a significant reduction in the primary endpoint of combined death or hospitalization for worsening HF in patients receiving digoxin therapy. Therapy was associated with a 28% reduction in the risk of at least one hospitalization for recurrent HF and a

6.5% reduction in total hospitalizations compared to placebo. Analysis of the mortality data indicates a reduction in death for worsening HF was offset by death from other causes, which many have presumed to be sudden death from arrhythmias related to digoxin toxicity. In addition, investigators determined that SDC could be reliably estimated in patients with normal serum creatinine (Table 11-6, Fig. 11-2).

Importantly, this study using prespecified subgroup analysis showed a reduction in total mortality and total hospitalizations during the first 2 years after randomization in patients with an EF of <25% or patients with moderate to severe symptoms of CHF (NYHA Class III–IV), and patients with cardiomegaly on chest x-ray.

▶ DIGITALIS IN HEART FAILURE AND PRESERVED SYSTOLIC FUNCTION

In the DIG trial, an additional 988 patients with EF >45% were randomized to digoxin or placebo in the same manner as the main trial.[54] For the combined endpoint of death or hospitalization for

► **Table 11-6** Outcomes of the Digitalis InveStigation Group trial

| Variable | n | Risk of all-cause mortality or all-cause hospitalization | | | Risk of HF-related mortality or HF-related hospitalization[*] | | |
		Placebo	Digoxin	Relative risk	Placebo	Digoxin	Relative risk
All patients (EF ≤0.45)	6801	604	593	0.94 (0.88–1.00)	294	217	0.69 (0.63–0.76)
NYHA I/II	4571	548	541	0.96 (0.89–1.04)	242	178	0.70 (0.62–0.80)
EF 0.25–0.45	4543	566	571	0.99 (0.91–1.07)	244	190	0.74 (0.66–0.84)
CTR ≤0.55	4455	561	569	0.98 (0.91–1.06)	239	180	0.71 (0.63–0.81)
NYHA III/IV	2224	719	696	0.88 (0.80–0.97)	402	295	0.65 (0.57–0.75)
EF <0.25	2258	677	637	0.84 (0.76–0.93)	394	270	0.61 (0.53–0.71)
CTR >0.55	2346	687	650	0.55 (0.77–0.94)	398	287	0.65 (0.57–0.75)
EF >0.45	987	571	585	1.04 (0.88–1.23)	179	136	0.72 (0.53–0.99)

[*]Number of patients with an event during the first 2 years per 1000 randomized patients

HF—heart failure; EF—ejection fraction; NYHA—New York Heart Association; CTR—cardiothoracic ratio

Source: Adapted from Eichhorn EJ, Gheorghiade M. Digoxin. *Prog in Card Dis.* 2002;44:251–256, with permission from Elsevier.

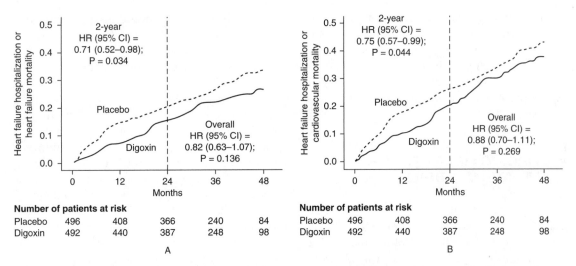

Figure 11-3 Kaplan-Meier plots for A) primary combined outcome of hospitalization for worsening heart failure or mortality resulting from HF and B) combined outcome of hospitalization for worsening heart failure or mortality from cardiovascular causes in diastolic heart failure patients randomized to digoxin or placebo in the DIG trial. HR—hazard ratio; CI—confidence interval. (Adapted with permission from: Ahmed A, et al. Effects of digoxin on morbidity and mortality in diastolic heart failure: The Ancillary Digitalis Investigation Group Trial. *Circulation.* 2006;114:397–403.)

worsening CHF, there was a decrease in the combined endpoint of heart failure hospitalization and cardiovascular mortality at 2 years, but this difference was not significant over the entire course of follow-up. The authors did note a trend toward reduction in hospitalization for worsening heart failure. The initial 2-year data from the DIG trial resulted in FDA approval of digoxin for patients with symptomatic heart failure regardless of LVEF; however, the endpoint reduction for patients with normal systolic function is less clear (Fig. 11-3). Accordingly, digoxin therapy should be considered in this population only after other therapies have failed. However, atrial fibrillation is common in the setting of diastolic dysfunction, and digoxin therapy can safely be initiated if needed for rate control.

▶ DIGITALIS IN WOMEN

A post-hoc subgroup analysis of the DIG trial sought to assess sex-based differences in the outcome of digoxin therapy. Women represented 22% of the patients enrolled in the DIG study, and an absolute mortality difference of 5.8% was found in favor of placebo.[35] This difference was not apparent in men, where there was no mortality difference between groups. Women were also found to have a smaller (but still significant) reduction in hospitalization for HF. Not surprisingly, these findings raised strong concern about the role of digoxin therapy for women with HF. The authors suggested that "women may not consider the potential increased risk of death associated with digoxin therapy worth the small reduction in the risk of hospitalization." However, further analysis has since revealed that for women with serum digitalis concentrations <1 ng/mL, there was no increase in mortality.[36] Some have hypothesized that data indicating increased mortality in women may be related to increased risk of toxicity due to overdosing and lower body weights; however, the DIG data do not support this conclusion. Further research is needed to examine sex-based differences in response to all common HF remedies, as women have always been underrepresented in important clinical trials. However, digoxin therapy at low doses remains safe and likely effective to improve symptoms and reduce the rate of hospitalizations for women with symptomatic, chronic HF and reduced systolic function.

▶ CHRONIC HEART FAILURE AND ATRIAL FIBRILLATION

Because it can be taken once daily, is well tolerated, and is inexpensive, digoxin remains an important drug for rate control in atrial fibrillation. However, in patients with normal AV node conduction in atrial fibrillation, digoxin alone will not control the rate of ventricular response, particularly during exercise unless very high doses are given. These doses have been shown to cause digoxin intoxication in a majority of patients. [37,38] Likewise, β-blockers and calcium channel blockers given as monotherapy are unlikely to control ventricular response unless given at doses likely to cause side effects.[39] The most likely combination to effectively control ventricular response in patients with atrial fibrillation and reduced systolic function is a combination of digoxin and β-blockers. In one randomized trial of patients with symptomatic heart failure and atrial fibrillation, the combination of carvedilol and digoxin was found to be superior to either drug alone in the management of atrial fibrillation in patients with HF and reduced systolic function.[52] This combination reduced symptoms, improved ventricular function, and achieved better ventricular rate control than either agent alone. Clinical experience with this combination has produced similar results, and should be considered the standard treatment for HF patients with reduced systolic function with persistent atrial fibrillation. In patients with atrial fibrillation and preserved systolic function, verapamil or diltiazem may be used, particularly in patients with reactive airway disease or in patients who are unable to tolerate β-blocker therapy. In addition, digoxin should be used to control ventricular response in atrial fibrillation even in patients without HF, unless there is intrinsic conduction disease.

Digoxin is not effective for rate control in patients with high sympathetic tone, low serum K levels, or in patients receiving sympathomimetic medications such as vasopressors or bronchodilators. In addition, digoxin therapy is not recommended for patients with atrial fibrillation and controlled ventricular response. These patients are more likely to have underlying conduction disease, and digoxin could worsen the condition. Digitalis has not been shown to promote conversion to normal sinus rhythm in patients with or without HF with decreased systolic function, but may reduce the frequency of symptomatic episodes.[40,41]

▶ DIGITALIS AND CORONARY ARTERY DISEASE

A significant number of patients with HF in the United States and Europe have coronary artery disease. Acute hypoxemia predisposes to the manifestations of digitalis intoxication, and myocardial ischemia itself may cause inhibition Na-K ATPase.[42,43] Digitalis in animal models has been shown to induce coronary vasoconstriction leading to ischemia, an effect postulated to be caused by α-adrenergic stimulation.[44,45] In several studies, digoxin has been reported to increase the early post-discharge mortality in patients who survive a myocardial infarction. In contrast, a regression analysis failed to show digitalis to be an independent predictor of mortality. In the DIG trial, 70% of patients had coronary artery disease. At the time of enrollment, 30% had angina and 60% had a previous myocardial infarction. Hospitalizations for acute coronary syndromes and ventricular arrhythmias were almost identical in the digoxin and placebo groups. However, when the digoxin effects in prespecified subgroups were examined, it appeared that the reduction in hospitalizations and mortality due to worsening HF was lower in patients with coronary artery disease. Similar results were seen in

▶ **Table 11-7** Digoxin use and mortality in postinfarction patients

Postinfarction studies	Mortality risk
Moss et al., 1981	Higher mortality among patients on digoxin overall, but differences compared with those not on digoxin are not significant. Statistically significant excess in retrospectively identified subgroup of patients with heart failure and couplet VPDs. This subgroup comprised only 8.4% of total population
Bigger et al., 1985	Nonsignificant higher mortality with digoxin overall and in the subgroup identified by Moss et al
Sweenet et al., 1991	Significant excess in sudden death in group receiving digitals. Overall mortality not provided
Byington and Goldstein, 1995	Nonsignificant higher mortality with digoxin overall and in several subroups examined
Muller et al., 1986	Nonsignificant higher mortality with digoxin overall
Madsen et al., 1984	Nonsignificant higher mortality with digoxin overall and in several subgroups examined
Leor et al., 1995	Higher mortality with digoxin

VPD—ventricular premature depolarization
Source: Adapted from Eichhorn EJ, Gheorghiade M. Digoxin. *Prog in Card Dis.* 2002. 44:251–256, with permission from Elsevier.

the RADIANCE and PROVED trials. During episodes of ischemia, the presence of digoxin may have a proarrhythmic effect and its beneficial effects in HF may be offset by its potential to cause malignant arrhythmias. If digoxin must be used in the setting of acute ischemia, there is experimental evidence that coadministration of β-blocker therapy will reduce the incidence of ventricular arrhythmias.[46] Digoxin therapy should be used with extreme caution, if at all, in patients with acute coronary syndromes. If used, serum concentration should be <0.9 ng/mL. The safety of digoxin may be increased by administration of β-blockers and aldosterone antagonists and decreased by the use of loop diuretics and other inotropic agents including dobutamine, dopamine, and milrinone (Table 11-7).

▶ SERUM DIGITALIS CONCENTRATION

There is increasing evidence that serum digitalis concentrations previously thought to be therapeutic may actually increase mortality. In the Prospective Randomized Milrinone Survival Evaluation (PROMISE) trial, SDC >1.1 ng/mL was associated with a 38% excess mortality rate.[48] Early post-hoc analysis of the DIG trial indicated an increased risk of cardiovascular mortality in patients with SDC >0.8 ng/dL.[47] More recently, a comprehensive post-hoc analysis was performed that analyzed 1687 patients from the digoxin group who had SDC measurements taken one month after randomization.[55] Compared to 3861 patients in the placebo group, it was found that while high SDC (>1.0 ng/mL) was associated with increased mortality, SDC of 0.5 to 0.9 ng/mL reduced overall mortality and hospitalization in all patients compared to placebo, including those with preserved systolic function (Fig. 11-4).[48] Although increasing digoxin dose within the therapeutic range may further improve cardiac performance, increasing the dose is not associated with an improvement in the neurohormonal profile.[49] These clinical trial data have led to the currently accepted practice of initiating low-dose digoxin therapy for patients with HF and decreased systolic function in sinus rhythm. In a separate analysis of the data from PROVED and

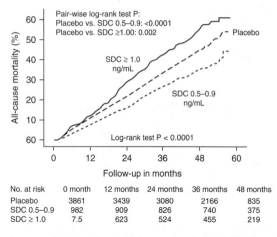

No. at risk	0 month	12 months	24 months	36 months	48 months
Placebo	3861	3439	3080	2166	835
SDC 0.5–0.9	982	909	826	740	375
SDC ≥ 1.0	7.5	623	524	455	219

Figure 11-4 Cumulative risk of death due to all causes by SDC from the DIG trial SDC—serum digitalis concentration. (Adapted with permission from Ahmed A, et al. Digoxin and reduction in mortality and hospitalization in heart failure: a comprehensive post hoc analysis of the DIG trial. *Eur Heart J.* 2006;27: 178–186.)

RADIANCE, there was no relationship between serum digitalis concentration and improvement in cardiovascular morbidity or mortality, perhaps further indication that low doses of digitalis are safe and equally effective. These clinical trial data have led to the currently accepted practice of initiating low-dose digoxin therapy for patients with HF and decreased systolic function in sinus rhythm. Low-dose digoxin resulting in SDC <0.9 ng/mL has beneficial hemodynamic, neurohormonal, and clinical effects. Accordingly, all patients receiving digoxin irrespective of underlying rhythm should receive a low dose that appears to be both safe and effective.

Since the development of the radioimmunoassay for digoxin by Dr Thomas Smith in 1969, there has been spirited debate regarding the levels of serum digoxin that result in clinical toxicity. There is significant overlap in SDC between patients who are intoxicated and those who are not. In the 30 years that SDC has been measured routinely, we have learned several important lessons. First, routine SDC should be obtained only under special circumstances—when toxicity is suspected or to monitor compliance, for monitoring of drug interactions, for example, quinidine, verapamil, and amiodarone, or in the setting of renal dysfunction. Levels should be measured just before daily administration to assure that a "trough" level is measured. Second, patients with systolic HF should be maintained on the lowest dose of digitalis, which is likely to provide a clinical effect, and large doses (>0.125 mg for women, >0.25 mg for men) should be reserved for patients with greater body mass and for patients in whom higher doses are needed for rate control in the setting of atrial fibrillation (Table 11-8).

▶ DIGITALIS IN THE SETTING OF MODERN THERAPY FOR CHRONIC HEART FAILURE

ACE Inhibitors

Analysis of PROVED and RADIANCE indicates that the combination of digoxin and an ACE inhibitor with diuretics is superior to either drug alone to prevent worsening HF and improve symptoms. These results were confirmed by the DIG trial,

▶ **Table 11-8** Possible factors affecting the safety of digoxin therapy

Increased safety	Decreased safety	Avoid use
Low dose (0.125 mg)	Loop diuretics	Cardiac amyloidosis
β–blockers	Hypomagnesemia	Hypertrophic obstructive cardiomyopathy
Spironolactone	SDC >1 ng/dL	First-degree AV block >0.3 sec or advanced AV block
	Hypokalemia	Acute coronary syndrome
	Renal failure	Hypercalcemia

SDC—serum digitalis concentration; AV—atrioventricular

leading to the acceptance of digoxin as standard therapy for symptomatic HF with reduced systolic function in patients stabilized on ACE inhibitor and diuretic therapy. Large randomized studies demonstrating the mortality benefits of ACE inhibitors have reported background digoxin therapy ranging from 50% to 90%. Retrospective analysis from the Assessment of Treatment with Lisinopril and Survival (ATLAS) study indicated that there was an incremental benefit of adding β-blocker therapy and digoxin to high dose ACE inhibitor therapy. Patients receiving high dose ACE inhibitors plus β-blockers plus digoxin had 12% fewer deaths and hospitalizations than patients receiving low-dose ACE inhibitors alone.[56]

β-Blockers

In recent large randomized studies demonstrating significant mortality benefit of β-blocker therapy in chronic heart failure, concurrent background digoxin therapy was reported. In a 1996 trial demonstrating the mortality benefit of carvedilol, 90% of patients were taking digoxin.[7] This percentage fell to 51% in a similar trial demonstrating the benefits of carvedilol published in 2001.[8] Digoxin may be safer in patients receiving β-blocker therapy, and useful particularly during the initiation of β-blocker therapy when there is an initial decrease in EF and cardiac output.

Aldosterone Blocking Agents

In the Randomized Aldactone Evaluation Study (RALES) trial, 75% of patients were receiving digoxin therapy.[50] Analysis of the mortality data indicates that patients receiving digoxin were more likely to benefit from aldactone therapy compared to placebo. In addition, the potential beneficial effects of aldosterone blockers on perivascular and myocardial fibrosis may be potentiated by the addition of digoxin therapy. Aldosterone-blocking agents also decrease the risk of digitalis toxicity by increasing serum potassium levels. Given these possible synergistic interactions, it is reasonable to recommend

continuation of digoxin therapy in patients with CHF receiving aldosterone-blocking agents.

Cardiac Resynchronization Therapy

The Cardiac Resynchronization in Heart Failure (CARE-HF) study was the first randomized study of CRT therapy in HF to demonstrate a clear mortality benefit in patients with reduced systolic function and severe symptoms.[51] In both the Comparison of Medical Therapy, Pacing, and Defibrillation in Heart Failure (COMPANION) and CARE-HF, digoxin was no longer considered as part of optimal pharmacological therapy.[51,52] Nevertheless, in CARE-HF, approximately 40% of patients received digoxin. Digoxin appears to significantly reduce mortality and hospitalization rate particularly in patients with severe symptoms and very low EF (those more likely to receive cardiac resynchronization therapy [CRT]). Accordingly, CRT therapy should be considered in patients who continue to have symptoms of HF despite standard therapy, including digoxin.

▶ RECOMMENDATIONS

Digoxin is inexpensive and has few side effects when dosed appropriately. Published clinical trial data support the current Class IIa recommendation of the ACC/AHA for its use in patients with symptomatic HF and reduced systolic function. It is the only available inotrope that decreases morbidity without increasing mortality. Current data indicate that its effect is enhanced, not diluted, in the presence of other proven therapies for chronic heart failure including β-blockers, aldosterone antagonists, and ACE inhibitors. This multidrug approach to the patient with HF is accepted as the standard of care. Until large randomized trials are performed that indicate the effectiveness of these medications persist in the absence of digoxin, continued use in this patient population should be considered to improve symptoms and prevent significant costs associated with repeated hospitalization. It is likely that digoxin will continue to play an important role in the

▶ **Table 11-9**   Recommendations for use of digoxin in heart failure

Digoxin should be used in patients with sinus rhythm who have signs and symptoms of heart failure and reduced systolic function while receiving standard therapy. Digoxin appears particularly useful in patients with NYHA Class III and IV symptoms, and/or increased cardiothoracic ratio on chest x-ray and/or LVEF <0.25

Digoxin should be used in patients with heart failure irrespective of their ejection fraction if atrial fibrillation and a rapid ventricular response is present. It is recognized; however, that digoxin therapy alone will not be sufficient to control ventricular response during exercise. The best results are noted when digoxin is combined with a β-blocker

In patients with sinus rhythm or atrial fibrillation, a relatively low dose of digoxin should be used (resulting in SDC <0.9 ng/dL) at least 12 hours after the dose. The usual dose in patients without renal failure not receiving medications that are likely to increase serum concentration (verapamil, amiodarone, quinidine) should be 0.125 mg for women and 0.25 for men

The loading dose or the use of intravenous digoxin should be discouraged in general and not be used in patients with coronary artery disease and active ischemia

NYHA—New York Heart Association; LVEF—left ventricular ejection fraction; SDC—serum digitalis concentration

future treatment of HF with and without atrial fibrillation (Table 11-9).

▶ REFERENCES

1. Hunt SA, Abraham WT, Chin MH, et al. ACC/AHA 2005 guideline update for the diagnosis and management of chronic heart failure in the adult: summary article. A report of the American College of Cardiology/American Heart Association Task Force on Practice Guidelines (Committee to revise the 2001 Guidelines for the Evaluation and Management of Heart Failure). *J Am Coll Cardiol.* 2005;46:1116–1143.
2. Adams KF Jr., Lindenfeld J, Arnold JM, et al. Executive summary: HFSA 2006 comprehensive heart failure practice guideline. *J Card Fail.* 2006; 12:10–38.
3. Rathore SS, Wang Y, Krumholz HM. Sex-based differences in the effect of digitalis for the treatment of heart failure. *N Engl J Med.* October 31, 2002;347(18):1403–1411.
4. Hunt SA, Abraham WT, Chin MH, et al. ACC/AHA 2005 Guideline Update for the Diagnosis and Management of Chronic Heart Failure in the Adult–Summary Article. *Circulation.* 2005;112: 1825–1852 and *J Am Coll Cardiol.* 2005;46: 1116–1143.
5. Withering W. *An account of the foxglove and some of its medicinal uses with practical remarks on dropsy and other diseases.* Swinney, Birmingham, England 1785.
6. Beller GA, Conroy J, Smith TW. Ischemia-induced alterations in myocardial Na/K-ATPase and cardiac glycoside binding. *J Clin Invest.* 1976;57: 341–350.
7. Packer M, Bristow M, Cohn J, et al. The Effect of Carvedilol on Morbidity and Mortality in Patients with Chronic Heart Failure. *NEJM.* 1996;334(21): 1249–1355.
8. Packer M, Coats J, Fowler M, et al. Effect of Carvedilol on Survival in Severe Chronic Heart Failure. *NEJM.* 2001;344(22):1651–1658.
9. The MERIT-HF Investigators. Effects of controlled-release metoprolol on total mortality, hospitalizations and well-being in patients with heart failure. *JAMA.* 2000;283(10):1295–1302.
10. CIBIS II Investigators and Committees. The Cardiac Insufficiency Bisoprolol Study II (CIBIS- II). *Lancet.* 1999;353:9–13.
11. Smith TW, Antman EM, Friedman PL, et al. Digitalis glycosides: mechanisms and manifestations of toxicity. *Prog Cardiovasc Dis.* 1984;26: 413–458, 495–530.
12. Wang W, Chen JS, Zucker IH. Carotid sinus baroreceptor sensitivity in experimental heart failure. *Circulation.* 1990;91:1959–1966.
13. Krum H, Bigger JT, Jr, Goldsmith RL, et al. Effect of long-term digitalis therapy on autonomic function in patients with chronic heart failure. *J Am Coll Cardiol.* September 1995;26(3):838.
14. Ferguson DW, Berg WJ, Sanders JS, et al. Sympathoinhibitory responses to digitalis glycosides in heart failure patients: direct evidence

from sympathetic neural recordings. *Circulation.* 1989;80:65–67.

15. van Veldhuisen DJ, Man in't Veld AJ, Dunselman PHJM, et al. Double-blind placebo controlled study of ibopamine and digoxin in patients with mild to moderate heart failure: results of the Dutch Ibopamine Multicenter Trial (DIMT). *J Am Coll Cardiol.* 1993; 22:155–161.

16. Zhang J, Sun Y, Weber K. Coronary fibrosis in hyperaldosteronism: prevention by digoxin. *Circulation.* 1999; 100 (suppl I):1–560.

17. Lown B, Grayboys TB, Podrid PJ, et al. Effect of digitalis drug on ventricular premature beats. *N Engl J Med.* 1977;296:301–306.

18. Gheorghiade M, St. Clair J, St. Clair C, et al. Hemodynamic effects of intravenous digoxin in patients with severe heart failure initially treated with diuretics and vasodilators. *J Am Coll Cardiol.* 1987:9:849–857.

19. Gheorghiade M, Hall VB, Jacobsen G, et al. Effects of increasing maintenance dose of digitalis on left ventricular function and neurohormones in patients with chronic heart failure treated with diuretics and angiotensin-converting enzyme inhibitors. *Circulation.* 1995;92:1801–1807.

20. Woodland C, Verjee Z, Giesbrecht E, et al. The digitalis-propafenone interaction: characterization of a mechanism using renal tubular cell monolayers. *J Pharmacol Exp Ther.* 1997;283:39–45.

21. Klein HO, Lang R, Weiss E, et al. The influence of verapamil on serum digitalis concentration. *Circulation.* 1982;65:998–1003.

22. Hager WD, Fenster P, Mayersohn M, et al. Digitalis-quinidine interaction pharmacokinetic evaluation. *N Engl J Med.* 1979;300:1238–1241.

23. Paladino JA, Davidson KH, McCall BB. Influence of spironolactone on serum digitalis concentration [letter]. *JAMA.* 1984;251:470–471.

24. Weeks CE, Conard GJ, Kvam DC, et al. The effect of flecainide acetate, a new antiarrhythmic, on plasma digitalis levels. *J Clin Pharmacol.* 1986; 26:27–31.

25. Robinson K, Johnston A, Walker S, et al. The digitalis-amiodarone interaction. *Cardiovasc Drugs Ther.* 1989;3:25–28.

26. Smith TW, Harber E. Digoxin intoxication: the relationship of clinical presentation toserum digoxin concentration. *J Clin Invest.* 1970;49: 2377–2386.

24. Yusuf S, Wittes J, Bailey K, et al. Digitalis – a new controversy regarding an old drug: the pitfalls of inappropriate methods. *Circulation.* 1986;73: 14–18.

27. Uretsky BF, Young JB, Shahidi FE, PROVED Investigative Group. Randomized study assessing the effect of digitalis withdrawal in patients with mild to moderate chronic congestive heart failure: results of the PROVED trial. *J Am Coll Cardiol.* 1993;22:955–962.

28. Packer M, Gheorghiade M, Young JB, et al. Withdrawal of digitalis from patients with chronic heart failure treated with angiotensin-converting-enzyme inhibitors. RADIANCE Study. *N Engl J Med.* 1993;329:1–7.

29. Digitalis Investigation Group. The effect of digitalis on mortality and morbidity in patients with heart failure. *N Engl J Med.* 1997;336:525–533.

30. The Captopril-Digitalis Multicenter Research Group. Comparative effects of therapy with captopril and digitalis in patients with mild to moderate heart failure. *JAMA.* 1988;259:539–544.

31. DiBianco R, Shabetai R, Kostuk W, et al. A comparison of milrinone, digitalis, and their combination in the treatment of patients with chronic heart failure. *N Engl J Med.* 1989;320: 677–683.

32. van Veldhuisen DJ, Man in't Veld AJ, Dunselman PH, et al. Double-blind placebo-controlled study of ibopamine and digoxin in patients with mild to moderate heart failure: results of the Dutch Ibopamine Multicenter Trial (DIMT). *J Am Coll Cardiol.* November 15, 1993;22(6):1564–1573.

33. Young, J, Gheorghiade M, Uretsky B, et al. Superiority of "triple" drug therapy in heart failure: insights from PROVED and RADIANCE Trials. *J Am Coll Cardiol.* 1998;3:686–692.

34. Ward RE, Gheorghiade M, Young JB, et al. Economic outcomes of withdrawal of digoxin therapy in adult patients with stable congestive heart failure. *J Am Coll Cardiol.* July 1995; 26(1): 93–101.

35. Rathore SS, Curtis JP, Wang Y, et al. Association of serum digitalis concentration and outcomes in patients with heart failure. *JAMA.* 2003;289: 871–878.

36. Adams KF, Patterson JH, Gattis WA, et al. Relationship of serum digoxin concentration to mortality and morbidity in women in the Digitalis Investigation Group Trial: a retrospective analysis. Moderated Poster at AHA Scientific Sessions, 2004.

37. Gold H, Cattell M, Greiner T, et al: Clinical pharmacology of digoxin. *J Pharmacol Exp Ther.* 1953; 109:45–57.

38. Redfors A. The effect of different digoxin doses on subjective symptoms and physical working capacity in patients with atrial fibrillation. *Acta Med Scand.* 1971;90:307–320.

39. Zarowitz BJ, Gheorghiade M. Optimal heart rate control for patients with chronic atrial fibrillation: are pharmacologic doses truly changing? *Am Heart J.* 1992;12:1401–1403.

40. Falk RH, Knowlton AA, Bernard SA, et al. Digoxin for converting recent-onset atrial fibrillation to sinus rhythm: a randomized, double-blinded trial. *Ann Intern Med.* 1987;106:503–506.

41. Murgatroyd FD, Gibson SM, Baiyan X, et al. Double-blind placebo controlled trial of digoxin in symptomatic atrial fibrillation. *Circulation.* 1999;99:2765–2770.

42. Beller GA, Conroy J, Smith TW. Ischemia-induced alterations in myocardial (Na$^+$-K$^+$)-ATPase and cardiac glycoside binding. *J Clin Invest.* 57:341–350.

43. Lynch JJ, Montgomery DG, Lucchesi BR. Facilitation of lethal ventricular arrhythmias by therapeutic digoxin in conscious postinfarction dogs. *Am Heart J.* 1986;111:883–890.

44. Mikkelsen E, Andersson KE, Ledeballe PE. Effects of digoxin on isolated human peripheral arteries and veins. *Acta Pharmacol Toxicol.* 1979; 45:249–256.

45. Vatner SF, Higgins CB, Franklin D, et al. Effects of digitalis glycosides on coronary and systemic dynamics in conscious dogs. *Circ Res.* 1971; 28:470–479.

46. Lynch JJ, Kitzen JM, Hoff PT, et al. Reduction in digitalis-associated postinfarction mortality with nadolol in conscious dogs. *Am Heart J.* 1988;115: 67–76.

47. Gheorghiade M, Pitt B. Digitalis Investigation Group (DIG) trial: a stimulus for further research. *Am Heart J.* 1997;134:3–12.

48. Mancini DM, Benotti JR, Elkayam U, the PROMISE Investigators and Coordinators. Antiarrhythmic drug use and high serum levels of digitalis are independent adverse prognostic factors in patients with chronic heart failure (Abstract). *Circulation.* 1991;84(II):243.

49. Benedict CR, Johnstone DE, Weiner DH, for the SOLVD Investigators. Relation of neurohormonal activation to clinical variables and degree of ventricular dysfunction: a report from the registry of studies of left ventricular dysfunction. *J Am Coll Cardiol.* 1994;23:1410–1420.

50. Pitt B, Zannad F, Remme W, et al. The effect of spironolactone on morbidity and mortality in patients with severe heart failure. *NEJM.* 1999;341:709–717.

51. Cleland JG, Daubert JC, Erdmann E, the Cardiac Resynchronization—Heart Failure (CARE-HF) Study Investigators. The effect of cardiac resynchronization on morbidity and mortality in heart failure. *N Engl J Med.* 2005;352(15):1539–1549.

52. Khand AU, Rankin AC, Martin W, et al. Carvedilol alone or in combination with digoxin for the management of atrial fibrillation in patients with heart failure? *J Am Coll Cardiol.* 2003;42: 1944–1995.

53. Eichhorn EJ, Gheorghiade M. Digoxin. *Prog in Card Dis.* 2002;44:251–256.

54. Ahmed A, Rich MW, Love TE, Lloyd-Jones DM, Aban IB, Colucci WS, Adams KF, Gheorghiade M. Digoxin and reduction in mortality and hospitalization in heart failure: a comprehensive post hoc analysis of the DIG trial. *Eur Heart Journal.* 2006; 27:178–186.

55. Ahmed A, Rich MW, Fleg JL, Zile MR, Young JB, Kitzman DW, Love TE, Aronow WS, Adams KF, Gheorghiade M. Effects of digoxin on morbidity and mortality in diastolic heart failure: The Ancillary Digitalis Investigation Group Trial. *Circulation.* 2006;114:397–403.

56. Majumdar SR, McAlister FA, Cree M, Chang W, Packer M, Armstrong PW. Do evidence-based treatments provide incremental benefits to patients with congestive heart failure already receiving angiotensin-converting enzyme inhibitors? A secondary analysis of one-year outcomes from the Assessment of Treatment with Lisinopril and Survival (ATLAS) Study. *Clin Ther.* 2004;26: 694–703.

CHAPTER 12

The Heart Failure Hospitalization

LYNNE WARNER STEVENSON, MD, FACC

▶ INTRODUCTION

Heart failure leads to over 1 million hospitalizations annually and is the most common diagnosis for hospitalization in patients over the age of 65 years. Readmission rates are 25–40% during the next 6 months. Death occurs in only 4% of hospital admissions, but in almost half of patients during the year after discharge. Although fewer than 1 in 5 patients who carry a heart failure diagnosis will be hospitalized each year, hospitalization accounts for over two-thirds of all health expenditures for heart failure in Western nations. As a marker of disease progression, worsening functional status, and poor prognosis, hospitalization can be considered a failure of the medical regimen. The major purposes of hospitalization are to establish stability and to design a regimen that will maintain it when the patient is at home.

▶ REASONS AND GOALS FOR HEART FAILURE HOSPITALIZATION

The most common precipitant for hospitalization with heart failure is worsening of congestive symptoms due to accumulation of excess circulating and total body volume (Table 12-1). However, decompensated heart failure may also be discovered during a hospitalization for other presenting symptoms such as tachyarrhythmias or angina in patients with low left ventricular ejection fraction (LVEF). For any patient presenting with new-onset heart failure, it is critical to review the primary etiology and potential exacerbating factors in order to address conditions that can be remedied, such as active ischemia and primary valve disease.

This chapter will focus on the approach to patients with chronic heart failure that has previously been evaluated. Hospitalization for patients with heart failure should address the fundamental goals of symptom relief, attention to potential exacerbating factors, clinical stabilization, and design of the discharge regimen, including education in connection with subsequent outpatient management (Table 12-2).

▶ PROFILES OF HOSPITALIZED PATIENTS

The typical patients hospitalized with heart failure have been well-defined recently by large registries. Previous information was gleaned from randomized controlled trials in which patients

▶ **Table 12-1** Typical indications for hospitalization of patient with heart failure

For Symptomatic Heart Failure
- Evaluation and therapy of new onset symptomatic heart failure in patient without prior diagnosis
- Severity of congestion
  - Respiratory distress in upright position
  - Anasarca
  - Persistent symptoms at rest or minimal exertion and
    - Failure to respond to elevation of outpatient loop diuretic doses, or
    - Limitation of diuresis by hypotension or worsening renal function
- Clinical "cold and wet" profile, as suggested by
  - Narrow pulse pressure
  - Systolic blood pressure confirmed <75 mm Hg
  - Cold extremities
  - Impaired mental status
  - New intolerance of neurohormonal antagonists

For Dysrhythmias
- Syncope
- Sustained ventricular tachycardia
- Repeated defibrillator discharges
- New-onset atrial fibrillation with decompensation
- Hyperkalemia (e.g., K $\geq$6 meq/L)

For Other Cardiovascular Events
- New or unstable angina
- Stroke, transient ischemic attack, or peripheral embolic event

For Noncardiac Conditions With Heart Failure Exacerbation
- Examples:
  - Severe pulmonary decompensation
  - Anemia requiring transfusion

▶ **Table 12-2** Goals of heart failure hospitalization

- Relief of symptoms
  - Focus on identification and therapy of elevated filling pressures (congestion)
  - Maintenance of adequate blood pressure to allow comfortable ambulation
- Attention to exacerbating factors, examples:
  - Tachyarrhythmia, bradycardia, or blocked heart rate reserve
  - Active coronary ischemia
  - Anemia
  - Infection
  - Thyroid imbalance
- Clinical stabilization
  - Achievement of optimal filling pressures
  - Weaning from intravenous vasodilator or inotropic infusions
  - Maintenance of adequate renal function
- Design of discharge regimen
  - Diuretics
    - Identification of routine oral dosing
    - First escalation level
    - Decision regarding spironolactone
  - Neurohormonal antagonists as tolerated
  - Consider adjunctive vasodilators
  - Therapy for coronary artery disease as indicated
  - Anticoagulation if indicated
- Readiness for discharge
  - Stability on oral regimen
  - Education and connection
  - Follow-up appointment within 2 weeks

were relatively young with few comorbidities and were felt sufficiently stable to undergo an active or placebo therapy. Centralized databases in Scotland and Canada have revealed the older age and almost 50% 1-year mortality of most populations hospitalized with heart failure.[1,2] Details of the initial clinical profiles and hospital events have been provided in the United States by the Acute Decompensated Heart Failure National Registry (ADHERE), including over 100,000 hospitalizations voluntarily reported by community and academic centers.[3] Recognizing the different hospitalized populations from communities and trials (Table 12-3), application of trial findings and the parallel guidelines should be carefully adapted for the profile of the individual patient.

Heart failure with a dilated ventricle and low ejection fraction (EF) is the basis for the major clinical trials and current heart failure guidelines. It has been increasingly recognized, however, that about half of heart failure hospitalizations occur in patients with an EF >40%, usually without significant dilation of the ventricle, often with left ventricular hypertrophy. Although often referred to as "diastolic dysfunction," accepted echocardiographic criteria for diastolic dysfunction are often found in patients with dilated heart failure and low EF and are not always present in patients with heart failure and preserved EF. The most typical clinical history for such a patient includes hypertension, diabetes, and advanced age, and about half of these patients are women, as discussed in Chap. 11.

Although much has been made of the distinctions between the pathophysiology of heart failure with low EF and with preserved EF, the

▶ **Table 12-3** Different hospitalized heart failure populations

	Preserved LVEF	Low LVEF	In-hospital β-blocker	Hospital IV trials	ESCAPE rehospitalization HF	REMATCH on oral therapy	REMATCH on IV inotropes
Age	70	74	68	63	56	68	67
EF	49	29	25	25	19	17	17
SBP	144	140	139	120	106	107	100
Creatinine	1.8	1.8	1.1	1.5	1.5	1.8	1.8
Na	138	138		138	137	137	134
% Previous diuretics	65	84	81	88	98	100	95
% ACEI/ARB	53	78	83	80	90	66	53
% β-blockers	45	46	0 initial	22	62	34	16
# Patients	34,000	35,000	363	1400	443	38	91

LVEF—left ventricular ejection fraction; IV—intravenous; HF—heart failure; ESCAPE—Evaluation Study of Congestive Heart Failure and Pulmonary Artery Catheterization Effectiveness; REMATCH—Randomized Evaluation of Mechanical Assistance for the Treatment of Congestive Heart Failure study; EF—ejection fraction; SBP—systolic blood pressure; ACEI—angiotensin-converting enzyme inhibitor; ARB—angiotensin receptor blocker

Source: Fonarow GC, Abraham WT, Yancy CW, et al. Risk stratification for in-hospital mortality in acutely decompensated heart failure: classification and regression tree analysis. *JAMA.* 2005;293:572–580.

ESCAPE Investigators and Coordinators. Evaluation study of congestive heart failure and pulmonary artery catheterization. *JAMA.* 2005;294:1625–1633.

VMAC Investigators. Intravenous nesiritide vs nitroglycerin for treatment of decompensated congestive heart failure: a randomized controlled trial. *JAMA.* 2002;287:1531–1540.

Cuffe MS, Califf RM, Adams KF, Jr, et al. Short-term intravenous milrinone for acute exacerbation of chronic heart failure: a randomized controlled trial. *JAMA.* 2002;287:1541–1547.

Gattis WA, O'Connor CM, Gallup DS, et al. Predischarge initiation of carvedilol in patients hospitalized for decompensated heart failure: results of the Initiation Management Predischarge: Process for Assessment of Carvedilol Therapy in Heart Failure (IMPACT-HF) trial. *J Am Coll Cardiol.* 2004;43:1534–1541.

Rose EA, Gelhjns AC, Moskowitz AJ, et al. Long-term use of a left ventricular assist device for end-stage heart failure. *N Engl J Med.* 2001;345:1435–1443.

presentation at the time of hospitalization is usually with similar symptoms. Blood pressure and cardiac output are less often low in the preserved EF patient, and ventricular tachyarrhythmias are rare, but renal dysfunction and atrial fibrillation are equally common. Furthermore, our current acute therapies are remarkably similar for the two populations, although some agents may be selected for different reasons. This chapter will focus on those considerations and therapies developed for patients with low LVEF, but will indicate those considerations that are appropriate to all patients hospitalized with heart failure regardless of EF (*all* EF).

Initial Evidence of Congestion (All Ejection Fraction)

The majority of patients hospitalized with symptoms of heart failure at rest or minimal exertion have elevation of both right- and left-sided filling pressures. Elevation of left-sided filling pressures can be reflected in symptoms of orthopnea and dyspnea on minimal exertion, such as walking to the bathroom or getting dressed. Shortness of breath relates primarily to stiffness of the lung interstitium limiting comfortable respiratory excursion. This is attributed most often to high hydrostatic pressure in the pulmonary veins, although may be exacerbated by impaired pulmonary lymphatic drainage into the right side, and by low serum proteins leading to reduced intravascular oncotic pressure. Elevation of right-sided systemic venous pressures can be associated with the discomfort of peripheral edema, hepatic congestion, and ascites, although can also cause anorexia and early satiety without detectable intra-abdominal fluid retention. Dominance of right-sided or left-sided symptoms does not necessarily define the relative elevation of pressure in these two venous circulations.

The relationship of right- to left-sided filling pressures has been delineated in chronic advanced heart failure with low EF by Drazner, indicating that right atrial pressure > or ≤10 mm Hg correlates with pulmonary wedge pressure ≥ or <22 mm Hg in 80% of patients.[4] In addition, for this population of patients from which severe intrinsic pulmonary disease was excluded, pulmonary artery systolic pressure was highly correlated with pulmonary capillary wedge pressure, pulmonary artery systolic pressure being about twice the wedge pressure, once elevated. These relationships have not been established for heart failure with preserved EF.

The clinical detection of high pulmonary capillary wedge pressures has been assessed specifically only for patients with low EF, but in the absence of other information, similar strategies should be used for the patient with heart failure and preserved EF. Rales and edema are relatively insensitive to the presence of chronic fluid elevation, and therapies targeted only for clear lungs and ankles will result in undertreatment.[5] In young patients, edema is very rare even with severe volume overload, while elderly patients often develop peripheral edema from local venous disease without elevated central filling pressures.

Jugular venous pressure remains the most important component of physical assessment for elevated filling pressures, both at baseline and through the course of changing therapies. Other measures that can be useful for experienced examiners include the Valsalva maneuver (which can be done approximately with a stethoscope and bedside blood pressure cuff or more precisely with a simple manometer device), and the leftward radiation of the pulmonic component of the second sound as indicative of elevated pulmonary artery systolic pressure in heart failure, most commonly due to elevated left-sided filling pressures.

Four Basic Hemodynamic Profiles

The concept of four major clinical hemodynamic profiles has been useful to triage patients both for initial therapy and for subsequent outcome (Fig. 12-1).[6] Some of the utility has been in the recognition that filling pressures are often severely elevated in the absence of clinical hypoperfusion,

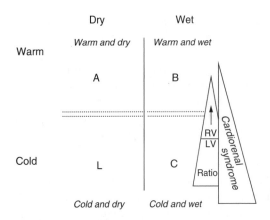

Figure 12-1 Modified hemodynamic profiles. The four basic hemodynamic profiles are defined in terms of wet and dry, in terms of evidence of excess perfusion, and warm or cold in terms of adequate perfusion. Patients with poor perfusion may have cool extremities but the "cold" label is more conceptual than palpable. Patients who appear warm and wet but do not respond well may fall into two groups who behave more like the "cold and wet" profile: patients with the RV profile in which RV filling pressures are approaching left ventricular filling pressures, and the cardiorenal syndrome, in which indices of renal function worsen during diuresis despite persistent volume in excess of that needed for optimal cardiac function. RV—right ventricular; LV—left ventricular.

although the converse is relatively uncommon. The four profiles are defined by the result of two binary questions regarding filling pressures and perfusion: Is there evidence of congestion? This question is answered as described above. Is there evidence of clinical hypoperfusion? Clues to hypoperfusion can be a proportional pulse pressure <25%, cool extremities, hypotension even to low-dose angiotensin-converting enzyme (ACE) inhibitors, and progressive renal dysfunction, although as discussed below, renal dysfunction is not primarily a result of low cardiac output. Although some patients with low perfusion may actually feel cold to palpation, the terms "cold and wet" or "cold and dry" are not meant to describe the actual physical temperature, but to conceptualize the circulatory status and guide initiation of therapy. Clinicians are less astute at recognizing cardiac index <2.2 L/min/m^2 than recognizing pulmonary wedge pressure >22 mm Hg.

Despite the limited accuracy of our estimates of cardiac output, the clinical profiles are important for prognosis. Outcome over the next 6- and 12-month period has been clearly linked to clinician determination of clinical profile at admission. Patients assessed to be warm and wet, which is the majority of hospitalizations in most series and the large majority of community hospitalizations, had twice the rate of death or urgent transplant at 1 year as those who appeared warm and dry. The cold and wet profile was associated with 3.7 times the 1-year mortality, while patients with the cold and dry profile had mortality similar to the warm and wet.[7] Patients with immediate compromise of organ perfusion due to life-threatening cardiogenic shock would fall within the cold and wet profile definition, but would require specific attention for definitive therapy beyond that for most cold and wet patients.

► WHAT IS THE GOAL FOR DRY?

The major goal for most hospitalized patients is to establish optimal filling pressures to maintain stability, regardless of the EF. Both excess circulating volume and high afterloads from systemic vasoconstriction and poorly compliant great arteries contribute to elevated filling pressures. The relative contribution of the volume overload and the decreased venous compliance and increased arterial tone vary between individuals. Before chronic use of ACE inhibitors, many patients with dilated low EF heart failure presented with severe vasoconstriction, which is now much less common than dominant volume overload.[8] For patients with preserved LVEF, volume overload is a major factor, but the contribution of inefficient ventriculo-vascular coupling into stiff vessels may be most important for chronic progression and acute decompensation. While the final goal for both warm-and-wet and cold-and-wet profiles is the warm and dry profile, initiation of therapy for the warm-and-wet is simplistically stated as "dry them out" while for cold-and-wet is to "warm up and then dry out," as discussed below under addition of vasoactive intravenous agents.

What is the target filling pressure in *dilated low EF heart failure*? At one time it was presumed that filling pressures needed to be high in order to maintain stroke volume from the chronically dilated ventricle. This arose in part as an extension from the observation that a pulmonary wedge pressure of 18 mm was optimal early after myocardial infarction; this, however, is a state characterized by acute reduction of compliance in a nondilated ventricle. It is now well-accepted that filling pressures can be reduced to near-normal levels while maintaining or even improving stroke volume in chronic dilated heart failure.[9] High filling pressures impair left ventricular function by imposing high oxygen demand, diminishing subendocardial perfusion, and increasing ventricular turgor by impairing coronary venous drainage against high right atrial pressures. They further detract from cardiac output through dynamic mitral regurgitation, which often consumes up to 75% of total stroke volume during decompensation. The regurgitant fraction is frequently reduced to only 25% of total stroke volume after effective therapy to reduce filling pressures, due to a decrease in the effective regurgitant orifice.[10]

Measured filling pressures remain robust predictors of survival in dilated low EF heart failure. They are much more predictive than indices of cardiac output, and the filling pressures measured after therapy tailored to reduce filling pressures are more important than those measured at admission.[11] It remains unclear, however, whether the achievement of the lowest filling pressures creates survivors, or merely identifies those with more favorable physiology regardless of therapy.

The target filling pressure in *preserved LVEF* heart failure has been assumed to be much higher, reflecting the relatively noncompliant left ventricle often characterized by left ventricular hypertrophy. The pressure-volume curves for these ventricles have not been well characterized, however. Some patients diagnosed with heart failure and preserved LVEF may have relatively little apparent abnormality of myocardial compliance, but instead have a fluid-retaining state with a high set point beyond that required for maintenance of cardiac output. For these patients, documentation of good cardiac output after diuresis to normal filling pressures can be helpful in guiding future adjustment of volume status. For almost all patients with resting symptoms from elevated left-sided filling pressures (in the absence of outflow gradients), fluid status can be reduced without compromise of cardiac output.

How Can Therapy Be Monitored?

Because it is the elevated filling pressures that lead to the symptoms of congestion at the time of heart failure hospitalization, therapy in a hospital is aimed at reduction of these filling pressures. Therapy is associated with improved symptoms, decreased clinical evidence of elevated filling pressures, decreased filling pressures measured invasively or estimated noninvasively, and decreased correlates of filling pressures, such as echocardiographic mitral regurgitation and natriuretic peptide levels. As the importance of lower filling pressures is recognized for relieving symptoms, for titrating β-blocking agents, and for limiting disease progression, further emphasis will likely be placed on strategies by which to monitor and adjust filling pressures. However at this time, the only two strategies that have been rigorously compared are the clinical evaluation and invasive measurement during hospitalization.

Symptoms and Signs of Congestion (All Ejection Fraction)

The most immediate goal of therapy for heart failure regardless of LVEF is relief from the symptoms of congestion that lead to hospital admission. As a gauge of therapy, however, symptom improvement is most useful at the beginning of therapy, to indicate progress in the right direction. For someone who has undergone gradual decompensation, the dramatic contrast after initial rapid reduction of filling pressures often is perceived by the patient as "back to normal," or "back to baseline," which is often still excessive compared to normal volume status. At this level, it requires very little fluid retention for symptomatic regression. Patients admitted with clinical fluid retention are at high risk for early readmission if they go home as soon as symptoms improve.

The adequacy of diuresis is tracked using resolution of orthopnea; hepatomegaly; peripheral edema; if present, and not due to local venous disease alone; and the most sensitive sign, jugular venous pressure ≤ 8 mm Hg. As discussed in the earlier paragraphs, clinical assessment of right atrial pressure provides a reasonable gauge of therapy. It correlates with left-sided filling pressures in almost 80% of patients with chronic dilated heart failure, and is assessed with reasonable accuracy by experienced clinicians (Table 12-4).[4] Although the accuracy of the physical signs discussed in the previous section have been better validated for single-time measurements than for the clinical assessment of changes in filling pressures, they appear to correlate reasonably well both at the beginning and end of therapy in the hospital.

▶ **Table 12-4** Relationship between physician-estimated and invasively measured right atrial pressures at time of heart failure hospitalization in 252 patients

	Measured RAP <8	Measured RAP 8–12	Measured RAP >12
Estimated RAP <8	9	1	1
Estimated RAP 8–12	20	29	18
Estimated RAP >12	12	22	80

Table courtesy of Drazner M. for the ESCAPE Investigators
Source: Drazner MH, Yancy C, Shah MR, et al. Utility of the history and physical examination in assessing hemodynamics in patients with advanced heart failure: the ESCAPE trial (abstract). *Circulation.* 2005;112:11–640.

Pulmonary Artery Catheters in Monitoring for Adjustment of Therapy

Direct measurement of hemodynamics during hospitalization may be useful for diagnosis of baseline hemodynamic profile in patients for whom the clinical assessment is ambiguous or discordant (Table 12-5). It may be particularly useful for determining the contribution of heart failure to a complex clinical picture such as sepsis, acute renal failure, or acute coronary syndrome in the setting of chronic heart failure. A common reason for determining left heart and pulmonary pressures is in the evaluation of concomitant pulmonary and cardiac disease in which the cause of dyspnea and elevation of right heart pressures could be due either to left-sided failure or intrinsic pulmonary disease.

In addition to diagnosis, hemodynamic monitoring has been used to guide ongoing adjustment of therapy for chronic decompensated heart failure.[12] For patients with the usual ratio of right atrial to wedge pressure <two-thirds, recommended hemodynamic goals of therapy tailored to reduce filling pressures are pulmonary capillary wedge pressure ≤16 mm Hg and right atrial pressure ≤8 mm Hg. Systemic vascular resistance is a target of therapy only as necessary to reduce the filling pressures, with a goal being 1100–1200 in normal size individuals in whom the wedge pressure is still high. If the filling pressures are not high, aggressive reduction of systemic vascular resistance is generally associated with symptomatic hypotension. Cardiac output and mixed venous saturation are useful for trending general circulatory status and usually improve with effective reduction of filling pressures. Beyond that, however, therapy targeted specifically to improve cardiac output has not been beneficial as part of a strategy for chronic management. (As mentioned above, hemodynamic monitoring to direct use of inotropic therapy in pressor doses in support of

▶ **Table 12-5** Potential use of pulmonary artery catheters during heart failure hospitalization

- Short-term management of inotrope and pressor support for cardiogenic shock until definitive therapy (Note: no controlled evidence that hemodynamic information improves outcome in shock)
- Evaluation of patients for cardiac transplantation or mechanical cardiac assistance
- Uncertainty regarding hemodynamic status, examples:
  - Concomitant pulmonary disease and heart failure
  - Acute coronary syndrome and chronic heart failure
  - Suspected dominance of right ventricular > left ventricular failure
  - Suspected very low or high systemic vascular resistance limiting other therapies
- Redesign of therapy for patients with recurrent or refractory symptoms of heart failure despite adjustment of standard therapy guided by clinical assessment
- Adjustment of diuretics and vasodilators to facilitate weaning from intravenous inotropic agents in patients with apparent dependence

cardiac output and blood pressure may be critical in the immediate management of cardiogenic shock during diagnosis and preparation for definitive therapy such as ventricular support device placement.)

The pulmonary artery catheter (PAC) was compared to clinical assessment during adjustment of therapy for a population of hospitalized patients with advanced chronic heart failure who either had one prior hospitalization during the past year or chronic high-dose diuretic therapy prior to the current admission (NHLBI-sponsored ESCAPE trial).[13] Adverse events specifically related to PAC occurred in 4% of patients, and there were twice as many infections in the patients with PAC as those treated based on clinical assessment alone. Both groups of patients had marked improvement in clinical status during hospitalization (Table 12-6). PAC had no effect on in-hospital mortality or the overall endpoint of days alive out of hospital over the next 6 months, although there was a strong trend for benefit in the higher volume centers (Fig. 12-2). Despite slightly higher overall net diuresis in patients whose therapy was monitored with the PAC (average 1.9 days of invasive monitoring),

there was significantly less deterioration in renal function by discharge. There was a consistent trend for better functional capacity and quality of life in the patients whose therapy was adjusted with the PAC (Fig. 12-3). Reduction in pulmonary capillary wedge pressure correlated with greater improvement in functional status, and the final pulmonary capillary wedge pressure was a strong predictor for the primary endpoint.

Based on the lack of benefit for the primary endpoint, PAC is not recommended during routine therapy of patients hospitalized with heart failure, nor is it recommended in centers that do not currently have extensive experience in the monitoring and therapy of this hospitalized population. It is reasonable, however, to consider the use of PAC monitoring to further adjust therapy in patients who demonstrate recurrent or refractory symptoms despite ongoing standard therapy adjusted according to clinical assessment (Table 12-5). Although randomized trial data do not address, nor are they likely to address in future, the potential benefit of PAC specifically for the small number of patients who appear dependent on intravenous inotropic agents, use of PAC

▶ **Table 12-6** Clinical improvement during hospitalization

Major clinical benefits achieved in both treatment groups during heart failure hospitalization		
	PAC n = 215	*Clinical Assessment n = 218*
Net weight loss, kg	4 (±5.4)	3.2 (±4.2)
JVP (average)	From 12 to 7 cm	From 12 to 7 cm
Edema >1 +	68% down to 4%	68% down to 5%
Orthopnea (0–4)	−1.4 (1.2)	−1.2 (1.2)
Improvement in worse symptom score (100)	25 (25)	24 (24)
RAP, mm Hg	14 down to 10 mm Hg	
PCW, mm Hg	25 down to 17	
SVR	1500 down to 1100	
Cardiac output	1.9 up to 2.4	

All changes during hospitalization are significant in each group
Source: Adapted from ESCAPE Investigators and Coordinators. Evaluation study of congestive heart failure and pulmonary artery catheterization. *JAMA.* 2005;294:1625–1633.

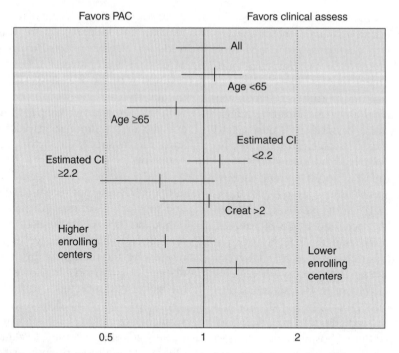

Figure 12-2   Days alive out of hospital during the 6 months after heart failure hospitalization during which therapy was guided by clinical assessment alone or clinical assessment in combination with PAC monitoring. The overall outcome was neutral, with a trend for benefit in patients who appeared to be in the "warm and wet" profile on admission. The benefit of PAC was more apparent in the high enrolling centers compared to the low enrolling centers (divided at the median site enrollment). PAC—pulmonary artery catheter.

for more precise adjustment of fluid status and vasodilator therapy seems warranted in view of the dismal prognosis if intravenous inotropic therapy is administered continuously for chronic palliation.

B-Type Natriuretic Peptide Levels

B-type natriuretic peptide (BNP) levels have been useful in the urgent evaluation of dyspnea in patients without previous diagnosis and in stratifying risk for patients in the peri-infarction period, at the time of hospital admission, and at the time of hospital discharge. BNP levels between 200 and 1000 characterize the majority of patients with chronic heart failure with low EF, slightly lower values characterize patients with heart failure and preserved EF, and persistent levels over 1300 predict highest risk for patients with known chronic heart failure.[14,15]

BNP levels tend to run higher with older age and worse renal dysfunction, and lower with obesity. They are correlated with filling pressures, and tend to change directionally with changes in filling pressures, but may continue to decline over time despite stable fluid balance. The baseline levels and the slopes of change for BNP levels vary widely between individuals. Current trials are testing whether BNP levels can be used as a target for adjusting therapy over time in the outpatient setting. At the present time, high BNP levels in the inpatient setting may identify patients at high risk for poor outcome, but are not therapeutic targets.

Echocardiographic Measurements

Multiple parameters that can be measured or estimated from echocardiography might become

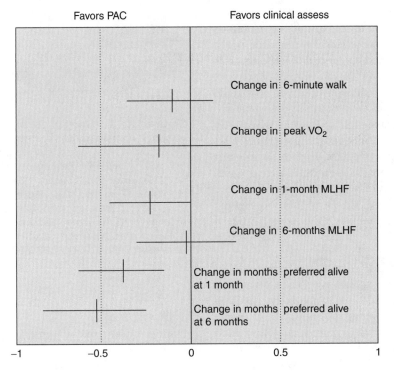

Figure 12-3 Demonstration of consistent trend for greater functional improvement in therapy guided by the PAC compared to therapy guided by clinical assessment alone. Patient preference for months alive was determined using the time trade-off tool, which asks patients how much time they would give up in order to feel better for their remaining time, and showed greater improvement in after PAC-guided therapy at all time points measured (1, 2, 3, and 6 months after discharge). PAC—pulmonary artery catheter; Peak VO_2—peak oxygen consumption during exercise; MLHF—Minnesota Living with Heart Failure questionnaire.

useful targets for acute adjustment of therapy, as serial echocardiography at the bedside and in the clinic becomes more feasible. Left-sided filling pressures can be estimated from the mitral regurgitation profile and simultaneous systolic blood pressure, right-sided venous pressures can be estimated from the inferior vena cava size and respiratory changes, pulmonary artery systolic pressure can be estimated from the tricuspid regurgitant velocity, and flow volumes can be estimated. Current calculations for absolute regurgitant volume are likely too cumbersome for rapid serial measurement by current techniques. The amount of mitral and tricuspid regurgitation can be qualitatively estimated, which may help confirm the directional change of clinical status, but at this time are not specific targets of therapy.

▶ SPECIFIC THERAPIES

Use of Diuretics—All Ejection Fraction

Assuming the presence of volume overload, escalating diuretic therapy is an early focus of hospitalization. Discussed in detail in Chap. 10, diuresis is often initiated with an intravenous bolus of at least the milligram equivalent of oral furosemide, with subsequent dose doubling until brisk diuresis is noted, then boluses two to three times daily in the hospital. Continuous furosemide infusion should be considered initially when the need for large volume diuresis is anticipated, or after initial boluses have not been effective. Supplementation with a thiazide diuretic, oral metolazone, or intravenous hydrodiuril frequently initiates brisk diuresis when loop diuretics alone are ineffective in a patient after chronic high-dose therapy. If diuresis remains ineffective, particularly in the setting of marginal blood pressure, it may be necessary to consider whether to reduce doses of neurohormonal antagonists until diuresis is achieved. Use of additional vasoactive infusion is discussed below.

Mechanical fluid removal may be considered when other efforts to remove excess fluid have been unsuccessful. This previously required cumbersome machinery and physical restriction of the patient by large catheters. Often fluid removal sufficient to relieve symptoms in diuretic resistance has been followed by progressive renal insufficiency. Now that fluid can be more easily removed in ambulatory patients without high volume circuits, ambulatory fluid removal devices are under investigation for use earlier in the hospital course. However, renal function and electrolytes should be monitored closely during any intervention that removes fluid rapidly.

Addition of Vasoactive Intravenous Agents

During hospitalizations for dilated low EF heart failure, intravenous vasodilators or inotropic agents are added in approximately 25% of patients (Fig. 12-4).[3] The major agents currently considered for addition to diuretic therapy during heart failure hospitalization are the vasodilators nesiritide and nitroglycerin, and the intravenous inotropic agents dobutamine, low-dose dopamine, or milrinone. A brief review of these intravenous vasoactive agents will be followed by discussion of situations in which they might be used.

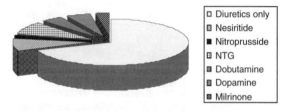

Figure 12-4 Current use of intravenous vasoactive therapy during heart failure hospitalization in the United States. Data are based on the ADHERE Registry. ADHERE—Acute Decompensated Heart Failure National Registry. (Fonarow GC, Abraham WT, Yancy CW, et al. Risk stratification for in-hospital mortality in acutely decompensated heart failure: classification and regression tree analysis. *JAMA.* 2005;293:572–580.)

Vasodilators

During chronic decompensation of dilated low EF heart failure, vasoconstriction is frequently present. In the previous era prior to the chronic use of ACE inhibitors, vasoconstriction was a more prominent part of decompensation, with systemic vascular resistance often above 1500–2000 dynes/s/cm.[5,16] Nitroprusside is a potent balanced vasodilator resulting in immediate reductions in systemic vascular resistance and venoconstriction. Pulmonary capillary wedge pressure falls and cardiac output increases, often by 30% or more. Nitroprusside remains the most effective and reliable vasodilator when systemic vascular resistances are high, but is limited by cyanide toxicity and diminishing physician familiarity with its use. The other nitrosovasodilator, nitroglycerin, has slightly less arterial vasodilation but is also effective when titrated to reduce vasoconstriction. The need for monitored titration of these nitrosovasodilators limited their use in favor of the more convenient inotropic agents except at experienced heart failure centers.

More recent hemodynamic studies indicate less vasoconstriction at the time of decompensation, even in advanced heart failure trial populations, perhaps related in part to the effects of chronic inhibition of the renin-angiotensin system in earlier stages of heart failure.[13] At the same time, the identification and recombinant technology for manufacture of the human BNP created enthusiasm for use of this endogenous vasodilator. Used in pharmacologic doses in heart failure patients, nesiritide is a modest arterial vasodilator that causes reductions of pulmonary capillary wedge and right atrial pressures, which were linked to improvement in heart failure symptoms. Nesiritide caused slightly greater reduction of pulmonary artery and pulmonary capillary wedge pressures with slightly less reduction in blood pressure than nitroglycerin titrated in a blinded protocol to relatively low doses.[17]

In addition to systemic vasodilation, the natriuretic peptides are renal vasodilators that increase renal blood flow. Their natriuretic effect is modest, but may allow a decrease in total diuretic dose. The clinical significance of these cardiorenal effects during heart failure hospitalization is controversial, and remains under investigation.

Administration of either nitroglycerin or nesiritide has been shown to accelerate improvement of heart failure symptoms after hospital admission.[17] Nitroglycerin causes headaches more often than nesiritide. All vasodilators can cause hypotension, which is generally well tolerated in supine patients, and responds to withdrawal of the vasodilator, although resolution takes longer with nesiritide due to the longer half-life. Both nitroglycerin and nesiritide occasionally cause hypotension associated with bradycardia. The biggest concern for the use of vasodilators is in patients who have been incorrectly assessed to have elevated volume status but actually are volume depleted or excessively vasodilated prior to administration.

Inotropic Agents

The most common intravenous inotropic agent used during heart failure hospitalization is dobutamine, which acts through β-adrenergic receptors to increase cyclic adenosine monophosphate

(AMP) production.[18] Cardiac output is increased, often with a slight increase in blood pressure. Stimulation of peripheral β-receptors without significant α-receptor stimulation leads to a slight decrease in systemic vascular resistance in most patients, but to a lesser degree than seen with intravenous vasodilators. Pulmonary capillary wedge pressure is modestly decreased. Heart rate usually increases, particularly in atrial fibrillation. Dobutamine increases the occurrence of atrial fibrillation and ventricular tachyarrhythmias. Clinical ischemic episodes are increased with dobutamine, which has also been associated with asymptomatic troponin leak. Due to these risks, and to the difficulty of weaning after intravenous inotropic therapy, doses used should be the lowest that provide the desired effect. Patients with chronic heart failure often respond well to doses as low as 2 μg/kg/min of dobutamine, and rarely need the 5 μg/kg/min that has often been used as a starting dose.

Dopamine binds to β-receptors but also stimulates α-adrenergic receptors and dopaminergic receptors located primarily in the kidney. Low-dose dopamine ($\leq$3 mcg/kg/min) sufficient to activate renal dopaminergic receptors is frequently said to be "renal-dose dopamine." At doses of 1–3 μg/kg/min for patients with heart failure, however, responses are very similar to those observed with dobutamine in terms of blood pressure and urine output. While there is little information regarding any selective renal effects, all doses of dopamine have detectable hemodynamic effects to increase cardiac output, heart rate, and potentially ischemia and tachyarrhythmias when used in patients with heart failure. As dopamine can release norepinephrine from nerve terminals, initiation may theoretically be associated more with tachycardia and ischemia than with dobutamine, but clinical events appear similar. Dopamine at a low dose is a reasonable drug to initiate in a patient in whom declining perfusion may necessitate escalation to pressor doses if early response is not favorable. Doses $\geq$5 mcg/kg/min usually increase systemic vascular resistance (Fig. 12-5), with

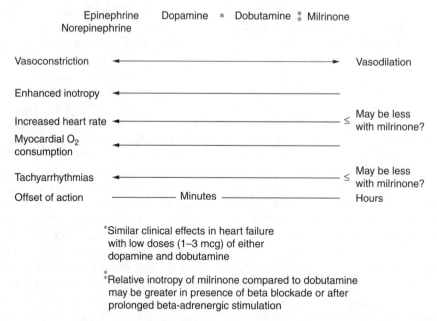

Figure 12-5 Qualitative comparison of perceived effects from current intravenous inotropic agents as clinically used for patients with heart failure. Relative effects are drawn in direction but not to scale. (Adapted from Stevenson LW. Clinical use of inotropic therapy for heart failure: looking backward or forward? Part I: inotropic infusions during hospitalization. *Circulation.* 2003;108:367–372.)

increasing inotropy and vasoconstriction up to doses of 15–20 mcg/kg/min, above which there is little further clinical effect.

In the rare cases of acute deterioration where blood pressure cannot be supported with escalating doses of dopamine, further inotropic and vasoconstrictor effect can be gained from the full agonist epinephrine, starting at doses of 1 μg/min (not usually dosed per kilogram). The most common time this is employed is in patients with acute fulminant myocarditis or shock post-infarction or cardiotomy. Norepinephrine is occasionally employed when abnormal vasodilation is suspected, because it has little effect on the vasodilatory β_2-adrenergic receptors and is thus an even more potent vasoconstrictor than epinephrine. It is also considered more likely to cause renal and peripheral ischemic injury. These two agents carry high risks of tachyarrhythmias and ischemia (Fig. 12-5), and their use is reserved only for imminent life-threatening situations while more definitive intervention is arranged.

Particularly for the vasoplegia that occasionally develops in severe circulatory compromise, vasopressin may provide additional support for blood pressure and potentiate the actions of the catecholamines. All of these agents have half-lives in minutes, and can be rapidly titrated and weaned.

Milrinone, often termed an "ino-dilator," is a phosphodiesterase inhibitor, the only one currently approved. It acts directly to inhibit the breakdown of cyclic AMP, bypassing the β-receptors that may become downregulated after prolonged stimulation. The phosphodiesterase inhibitors, however, do appear to cause other downregulatory adaptations. As with other inotropic agents, the risks of tachycardia and ischemia are increased by milrinone. Compared to the other inotropic agents, the phosphodiesterase inhibitors cause more vasodilation, which in some patients may be the dominant effect. Milrinone should *not* be used when the primary concern is hypotension, which can be aggravated. Clinical hypotensive episodes occurred more commonly with milrinone than with placebo infusion in one trial.[19] This is particularly concerning as the pharmacologic half-life of milrinone is 2–4 hours, and is prolonged by impaired renal excretion. The physiological offset may be further prolonged, often lasting up to a day after discontinuation of chronic use.

Because milrinone bypasses the β-receptors, it is often considered for patients felt to need inotropic support in the presence of β-adrenergic blockade. If the major concern is hypotension, milrinone should still not be the first choice for the reasons above, as blood pressure may fall further. β-Adrenergic antagonism is rarely complete in these patients, who will generally respond to dobutamine and dopamine, although higher doses may be required. In general, there is no consistent rationale for patients requiring urgent inotropic support to be maintained on previous

β-blockers, particularly when the situation may be deteriorating.

Levosimendan, an intravenous inotropic agent, is a calcium sensitizer that increases contractility, lowers filling pressures, and also acts on potassium sensitive channels to cause vasodilation.[20] It appears to be as safe as dobutamine as used in clinical trials, and is currently approved in some European countries for acute therapy of heart failure.

Vasodilators Compared to Inotropic Agents

When vasoconstriction is marked, increases in cardiac output are often comparable between the inotropic agents dobutamine and milrinone and the nitrosovasodilators nitroprusside and nitroglycerin (Fig. 12-6). While cardiac output increased to a similar degree with all three agents, there were greater decreases in systemic

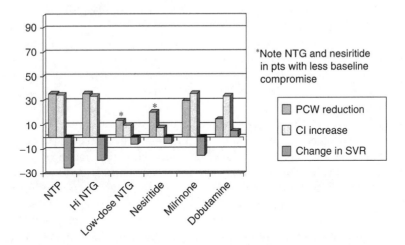

Figure 12-6 Hemodynamic effects of nitrosovasodilators (NTP and NTG) and current intravenous inotropic therapy as described in different studies. The populations in which nitroprusside, dobutamine, and milrinone were compared had more severe hemodynamic compromise and more striking hemodynamic changes during therapy than the patients receiving low-dose NTG and nesiritide in the VMAC trial, as described by Monrad et al. The high-dose nitroglycerin study was reported by Elkayam et al. NTP—nitroprusside; NTG—nitroglycerin; VMAC—Vasodilation in the Management of Acute Congestive Heart Failure. (VMAC Investigators. Intravenous nesiritide vs nitroglycerin for treatment of decompensated congestive heart failure: a randomized controlled trial. *JAMA.* 2002;287:1531–1540. Monrad ES, Baim DS, Smith HS, et al. Milrinone, dobutamine, and nitroprusside: comparative effects on hemodynamics and myocardial energetics in patients with severe congestive heart failure. *Circulation.* 1986;73:III168–III174. Elkayam U. Nitrates in the treatment of congestive heart failure. *Am J Cardiol.* 1996;77:C41–C51.)

vascular resistance and pulmonary capillary wedge pressure with nitroprusside and milrinone compared to dobutamine when they were compared directly.[21] Milrinone and nitroglycerin titrated up to effect also had a similar hemodynamic impact. For patients with normal systemic vascular resistance, there are few comparative data, but it is likely that dobutamine would increase cardiac output more than the vasodilators and be more likely to maintain blood pressure. Experience with the vasodilator nesiritide demonstrates lower incidence of ventricular arrhythmia and ischemia than with dobutamine in patients hospitalized with heart failure. Heart rate and blood pressure are both lower with nesiritide than with inotropic agents.

Initiation of inotropes is often considered more convenient, as there is less concern about initial responses than with intravenous vasodilators. However, after initial stabilization, continued use of these infusions may mask inadequacy or intolerability of the oral regimen. It is thus recommended that these infusions be stopped at least 24–48 hours prior to discharge to determine stability on oral therapy.[22] Although requiring more supervision to initiate, vasodilator infusions are more convenient once it is time to wean onto oral therapies. Failure of weaning is much less common with vasodilator than with inotropic therapy, unless diuresis has been inadequate prior to weaning. The effects of intravenous vasodilators can more easily be matched with available oral therapies.

Randomized trial data are very limited regarding these agents in hospitalized populations. In a randomized trial of patients without baseline hypotension, the addition of milrinone was associated with more hypotension, tachyarrhythmias, and other cardiac events than placebo infusion, with no benefit for subsequent outcomes.[19] Nitroglycerin and nesiritide caused earlier symptom relief and lower wedge pressures than placebo infusions.[17] Most information comparing inotropes and vasodilator agents derives from retrospective review, in which it is not possible to capture all of the reasons leading to use of inotropic therapy, vasodilator therapy, or neither. Attempts to determine the factors leading to selection of inotropic therapy suggest that the

practice at a given site dominates over physiologic variables. Nonetheless, a consistent theme emerges of worse in-hospital and subsequent outcomes in patients who have received intravenous inotropic therapy while in hospital. These differences persist when adjusted for all recognized clinical factors contributing to outcome, such as renal function, blood pressure, serum sodium, and diuretic dose. Patients receiving intravenous vasodilators in actual practice have baseline profiles indicative of more compromise than patients not receiving any intravenous therapy except diuretics. Outcomes with intravenous vasodilator therapy in these analyses have not been significantly different from outcomes with no vasoactive therapy, with or without adjustment for baseline characteristics.

▶ COMBINING THERAPIES FOR PROFILES

Wet and Warm—Diuretics Only? (All Ejection Fraction)

The first decision regarding intravenous vasoactive therapy is made at the time of admission. Most patients will demonstrate moderate decompensation with congestive symptoms without evidence of acute circulatory compromise. Diuretic therapy would be initiated during continuation of the usual outpatient heart failure regimen, with consideration of additional vasoactive therapy if the response to escalating diuretic doses was inadequate over the next 48–72 hours. Patients who have required additional intravenous therapy for adequate response on previous admissions, or those in whom effective therapy was previously limited by poor renal function, might be considered for earlier use of these adjunctive intravenous agents but should also undergo frank discussions about prognosis and the appropriate goals of subsequent care.

Occasionally patients will present with frank pulmonary edema, often due to sudden severe elevation of filling pressures, particularly in the presence of severe hypertension or relatively low plasma oncotic pressure. This presentation is more common in patients with preserved than reduced LVEF. In this emergency setting of impending respiratory failure, intravenous vasodilators should be started along with diuretics for rapid relief of symptoms, improved oxygenation, and hopefully avoidance of intubation. Assuming that systolic blood pressure is adequate, intravenous nitroglycerin or nesiritide may be used. Nitroprusside is generally avoided in the emergency setting where myocardial ischemia may be present, due to concern that nitroprusside may produce coronary steal.

Intravenous vasoactive therapy is not currently considered necessary for most wet and warm patients, but it may allow lesser total diuretic dose. There is increasing concern that high doses of diuretics not only identify patients with poor underlying renal compensation, but may actually aggravate renal dysfunction during diuresis. It is not known whether patients requiring high doses to overcome diuretic "resistance" would benefit from earlier use of intravenous therapies that might improve renal blood flow and decrease diuretic requirements, to "spare" the kidney.

Definition of Two Limiting Profiles—All Ejection Fraction

During therapy directed to relieve congestion as clinically assessed, some patients who initially appear to fit the above profile of warm and wet do not respond as anticipated. Two recognized patterns that limit efficacy of the usual hierarchy of diuretic therapies are disproportionate right ventricular (RV) dysfunction and the cardiorenal syndrome (Fig. 12-1). Intravenous vasoactive infusions are frequently added to facilitate diuresis for these limiting profiles.

Right Ventricular > Left Ventricular Failure

Most patients with chronic heart failure have RV filling pressures that are less than half of the left-sided ventricular filling pressures, although they generally change in parallel. In the hemodynamic study of 1000 patients by Drazner, only 6% of patients had right atrial pressures >10 if the pulmonary wedge pressure was <22 mm Hg.[4] As outcomes improve with heart failure, however, there is the clinical impression that more patients

are surviving to develop progressive right heart failure. It should be emphasized that the distinction is not necessarily apparent from clinical assessment, as many patients with the average right-left relationship of elevated filling pressures will nonetheless have their clinical presentation dominated by symptoms of systemic venous congestion rather than dyspnea.

For patients in whom the right-sided pressures are more than two-thirds the left, it is more difficult to gauge optimal volume status. If the jugular venous pressure is reduced to the usual near-normal targets, the left-sided filling pressures could be excessively reduced, leading to a fall in cardiac output, hypotension, and renal dysfunction. More commonly, it is not possible to reduce the right atrial pressures, leading to escalating interventions with their own risks. Patients in whom diuresis is ineffective or limited by hypotension while jugular venous pressures are still elevated may benefit from invasive measurement of hemodynamics in order to establish modified filling pressure targets.

For the RV profile, vasodilation can be helpful if left-sided filling pressures are also markedly elevated, as the reduction of systemic vascular resistance, mitral regurgitation, and pulmonary pressures should allow better RV performance. Often, however, inotropic therapy is used to increase cardiac output and improve hemodynamic status. It is generally difficult to maintain improvement once inotropic therapy is weaned. If left ventricular assist device support is being considered, these patients need thoughtful evaluation regarding the potential need for added RV support.

The Cardiorenal Syndrome (All Ejection Fraction)

Whether LVEF is low or preserved, renal function becomes the major limiting factor in effective therapy during at least 25% of heart failure hospitalizations. The cardiorenal syndrome is variously defined, but might be considered the worsening of renal function (e.g., ≥0.3 mg or 25% increase of creatinine) during diuresis for symptomatic heart failure, despite persistence of clinical volume overload.[23] While little is known about the specific causes and therapeutic targets of the cardiorenal syndrome, the major advance that has been made in understanding is the growing recognition that the acute decline in renal function is *not* usually the result of an acute decline in cardiac output.[24] This has been appreciated from direct hemodynamic studies, but also from the prevalence of the same clinical syndrome in patients with preserved LVEF in whom resting cardiac output is not reduced. For patients with low EF, the contribution of chronically impaired renal perfusion is assumed. For patients with preserved EF, additional components may be the greater prevalence of diabetes and baseline renal dysfunction, often in the setting of hypertension. Additional risk factors for all LVEF groups include chronic high diuretic dosage, duration of heart failure, and baseline renal dysfunction.[25] Although the data are not well-established, there may be a major overlap between the disproportionate RV profile and the cardiorenal syndrome.

The pathophysiology is now agreed to include direct cardiorenal connections beyond those provided by central cardiac output (*http:// www.nhlbi.nih.gov/meetings/workshops/cardiorenal-hf-hd.htm*). Low pressure baroreceptors within the atria and pulmonary circuit may become desensitized by chronic distention, such that beneficial volume reduction is transduced as volume depletion. Changes in vasopressin and other circulating neurohormones are tightly influenced by cardiac distention, vascular baroreceptors, and intrarenal hemodynamics. Multiple responses in the glomeruli, afferent and efferent arterioles, and tubules likely contribute to the diminution in effective renal blood flow and increase in fluid retention in chronic heart failure. There is increasing concern that the high doses of diuretics used to achieve clinical targets may themselves be contributing to progressive renal dysfunction. Nonetheless, the robust relationship between elevated filling pressures and adverse outcomes mandate continued focus on volume reduction, hopefully with newer strategies.

The cardiorenal syndrome is generally treated with agents that could improve renal blood flow.

One method is to increase renal blood flow by increasing total cardiac output. This can be accomplished by low-dose inotropic therapy with dobutamine or dopamine, without evidence that any selective dopaminergic effect of dopamine is clinically useful. For some patients with marked volume overload, the progressive improvement that can occur in cardiac performance, peripheral perfusion, nutrition, and activity with diuresis may be adequate to maintain better renal function even after the inotropic therapy is discontinued.

The development of selective agents to enhance renal vasodilation remains a focus of new investigation. The natriuretic peptides can enhance renal blood flow as well as inhibit tubular reabsorption in multiple experimental settings. It has been difficult to show these effects in clinical practice for patients with the cardiorenal syndrome. BNP, nesiritide, has been associated with improved renal function in acute renal failure and is currently being studied in postoperative settings as well as in patients hospitalized with risk factors for the cardiorenal syndrome. Combinations of natriuretic peptides are also under investigation for this condition. Specific inhibitors of vasopressin and adenosine are also being evaluated.

Wet and Cold—How Acute?

The patient presenting with chronic decompensation and a cold and wet profile would generally be considered early for initiation of additional vasoactive therapy "to warm up" in order to "dry out."[22] As the "cold and wet" profile is an imprecise clinical definition, it would also be reasonable in some cases to observe the initial response to intravenous diuretic therapy before adding other therapy, particularly if there is an obvious factor to be addressed, such as recent increase in β-blocker dose or anemia requiring transfusion. The choice of vasodilators or inotropic agents in this population depends upon the adequacy of blood pressure and the assumption regarding systemic vascular resistance. When perfusion appears inadequate, it is important to reevaluate the level of neurohormonal antagonist therapy. Patients who have recently had initiation or escalation of β-blocker therapy should return to the previous level until stabilized. Inhibition of the renin-angiotensin system can also decrease perfusion in patients whose clinical compromise is so severe that angiotensin is potentiating maintenance of systolic blood pressure. These inhibitors may occasionally need to be stopped or decreased when adequate perfusion cannot be maintained. It remains controversial when or whether it is preferable to continue neurohormonal antagonism when the price includes the addition of inotropic therapy with its inherent risks.

Patients with dilated low EF heart failure who are initially without evidence of hypoperfusion may occasionally move into the cold and wet profile during observation, particularly in conjunction with the cardiorenal syndrome. Inotropic therapy is generally chosen over vasodilator therapy in the presence of severe hypotension (systolic blood pressure <80 mm Hg), for which vasodilator therapy should be administered only with extreme caution, usually with invasive monitoring.

It is critical to identify the patient in whom hypoperfusion is acutely progressive, with imminent compromise of organ function. This is the patient who presents a hemodynamic cold and wet profile together with additional components of life-threatening circulatory compromise such as lactic acidosis, anuria, declining mental status, or systolic blood pressure <70 mm Hg. The initial therapy for this patient will include inotropic stimulation with blood pressure support, usually with dopamine at pressor (vasoconstriction) doses. In the occasional patient who fails to respond, addition of epinephrine provides additional inotropic stimulation, although at high cost of tachyarrhythmias and ischemia.[18] At this level of circulatory compromise, mechanical support should be considered immediately if appropriate in terms of the longer term outlook. It should be recognized that only a small minority of patients are appropriate candidates for urgent support with current mechanical devices. For patients in whom circulatory compromise is not rapidly resolving, decisions will need to be made expeditiously regarding the appropriate escalation of intervention or shift to emphasis on comfort over life-sustaining measures.

▶ DESIGN FOR DISCHARGE

Design of the regimen for discharge should be a topic of consideration as soon as the patient is admitted (Table 12-2). At that time, consideration of the factors leading to hospital admission should include not only the medication regimen, but patient understanding and compliance, and potential exacerbating factors to be addressed during hospitalization, such as hypothyroidism or atrial fibrillation with rapid ventricular rates.

Neurohormonal Antagonists and Vasodilators

Once the patient has reached optimal volume status, neurohormonal antagonist therapy should be adjusted. Neurohormonal inhibition is generally not increased while volume overload persists, as transient decreases in cardiac output and blood pressure may impair effective diuresis. (For patients admitted with heart failure and hypertension, neurohormonal antagonists may be titrated up immediately as needed for blood pressure control, with close monitoring of renal function.) On the other hand, doses of renin-angiotensin system antagonists tolerated during volume overload may cause too much vasodilation when volume status is restored to normal and the peripheral vasculature is more responsive.

Initiation of β-blockade in hospital has been shown to be well-tolerated and effective in many patients with good baseline blood pressure who have responded well to diuretic therapy without evidence of hypoperfusion or the need for inotropic support (Table 12-3).[26] If such patients were previously stable on β-blocker therapy before admission, most can be discharged on the same doses. Patients with recent escalation in dose prior to admission should in general be discharged on the earlier dose. For patients with recent need for inotropic support, severely reduced renal function, or systolic blood pressures <90 mm Hg, β-blockers would generally not be started until stability was demonstrated in the first few weeks after discharge. The striking benefit of β-blockers to decrease mortality, hospitalizations, and disease progression mandates that they be considered for all patients with heart failure, including the elderly. Despite vigorous efforts, however, β-blocker therapy is successfully initiated in only 65–80% of patients requiring hospitalizations for advanced heart failure. Patients admitted on β-blockers in whom they have to be discontinued by the time of hospital discharge have a 6-month mortality over twice as high as those who can tolerate β-blocker therapy.

The majority of patients tolerate ACE inhibitors or angiotensin receptor blockers even in late-stage heart failure. However, some patients develop circulatory-renal limitations of hypotension, progressive renal dysfunction, or hyperkalemia that lead to discontinuation of ACE inhibitors. While the relative risks and benefits of ACE inhibitors in such patients have not been established, those who discontinue ACE inhibitors for these reasons have a 1-year mortality that exceeds 50%.[27]

Spironolactone has been shown to improve survival and decrease hospitalizations when patients are carefully selected and monitored to reduce the risk of life-threatening hyperkalemia.[28,29] Particular care is required when initiating this potassium-sparing diuretic during periods of changing volume status and renal function. Of particular concern is the patient with fluctuating renal function who tolerates spironolactone initiated in the hospital during active diuresis and kaliuresis, in whom hyperkalemia may not manifest until after discharge.

Combinations of hydralazine and nitrates, or, in some patients, high-dose nitrates alone, represent alternative therapy for patients no longer able to tolerate ACE inhibitors. Nitrates have often been added to ACE inhibitors in patients to treat persistent exertional dyspnea or marked vasoconstriction. Recent information on the benefit of adding the hydralazine-nitrate combination to ACE inhibitors in moderate-severe ambulatory heart failure indicates that these three agents in combination can produce further benefit in survival and quality of life.[30]

Risk Assessment During Hospitalization

Multiple parameters predict clinical outcome during and after hospitalization with heart failure. At the time of admission, risk for long length of stay and in-hospital mortality has been analyzed from the ADHERE database of routine clinical information for over 100,000 hospitalizations, both with reduced and preserved EFs.[3] The strongest adverse predictive factor was admission blood urea nitrogen of >43 mg/dL. Once knowing that, the next stratification was systolic blood pressure > or <115 mm Hg. For populations with more advanced disease and rehospitalizations (Table 12-3), high blood urea nitrogen or creatinine and low systolic blood pressure also predict worse outcome.[3,13] Additional information is provided in that population by elevated right atrial filling or pulmonary capillary wedge pressures, with the most predictive measurements being those obtained after best efforts to optimize therapy. High BNP levels at admission predict longer stay and higher in-hospital mortality. Discharge BNP levels are even more predictive, indicating that those patients whose BNP decreases during in-hospital therapy have a better outcome than those whose BNP remains higher.[15] In the advanced heart failure population, short 6-minute walk distance at discharge, or the inability to do the 6-minute walk test, additionally predicts rehospitalization and mortality. The discharge regimen itself is predictive, with those patients on β-blockers, ACE inhibitors, and low diuretic doses having the best outcome. Patients at high risk for rehospitalization and death should be carefully evaluated for further intervention.

A few selected patients may have options for cardiac transplantation or left ventricular assist devices. Others may benefit from enrollment in intensive heart failure management programs, some with options for home monitoring in addition to daily weights and frequent phone calls. For patients without definitive replacement options, discussions should take place regarding patient preferences and increasing emphasis on palliation of symptoms.[31]

Patients with LVEF ≤30% have a significant risk of sudden death that increases with the clinical severity of disease. Patients with a prior history of sudden death, ventricular tachycardia, or syncope are at highest risk. Patients with this history and otherwise good prognosis for 1–2-year survival should undergo defibrillator implantation during the related hospitalization or as soon as possible thereafter. For patients who have not had prior events, the risk for sudden death increases in parallel with the risk for terminal hemodynamic decompensation, which is now the dominant mode of death for patients with heart failure. The risk factors discussed above identify patients who are most likely to have recurrent heart failure events. A robust predictor of poor outcome remains Class IV symptoms, defined as symptoms at rest or with minimal exertion. These are the indications for most heart failure hospitalizations, and constitute a contraindication to defibrillator implantation.

Stability at a better functional class cannot be determined until patients return for follow-up after hospitalization. Furthermore, there is some concern that defibrillator implantation after a recent event such as myocardial infarction may itself be associated with increased nonsudden death.[32] With these considerations, it is reasonable to defer decisions regarding implantable cardioverter defibrillator (ICD) implantation for primary prevention to the outpatient setting.

Criteria for Discharge

With rising concern for hospital costs associated with length of stay, there is frequently pressure to discharge patients as soon as symptoms have improved. Failure to address all of the goals of hospitalization is a common cause for hospital readmission. It is frequently said that the first day of readmission is a more costly one than an extra day to ensure stability at the end of the initial hospitalization. Most crucial are the goals of stability (Table 12-7). Specifically, patients should demonstrate stability of fluid balance and blood pressure for at least 24 hours on the regimen planned for discharge.[22] If intravenous therapy has been used, patients should not be discharged until at least 24 hours from the last intravenous therapy, or at least 48 hours after discontinuing an agent with prolonged physiological effects such as milrinone.

▶ **Table 12-7** Clinical stability

- ≥24 hours on oral regimen for discharge
  - Off short-acting intravenous agents ≥24 hours
  - Off long-acting agents ≥48 hours
  - No planned medication doses held
  - Stable blood pressure (systolic usually ≥80 mm Hg) without postural decline
- Stable fluid balance/renal function
- Ambulation without dyspnea or dizziness
- Demonstrated comprehension of fluid maintenance
  - Sodium and fluid intake
  - Weight monitoring
  - Symptoms of fluid overload
  - Flexible diuretic plan

Education should begin early during hospitalization, with involvement of both patient and family. Key components include the major symptoms of heart failure and the elements of stable fluid balance regarding salt, fluid intake, daily weights, and the flexible diuretic regimen. Connection to follow-up care is critical, both for scheduled follow-up and for early changes noted at home. The benefits of specific heart failure management after heart failure hospitalization have been clearly shown, reducing rehospitalization and mortality, within those programs where a specialized nurse or nurse practitioner with ongoing knowledge of the patient can implement treatment changes within specified ranges.[33] They have not been realized with centralized call centers isolated from patients and clinical decision makers.

Heart failure is a chronic undulating disease with periods of good clinical stability and periods of decompensation. Presentation to the hospitalization serves as a warning that the clinical condition is no longer stable. Heart failure hospitalization must be viewed not as a challenge for rapid discharge, but as an opportunity to reevaluate, revise the medical regimen, and improve the clinical course. The hospital plays a central role in the overall continuum of inpatient and outpatient care, which must be coordinated and integrated in order to maximize the quality and length of life for patients with heart failure.

▶ REFERENCES

1. Lee DS, Austin PC, Rouleau JL, et al. Predicting mortality among patients hospitalized for heart failure: derivation and validation of a clinical model. *JAMA*. 2003;290:2581–2587.

2. MacIntyre K, Capewell S, Stewart S, et al. Evidence of improving prognosis in heart failure: trends in case fatality in 66 547 patients hospitalized between 1986 and 1995. *Circulation*. 2000;102:1126–1131.

3. Fonarow GC, Abraham WT, Yancy CW, et al. Risk stratification for in-hospital mortality in acutely decompensated heart failure: classification and regression tree analysis. *JAMA*. 2005;293:572–580.

4. Drazner MH, Yancy C, Shah MR, et al. Utility of the history and physical examination in assessing hemodynamics in patients with advanced heart failure: the ESCAPE trial (abstract). *Circulation*. 2005;112:11–640.

5. Stevenson LW, Perloff JK. The limited reliability of physical signs for estimating hemodynamics in chronic heart failure. *JAMA*. 1989;261:884–888.

6. Nohria A, Lewis E, Stevenson LW. Medical management of advanced heart failure. *JAMA*. 2002;287:628–640.

7. Nohria A, Tsang SW, Fang JC, et al. Clinical assessment identifies hemodynamic profiles that predict outcomes in patients admitted with heart failure. *J Am Coll Cardiol*. 2003;41:1797–1804.

8. Stevenson L, Bellil D, Grover-McKay M, et al. Effects of afterload reduction (diuretics and vasodilators) on left ventricular volume and mitral regurgitation in severe congestive heart failure secondary to ischemic or idiopathic dilated cardiomyopathy. *Am J Cardiol*. 1987;60:654–658.

9. Stevenson LW, Tillisch JH. Maintenance of cardiac output with normal filling pressures in patients with dilated heart failure. *Circulation*. 1986;74:1303–1308.

10. Rosario LB, Stevenson LW, Solomon SD, et al. The mechanism of decrease in dynamic mitral regurgitation during heart failure treatment: importance of reduction in the regurgitant orifice size. *J Am Coll Cardiol*. 1998;32:1819–1824.

11. Stevenson LW, Tillisch JH, Hamilton M, et al. Importance of hemodynamic response to therapy in predicting survival with ejection fraction less than or equal to 20% secondary to ischemic or nonischemic dilated cardiomyopathy. *Am J Cardiol*. 1990;66:1348–1354.

12. Stevenson LW. Tailored therapy to hemodynamic goals for advanced heart failure. *Eur J Heart Fail*. 1999;1:251–257.

13. ESCAPE Investigators and Coordinators. Evaluation study of congestive heart failure and pulmonary artery catheterization. *JAMA*. 2005; 294:1625–1633.

14. Johnson W, Omland T, Hall C, et al. Neurohormonal activation rapidly decreases after intravenous therapy with diuretics and vasodilators for class IV heart failure. *J Am Coll Cardiol*. 2002;39:1623–1629.

15. Logeart D, Thabut G, Jourdain P, et al. Predischarge B-type natriuretic peptide assay for identifying patients at high risk of re-admission after

decompensated heart failure. *J Am Coll Cardiol.* 2004;43:635–641.

16. Fonarow GC, Chelimsky-Fallick C, Stevenson LW, et al. Effect of direct vasodilation with hydralazine versus angiotensin-converting enzyme inhibition with captopril on mortality in advanced heart failure: the Hy-C trial. *J Am Coll Cardiol.* 1992;19:842–850.

17. VMAC Investigators. Intravenous nesiritide vs nitroglycerin for treatment of decompensated congestive heart failure: a randomized controlled trial. *JAMA.* 2002;287:1531–1540.

18. Stevenson LW. Clinical use of inotropic therapy for heart failure: looking backward or forward? Part I: inotropic infusions during hospitalization. *Circulation.* 2003;108:367–372.

19. Cuffe MS, Califf RM, Adams KF, Jr, et al. Short-term intravenous milrinone for acute exacerbation of chronic heart failure: a randomized controlled trial. *JAMA.* 2002;287:1541–1547.

20. Follath F, Cleland JG, Just H, et al. Efficacy and safety of intravenous levosimendan compared with dobutamine in severe low-output heart failure (the LIDO study): a randomised double-blind trial. *Lancet.* 2002;360:196–202.

21. Monrad ES, Baim DS, Smith HS, et al. Milrinone, dobutamine, and nitroprusside: comparative effects on hemodynamics and myocardial energetics in patients with severe congestive heart failure. *Circulation.* 1986;73: III168–III174.

22. Stevenson LW, Massie BM, Francis GS. Optimizing therapy for complex or refractory heart failure: a management algorithm. *Am Heart J.* 1998;135:S293–S309.

23. Gottlieb SS, Abraham W, Butler J, et al. The prognostic importance of different definitions of worsening renal function in congestive heart failure. *J Card Fail.* 2002;8:136–141.

24. Weinfeld MS, Chertow GM, Stevenson LW. Aggravated renal dysfunction during intensive therapy for advanced chronic heart failure. *Am Heart J.* 1999;138:285–290.

25. Forman DE, Butler J, Wang Y, et al. Incidence, predictors at admission, and impact of worsening renal function among patients hospitalized with heart failure. *J Am Coll Cardiol.* 2004;43:61–67.

26. Gattis WA, O'Connor CM, Gallup DS, et al. Predischarge initiation of carvedilol in patients hospitalized for decompensated heart failure: results of the Initiation Management Predischarge: Process for Assessment of Carvedilol Therapy in Heart Failure (IMPACT-HF) trial. *J Am Coll Cardiol.* 2004;43:1534–1541.

27. Kittleson M, Hurwitz S, Shah MR, et al. Development of circulatory-renal limitations to angiotensin-converting enzyme inhibitors identifies patients with severe heart failure and early mortality. *J Am Coll Cardiol.* 2003;41:2029–2035.

28. Pitt B, Zannad F, Remme WJ, Randomized Aldactone Evaluation Study Investigators. The effect of spironolactone on morbidity and mortality in patients with severe heart failure. *N Engl J Med.* 1999;341:709–717.

29. Bozkurt B, Agoston I, Knowlton AA. Complications of inappropriate use of spironolactone in heart failure: when an old medicine spirals out of new guidelines. *J Am Coll Cardiol.* 2003;41:211–214.

30. Taylor AL, Ziesche S, Yancy C, et al. Combination of isosorbide dinitrate and hydralazine in blacks with heart failure. *N Engl J Med.* 2004;351: 2049–2057.

31. Stevenson LW. Rites and responsibility for resuscitation in heart failure: tread gently on the thin places. *Circulation.* 1998;98:619–622.

32. Hohnloser SH, Kuck KH, Dorian P, et al. Prophylactic use of an implantable cardioverter-defibrillator after acute myocardial infarction. *N Engl J Med.* 2004;351:2481–2488.

33. McAlister FA, Stewart S, Ferrua S, et al. Multidisciplinary strategies for the management of heart failure patients at high risk for admission: a systematic review of randomized trials. *J Am Coll Cardiol.* 2004;44:810–819.

CHAPTER 13

Ancillary Pharmacologic Therapies for Heart Failure

HENRY KRUM, MBBS, PHD, FRACP

▶ INTRODUCTION

There have been considerable advances in the pharmacologic management of chronic heart failure (CHF) over the past 20 years. Both angiotensin-converting enzyme (ACE) inhibitors and β-adrenoceptor blockers have been shown to reduce mortality and improve symptom status in patients with systolic CHF. In patients with mild-to-moderate CHF, ACE inhibitors reduce absolute annual mortality by around 1.5%, β-blockers by 3.6%, and the two agents combined by 4.9%.[1] Angiotensin receptor blocking agents may confer additional mortality benefit. Nevertheless, mortality remains high in such patients (around 8% annual mortality) despite optimal use of current agents. Mortality remains very high in patients with more advanced disease despite use of ACE inhibitors, β-blockers, and aldosterone receptor antagonists. Furthermore, CHF is a debilitating condition with high morbidity, frequent hospitalization, and poor quality of life. Therefore, the need for new pharmacologic agents in addition to the above therapies continues to be a priority.

Novel therapies have emerged from our improved understanding of the pathophysiology of CHF. The benefits of blocking activated neurohormonal vasoconstrictor systems in CHF are now well-recognized. This has been supported by the success of treatment strategies involving blockade of the renin-angiotensin-aldosterone system (RAAS) (specifically with ACE inhibitors and aldosterone receptor antagonists) and the sympathetic nervous system (SNS) (specifically with β-blockers, angiotensin receptor blockers (ARBs), and aldosterone receptor antagonists). More recently, further understanding of other key systems involved in pathophysiologic responses to myocardial injury (Fig. 13-1) have led to promising new avenues for pharmacologic intervention that may be of therapeutic benefit in this condition.

This chapter focuses on new pharmacologic approaches to the perturbation of a number of these pathways of disease progression. Because

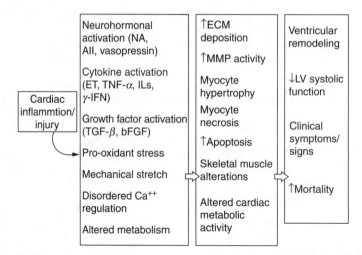

Figure 13–1   Key systems involved in pathophysiologic responses to myocardial injury. ET—exercise test; TNF—tumor necrosis factor; TGF—transforming growth factor; ECM—extracellular matrix; MMP—matrix metalloproteinase; LV—left ventricular; BFGF—basic fibroblast growth factor; NA—noradrenaline; AII—angiotensin II; ILS—interleukins; γ-IFN—interferon-gamma

of the large number of candidate drugs under investigation, this chapter focuses on agents that are currently in clinical development for the specific indication of CHF.

► RECENT TRIALS OF ANCILLARY THERAPIES

In the development of novel agents for the treatment of heart failure, it is important to consider the results of recent trials in the development of promising drug classes for this indication. These recent trials include studies of vasopeptidase inhibitors (Omapatrilat Versus Enalapril Randomized Trial of Utility in Reducing Events

[OVERTURE]), endothelin receptor antagonists (Endothelin Antagonist Bosentan for Lowering Cardiac Events in Heart Failure [ENABLE]), and tumor necrosis factor (TNF)-α inhibitory agents (Randomized Etanercept Worldwide Evaluation [RENEWAL]), Anti-TNF Therapy Against Congestive Heart Failure (ATTACH).[2–5] These studies were all based on compelling preclinical data and a strong mechanistic rationale. Furthermore there were supportive early phase data that led to these Phase III programs. The results of these study programs are summarized in Table 13-1.

It is therefore worth speculating, in the context of discussion of novel and emerging therapies, to consider why these strategies might have failed.

► **Table 13-1**   Recent trials of ancillary therapies

Trial	Drug/comparator	Class	Result
RENEWAL	Etanercept/placebo	TNF blockade	No significant ↓ death/HF hospitalization
ENABLE	Bosentan/placebo	Endothelin blockade	Early excess death/HF hospitalization with bosentan; no significant ↓ by study end
OVERTURE	Omapatrilat/enalapril	Vasopeptidase inhibition	Nonsignificant 6% death/HF hospitalization cf enalapril; noninferior to enalapril

A number of possibilities exist as to the failure of these agents in heart failure. First, it has been suggested that there may be a threshold for benefit of pharmacological therapy. Next, the patient population studied may have been too broad-based. Specific subgroups within the total heart failure population may have benefited the most. For example, with TNF antagonists, patients with evidence of cardiac cachexia and/or elevated baseline TNF levels may *a priori* be considered to be those most likely to benefit.

Further, some degree of target system activity may be required for maintenance of normal cardiac function. Therefore, even though the target system may be activated within the failing heart, complete inhibition may have contributed to lack of benefit. There is some evidence to support this from within the TNF literature.

Next, the target for drug therapy may have been too specific to be of benefit in the setting of a broad-based response to myocardial injury. Again, using the example of TNF-α blockade, these biologicals potently inhibit TNF without necessarily acting on other activated proinflammatory cytokines. In this way, only TNF and not other activated cytokines are inhibited and indeed there may be a negative feedback loop operative, which may further activate non-TNF-α proinflammatory cytokines.

Finally, there exists the concept of "regression to the truth" whereby therapies producing false-positive results in the early phase go on to be studied in the late phase with the therapy proving to be nonbeneficial when definitively tested.[6]

All the above are critical considerations in the planning of trials of novel therapies and will need to be considered in the development of new drugs as outlined in the remainder of this chapter.

► ANCILLARY THERAPIES IN CLINICAL DEVELOPMENT

Neurohormonal Blockade

It is well-recognized that blockade of the RAAS and SNS are the cornerstone of therapy for the treatment of heart failure. Therefore, it is not surprising that other, more recently discovered, neurohormonal systems may also be a target for pharmacological intervention in heart failure.

Development of these new therapies has proven more difficult than expected (as outlined above), for example, with regard to the development of endothelin antagonists. However, there are a number of other activated neurohormonal systems recently described that appear to play a role in heart failure disease progression.

Renin Blockade

Renin is the upstream substrate for RAAS activity and agents that block the biological activity of renin have been developed. The most advanced of these is the Novartis compound aliskerin. A highly bioavailable renin activity from Actelion is also soon to enter clinical development.

Despite low bioavailability, studies with the Novartis compound have demonstrated improved hemodynamic parameters and are about to enter an extensive clinical trial program in heart failure.[7]

The major drug development issue to be considered is whether renin blockade may offer therapeutic benefit over and above that observed with other neurohormonal blocking strategies directed towards the RAAS such as ACE inhibitors, ARBs, and aldosterone receptor antagonists. What can be offered by direct renin inhibitors are the benefits of blocking a system upstream rather than downstream. In this way, there is no reflex activation of renin, angiotensin I, and angiotensin II with the potential for direct adverse effects of activation of these peptides. Against this argument is the increasing recognition that the AT_2 receptor subtype of the angiotensin II receptor mediates potentially beneficial actions upon activation and is generally vasodilatory and anti-proliferative.[8] With upstream blockade of angiotensin II production by renin inhibitors, those beneficial effects may be diminished or lost. Whether the net effect of these actions translates into overall clinical benefit remains uncertain but is currently being explored.

Vasopressin Receptor Antagonism

The vasopressin system is well known to be activated in heart failure. This system comprises $V1_A$ receptors that mediate vasoconstriction primarily, as well as V_2 receptors that inhibit aquaresis. Agents have been developed that block either or both receptor subtypes. A number of these agents, for example, tolvaptan and conivaptan, are in clinical development for the treatment of heart failure. These agents are selective V_2 receptor antagonists. It is unclear whether blockade of one or both receptor subtypes may confer the greatest clinical benefit.

Much of the initial approach to this development has been focused on patients who are acutely decompensated with evidence of fluid overload. Early trials have shown that these agents are effective at inducing a diuresis with concomitant improvement in clinical status and body weight toward the euvolemic range.[9,10] There is also a suggestion of clinical benefit from at least one study, and ongoing studies are currently being conducted for this indication.[9]

Urotensin II Antagonism

Urotensin II (UII) is an amino acid peptide that, in certain vascular beds, is the most potent vasoconstrictor yet described.[11] The peptide appears to have multiple and sometimes opposing vascular actions in various vascular beds, including constriction, dilatation, and no vasoactivity. In the setting of heart failure, increased gene expression of both the ligand and receptor have been observed in failing human myocardium.[12] Also observed has been a paradoxical response in heart failure patients whereby skin microcirculation is constricted by UII in heart failure patients in contrast to vasodilation in normal subjects.[13] Therefore, UII may be contributory to the increased vascular tone of heart failure. Furthermore, plasma levels of UII have been found to be elevated in some (but not all) studies of CHF patients.[14]

UII receptor antagonists had been developed that selectively block this system. They have already entered clinical trials for the indication of diabetic nephropathy. CHF is clearly another target.

Neurohormonal Augmentation

A number of vasodilator systems may also be augmented to enhance natriuresis and reduce afterload.

Adrenomedullin is a potential therapy based on its known vasodilatory and antifibrotic actions.[15] In this way, adrenomedullin is similar to earlier neutral endopeptidase inhibitors, which augmented natriuretic peptides. These peptides appear to share some of the physiological actions of adrenomedullin. Based on this profile, this is clearly another potentially useful approach to neurohormonal modulation. As with the natriuretic peptides, perhaps a combination of vasoconstrictor inhibitory and vasodilator augmentory approaches may be optimal, although this remains to be formally tested. First time in man studies have demonstrated vasodilatory actions in heart failure.

Modulation of Immune Activation

Despite the disappointment of TNF-α receptor inhibition with etanercept and infliximab, there is still considerable interest in pursuing immune blockade as a therapeutic strategy in CHF. This is based on the pathophysiological consequences of activation of a cascade of proinflammatory cytokines in response to the initial myocardial injury. These activated cytokines include TNF-α, various interleukins (interleukin-1-β, interleukin-2, interleukin-6, interleukin-12, interleukin-17, and interleukin-18), as well as a number of other markers of a proinflammatory state, including c-reactive protein (CRP).[16] As mentioned earlier, one hypothesis is that to be effective against this broad-based proinflammatory immune activation in heart failure, broad-based immune inhibition may be necessary.

Intravenous Immunoglobulin Therapy

Intravenous immunoglobulin (IVIG) provides a rich source of buffers against proinflammatory cytokine immune activation. This has been utilized in a number of inflammatory disorders and also studied in heart disease. Data with IVIG from patients with established heart failure are encouraging based on the trial of Gullestad and colleagues.[17] In that trial, there was a significant improvement in ejection fraction in IVIG-treated heart failure patients but not in those receiving placebo. However, the study was somewhat underpowered and the between-group difference was not significant. In contrast, a study in patients with recent-onset dilated cardiomyopathy failed to discern differences between IVIG and placebo.[18] There were large increases in ejection fraction in the IVIG group but this was also observed in the placebo group, reflecting the spontaneous recovery observed in patients with acute myocarditis manifesting as dilated cardiomyopathy.

Immune Modulation Therapy

This approach involves removal of blood, application of oxidant stress, heat and light, and then reinjection of this autologous blood.[19] The *ex-vivo* processes as described are said to induce an anti-inflammatory cytokine action upon the circulation. A Phase II clinical trial did not meet its primary endpoint of improvement in exercise time.[20] However, there was a significant reduction in major clinical endpoint events.[20] On this basis, a major outcome trial for registration is currently being undertaken in North America and Europe.

HMG CoA Reductase Inhibitors

Although statins are widely utilized for primary and secondary prevention of cardiovascular disease (primarily in hypercholesterolemic patients), these agents also have potent anti-inflammatory effects. Blockade of TNF-α and interleukin-6 has been demonstrated in man with these agents, both in circulating levels in plasma and in gene expression in mononuclear cells.[21]

On the basis of this and a number of additional pharmacological properties of these agents, statins have been postulated to be of benefit in patients with heart failure independent of anti-ischemic effects.[22]

However, there are also theoretical reasons to suggest that statins may not be beneficial in heart failure. Epidemiologically, patients with low-density lipoprotein (LDL) cholesterol levels have the worst outcomes in established heart failure.[23] The endotoxin-lipoprotein hypothesis suggests that lipoproteins are required to "mop up" excess endotoxin and thus reduce activation of proinflammatory cytokines such as TNF-α.[24] Finally, coenzyme Q is depleted by statins and this may be important in the function of cardiac cells in left ventricular (LV) dysfunction.[25]

Therefore, like many agents, statins may have positive and negative effects in CHF. The net effect of those actions needs to be definitively elucidated but overall appears to be one of benefit. Several post-hoc analyses of large heart failure databases suggest beneficial effects of statins. However, in none of these were patients prospectively randomized to statins. Preclinical studies support the anti-remodeling benefits of these agents. These findings have recently been supported by a small Japanese study of patients with dilated cardiomyopathy treated with simvastatin for 13 weeks. In that study, potent anti-inflammatory effects of simvastatin were noted, together with anti-remodeling effects as assessed by echocardiography.[26]

A number of large-scale clinical trials of statin therapy in heart failure are currently being undertaken (CORONA, GISSI HF). Given the large number of patients who are receiving statins by virtue of background ischemic heart disease, the results of these studies are of considerable importance.

Kinase Inhibitors

A number of kinases are involved in mediating the actions of proinflammatory cytokines and inducing downstream cytokine activation. Prominent amongst these are p38 mitogen-activated protein (MAP)-kinase inhibitors. The p38 MAP-kinase inhibitor RWJ-67657 has been demonstrated to reduce remodeling and pathological fibrosis in rats with permanent coronary ligation myocardial infarction (MI).[27] These agents have been shown to be potent inhibitors of TNF and other proinflammatory cytokines in man. Indeed, clinical trials are currently underway with these agents for noncardiovascular indications such as rheumatoid arthritis and Crohn's disease as well as cardiovascular indications such as atherosclerosis.

Other Targets and Agents

Cardiac Metabolic Agents

These agents address defects in cardiac metabolism that occur in the setting of myocardial dysfunction. Metabolism of fatty acids is the major source of adenosine triphosphate (ATP) production in the heart. However, fatty acids require more oxygen than glucose to produce an equivalent amount of ATP. As a result, fatty acids are not as efficient as glucose as a source of energy. In addition, in the setting of myocardial ischemia and dysfunction, products of glycolysis (i.e., lactate and protons) can accumulate and promote an increase in intracellular sodium and calcium, which in turn requires more ATP to reestablish ionic homeostasis.

During LV dysfunction, the oxidation of both fatty acids and carbohydrates is limited by relative myocardial ischemia. Therefore, the ratio of anaerobic glycolysis to ATP production increases, and high concentrations of fatty acid further inhibit, glucose oxidation.

In general, cardiac metabolic agents switch metabolism from fatty acid to that of glucose and this involves more efficient utilization of ATP and thus improved actin-myosin contractility per unit ATP expended.

Agents in this category include ranolazine, a partial fatty acid oxidase inhibitor, perhexiline, a carnitine palmitoyl transferase (CPT1) inhibitor, and trimetazidine, an inhibitor of mitochondrial long chain 3-cetoaryl coenzyme (CoA) thiolase, a fundamental enzyme in cardiac metabolism. Another agent within this group of drugs, etomoxir, has recently yielded disappointing results and is not being further developed for heart failure.

Modulation of Collagen Deposition and Crosslinking

Pathological fibrosis has emerged as a key target for pharmacological intervention in heart failure.[28] Renin-angiotensin system blocking agents such as ACE inhibitors, ARBs, and particularly aldosterone

receptor antagonists have all been demonstrated to reduce pathological fibrosis, both indirectly via improved hemodynamics but also directly via direct effects on collagen synthesis. Many of these effects are mediated via growth factors and cytokines such as transforming growth factor beta (TGF-β), p38 MAP-kinase, and protein kinase C. Similarly, β-blockers have also been demonstrated to have antifibrogenic properties.

There are a number of agents where antifibrotic effects are the predominant pharmacological property of the drug. One such agent is tranilast. Tranilast was disappointing in the PRESTO study for post-percutaneous transluminal coronary angioplasty (PTCA) restenosis prevention.[25] However, antifibrotic actions have been demonstrated with tranilast in a number of animal models including the Ren-2 diabetic model of cardiomyopathy and the permanent ligation post-MI model.[30] Reductions in fibrosis were associated with improvements in the ventricular function in these models.

Other antifibrotic strategies currently being studied including agents that inhibit phosphorylation of TGF-β and blockers of the actions of connective tissue growth factor, the latter a commonly activated factor in the ventricular remodeling process.

Diastolic heart failure is characterized by an increase in advanced glycation end products (AGEs). The biochemical steps of AGE formation are irreversible, leading to accumulation in long-lived proteins such as collagen. Serum concentration of AGEs has been correlated with echocardiographic indices of cardiac stiffness. The AGE cross-link breaker ALT711 has been demonstrated to reduce myocardial stiffness in animal models.[31] Clinical trials are ongoing in diastolic heart failure patients, with and without associated diabetes mellitus.

Direct Sinus Node Inhibitors

The I_F channel has been identified as a major pathway of sinus node electrical activity, which can be blocked by specific agents, such as ivabradine.

It is unclear whether slowing of heart rate alone results in significant improvements in ventricular function. Preclinical studies do suggest that this is indeed the case with improvements in ventricular function and early clinical evidence of improved cardiac hemodynamics through rate reduction alone.[32] Whether this benefit can be observed incremental to background β-blocker therapy in heart failure is currently unclear. Nevertheless, a significant percentage of patients are either ineligible to receive or unable to tolerate β-blockers and these patients may benefit from alternative forms of heart rate reduction. A large-scale clinical trial in patients with ischemic heart disease and systolic LV dysfunction (with and without background β-blockade) is currently underway (BEAUTIFUL study).

Direct Myosin Activators

Cardiac myosin activators directly address the major deficit in myocardial contractile function: defective myosin motor protein activity. Preclinical studies demonstrate increased cardiac contractility without CAMP activation or increasing intracellular calcium. Such agents are about to enter clinical trials.[33]

Agents Augmenting Renal Function in CHF

Adenosine A_1-receptor antagonists decrease different arteriolar pressure, increase urine flow, and enhance sodium excretion in CHF patients. Diuretic actions are achieved via inhibition of sodium reabsorption in tubular sites. The net effect is diuresis with improved or maintained glomerular filtration rate, an attractive pharmacological profile in CHF.[34] These agents are currently in clinical development.

▶ SUMMARY

As has been described in this chapter, a number of novel pharmacological approaches have been employed to improve outcomes in patients with heart failure additional to background standard therapies. It is clear that the greatest overall health care gains are to be made in widespread public health campaigns to ensure that all eligible patients are able to receive optimal best practice therapies. However, we should continue to strive to improve outcomes in such patients. This includes not only ancillary drug therapy but also nonpharmacological measures and multidisciplinary supports as described elsewhere in this textbook. More recently, use of devices in selected patients has resulted in improved outcomes. However, for the majority of patients such devices are either clinically inappropriate or unaffordable. For this reason alone we should continue to pursue drug therapies, which are affordable, directed toward appropriate patients, and capable of providing either alternative or complementary benefit to existing therapies. Some have argued that we have reached the limits of clinical benefit that can be obtained from pharmacological therapy in heart failure. It is far from certain, however, that this is the case and we must continue to pursue novel drug therapies for the reasons described above. Clearly, however, these will need to be more carefully targeted to avoid the disappointments with recent trials as described at the beginning of this chapter.

▶ REFERENCES

1. Swedberg K, Cleland J, Dargie H, Task Force for the diagnosis and treatment of chronic heart failure of the European Society of Cardiology. Guidelines for the diagnosis and treatment of chronic heart failure: executive summary (update 2005). *Eur Heart J.* 2005;26:1115–1140.
2. Packer M, Califf RM, Konstam MA, et al. Comparison of omapatrilat and enalapril in patients with chronic heart failure: the Omapatrilat Versus Enalapril Randomized Trial of Utility in Reducing Events (OVERTURE). *Circulation.* 2002;106:920–926.
3. Kalra PR, Moon JC, Coats AJ. Do results of the ENABLE (Endothelin Antagonist Bosentan for Lowering Cardiac Events in Heart Failure) study spell the end for non-selective endothelin antagonism in heart failure? *Int J Cardiol.* 2002;85: 195–197.
4. Mann DL, McMurray JJ, Packer M, et al. Targeted anticytokine therapy in patients with chronic heart failure: results of the Randomized Etanercept

Worldwide Evaluation (RENEWAL). *Circulation*. 2004;109:1594–1602.

5. Chung ES, Packer M, Lo KH, Anti-TNF therapy against congestive heart failure investigators. Randomized, double-blind, placebo-controlled, pilot trial of infliximab, a chimeric monoclonal antibody to tumor necrosis factor-alpha, in patients with moderate-to-severe heart failure: results of the anti-TNF Therapy Against Congestive Heart Failure (ATTACH) trial. *Circulation*. 2003;107:3133–3140.

6. Krum H, Tonkin A. Why do phase III trials of promising heart failure drugs often fail? The contribution of "regression to the truth." *J Card Fail*. 2003;9:364–367.

7. Stanton A. Therapeutic potential of renin inhibitors in the management of cardiovascular disorders. *Am J Cardiovasc Drugs*. 2003;3:3 89–394.

8. Matsubara H. Pathophysiological role of angiotensin II type 2 receptor in cardiovascular and renal diseases. *Circ Res*. 1998;83:1182–1189.

9. Gheorghiade M, Gattis WA, O'Connor CM, Acute and Chronic Therapeutic Impact of a Vasopressin Antagonist in Congestive Heart Failure (ACTIV in CHF) investigators. Effects of tolvaptan, a vasopressin antagonist, in patients hospitalized with worsening heart failure: a randomized controlled trial. *JAMA*. 2004;291:1963–1971.

10. Goldsmith SR, Gheorghiade M. Vasopressin antagonism in heart failure. *J Am Coll Cardiol*. 2005; 46:1785–1791.

11. Gilbert RE, Douglas SA, Krum H. Urotensin-II as a novel therapeutic target in the clinical management of cardiorenal disease. *Curr Opin Investig Drugs*. 2004;5:276–282.

12. Douglas SA, Tayara L, Ohlstein EH, et al. Congestive heart failure and expression of myocardial urotensin II. *Lancet*. 2002;359:1990–1997.

13. Lim M, Honisett S, Sparkes CD, et al. Differential effect of urotensin II on vascular tone in normal subjects and patients with chronic heart failure. *Circulation*. 2004;109:1212–1214.

14. Richards AM, Nicholls MG, Lainchbury JG, et al. Plasma urotensin II in heart failure. *Lancet*. 2002;360: 545–546.

15. Rademaker MT, Cameron VA, Charles CJ, et al. Adrenomedullin and heart failure. *Regul Pept*. 2003;112:51–60.

16. Aukrust P, Gullestad L, Ueland T, et al. Inflammatory and anti-inflammatory cytokines in chronic heart failure: potential therapeutic implications. *Ann Med*. 2005;37:74–85.

17. Gullestad L, Aass H, Fjeld JG, et al. Immuno-modulating therapy with intravenous immunoglobulin in patients with chronic heart failure. *Circulation*. 2001;103:220–225.

18. McNamara DM, Holubkov R, Starling RC, et all. Controlled trial of intravenous immune globulin in recent-onset dilated cardiomyopathy. *Circulation*. 2001;103:2254–2259.

19. Torre-Amione G, Sestier F, Radovancevic B, et al. Broad modulation of tissue responses (immune activation) by celacade may favorably influence pathologic processes associated with heart failure progression. *Am J Cardiol*. 2005; 95:C30–C37.

20. Torre-Amione G, Sestier F, Radovancevic B, et al. Effects of a novel immune modulation therapy in patients with advanced chronic heart failure: results of a randomized, controlled, phase II trial. *J Am Coll Cardiol*. 2004;44:1181–1186.

21. Marz W, Koenig W. HMG-CoA reductase inhibition: anti-inflammatory effects beyond lipid lowering? *J Cardiovasc Risk*. 2003;10:169–277.

22. Krum H, McMurray JJ. Statins and chronic heart failure: do we need a large-scale outcome trial? *J Am Coll Cardiol*. 2002;39:1567–1573.

23. Fonarow GC, Horwich TB. Cholesterol and mortality in heart failure: the bad gone good? *J Am Coll Cardiol*. 2003;42:1941–1943.

24. Rauchhaus M, Coats AJ, Anker SD. The endotoxin-lipoprotein hypothesis. *Lancet*. 2000;356: 930–933.

25. Hargreaves IP, Duncan AJ, Heales SJ, et al. The effect of HMG-CoA reductase inhibitors on coenzyme Q10: possible biochemical/clinical implications. *Drug Saf*. 2005;28:659–676.

26. Node K, Fujita M, Kitakaze M, et al. Short-term statin therapy improves cardiac function and symptoms in patients with idiopathic dilated cardiomyopathy. *Circulation*. 2003;108:839–843.

27. See F, Thomas W, Way K, et al. p38 mitogen-activated protein kinase inhibition improves cardiac function and attenuates left ventricular remodeling following myocardial infarction in the rat. *J Am Coll Cardiol*. 2004;44:1679–1689.

28. See F, Kompa A, Martin J, et al. Fibrosis as a therapeutic target post-myocardial infarction. *Curr Pharm Des*. 2005;11:477–487.

29. Savage M, LaBlanche JM, Grip L, et al. Results of Prevention of REStenosis with Tranilast and its

Outcomes (PRESTO) trial. *Circulation*. 2002;106:1243–1250.

30. Martin J, Kelly DJ, Mifsud SA, et al. Tranilast attenuates cardiac matrix deposition in experimental diabetes: role of transforming growth factor-beta. *Cardiovasc Res*. 2005;65:694–701.

31. Candido R, Forbes JM, Thomas MC, et al. A breaker of advanced glycation end products attenuates diabetes-induced myocardial structural changes. *Circ Res*. 2003;92:785–792.

32. Mulder P, Barbier S, Chagraoui A, et al. Long-term heart rate reduction induced by the selective I(f) current inhibitor ivabradine improves left ventricular function and intrinsic myocardial structure in congestive heart failure. *Circulation*. 2004;109:1674–1679.

33. Morkin E. Regulation of myosin heavy chain genes in the heart. *Circulation*. 1993;87:1451–1460.

34. Gottlieb SS, Skettino SL, Wolff A, et al. Effects of BG9719 (CVT-124), an A1-adenosine receptor antagonist, and furosemide on glomerular filtration rate and natriuresis in patients with congestive heart failure. *J Am Coll Cardiol*. 2000;35:56–69.

CHAPTER 14

Devices for the Treatment of Heart Failure

WILLIAM T. ABRAHAM, MD, FACP, FACC, FAHA

From the mid-1980s through the late 1990s, great advances were made in the pharmacological management of chronic systolic heart failure. During that time, several drugs or drug combinations were shown to substantially improve functional status and to reduce morbidity and mortality in heart failure patients. Since then, however, no additional gains have been made in improving heart failure clinical status or outcomes with newer (investigational) drug therapies, and heart failure morbidity and mortality have remained high. In the year 2001, a new era of implantable device therapies for the treatment of heart failure began with the U.S. Food and Drug Administration (FDA) approval of the first cardiac resynchronization therapy (CRT) device. Over the subsequent 4 years, implantable cardioverter defibrillators (ICDs) and combined CRT-ICD devices were also approved for the management of heart failure. In the former case, ICDs became indicated for the primary prevention of death in patients with heart failure and reduced ejection fractions, in addition to the previous secondary prevention indication for these devices. In the latter instance, combined CRT-ICD devices were shown to reduce morbidity and mortality in heart failure patients with ventricular dyssynchrony. In acknowledgement of the evidence-based benefits of these devices, the 2005 update to the American College of Cardiology/American Heart Association (ACC/AHA) heart failure guideline strongly supports, with Class I indications, the use of an ICD or CRT device in the management of eligible heart failure patients.[1]

Left ventricular assist devices (LVADs) represent another approved approach to treating highly selected patients with end-stage heart failure. These devices may be used as a bridge to cardiac transplant, as so-called destination (or permanent) therapy, or as means to support patients with reversible causes of heart failure temporarily as they recover left ventricular function. The use of an LVAD as a surgical approach to heart failure is discussed in Chap. 15. While not therapeutic per se, implantable devices that monitor physiological parameters such as patient activity level, heart rate variability, intrathoracic impedance, and/or hemodynamics have been developed. In some instances, these data are already available in currently implantable CRT and ICD devices. The exact utility of such device-based diagnostic or monitoring features is unknown and currently under investigation. Other promising novel implantable therapeutic devices are also under investigation for the treatment of heart failure. This chapter reviews the use of CRT and ICDs for the management of heart failure, discusses the potential utility of implantable heart failure monitoring devices, and previews some other investigational device therapies for heart failure.

▶ VENTRICULAR DYSSYNCHRONY IN HEART FAILURE

Several conduction abnormalities are commonly seen in association with chronic heart failure. Among these are abnormalities of ventricular conduction such as bundle branch blocks that alter the timing and pattern of ventricular contraction so as to place the already failing heart at a further mechanical disadvantage. Specifically, these ventricular conduction delays produce suboptimal ventricular filling, a reduction in left ventricular contractility, prolonged duration of mitral regurgitation, and paradoxical septal wall motion.[2–5] Collectively, these mechanical manifestations of altered ventricular conduction have been termed ventricular dyssynchrony. Classically, ventricular dyssynchrony has been defined by QRS duration ≥120 msec. By this definition, about one-third of patients with systolic heart failure have ventricular dyssynchrony.[6,7] In addition to reducing the ability of the failing heart to eject blood, ventricular dyssynchrony has also been associated with increased mortality in heart failure patients.[8–11]

After several attempts during the mid-1990s to improve heart failure with pacing therapies, atrial-synchronized biventricular pacing emerged as the most promising approach for the treatment of ventricular dyssynchrony. This form of pacing therapy has come to be known as CRT. The history of CRT began with a single case report of encouraging results.[12] Such favorable single-case experiences led to small observational studies evaluating the acute effects of biventricular pacing on hemodynamics and on other measures of cardiac performance.[4,13] These studies provided additional support for the concept of CRT. Several uncontrolled or unblinded studies soon followed to further evaluate the acute and longer term effects of CRT on clinical status in heart failure patients.[14–22] The results of these trials were equally encouraging, with patients demonstrating consistent and sustained improvement in exercise tolerance, quality of life, and New York Heart Association (NYHA) functional class. Finally, large-scale randomized controlled trials of CRT confirmed the beneficial effects of this therapy in heart failure patients with ventricular dyssynchrony.

▶ RANDOMIZED CONTROLLED TRIALS OF CARDIAC RESYNCHRONIZATION THERAPY

More than 4000 patients have been evaluated in randomized single- or double-blinded controlled trials of CRT in heart failure. The following randomized controlled trials are considered among the landmark studies of CRT: the Multisite Stimulation in Cardiomyopathy (MUSTIC) studies, the Multicenter InSync Randomized Clinical Evaluation (MIRACLE) trial, MIRACLE ICD, the CONTAK CD trial, the Cardiac Resynchronization in Heart Failure (CARE HF) trial, and the Comparison of Medical Therapy, Pacing and Defibrillation in Heart Failure (COMPANION) trial.[23–32] To understand the clinical benefits, risks, and limitations of CRT with or without an ICD, these studies will be reviewed.

Multisite Stimulation in Cardiomyopathy Trials

The MUSTIC trials were designed to evaluate the safety and efficacy of cardiac resynchronization in patients with advanced heart failure, ventricular dyssynchrony, and either normal sinus rhythm or atrial fibrillation.[23,24] They represent the first randomized single-blinded trials of CRT for heart failure. The first study involved 58 randomized patients with NYHA Class III heart failure, normal sinus rhythm, and QRS duration of at least 150 msec. All patients were implanted with a CRT device, and after a run-in period, patients were randomized in a single-blind fashion to either active pacing or to no pacing. After 12 weeks, patients were crossed over and remained in the alternate study assignment for 12 weeks. After completing this second 12-week period, the device was programmed to the patient's preferred mode of therapy. The second MUSTIC study involved fewer patients (only 37 completers) with atrial fibrillation and a slow ventricular rate (either

spontaneously or from radiofrequency ablation). A VVIR biventricular pacemaker and leads for each ventricle were implanted and the same randomization procedure described above was applied; however, biventricular VVIR pacing versus single site right ventricular VVIR pacing (rather than no pacing) were compared in this group of patients with atrial fibrillation.

The primary endpoints for MUSTIC were exercise tolerance assessed by measurement of peak VO_2 or the 6-minute hall walk test and quality of life determined using the Minnesota Living with Heart Failure questionnaire. Secondary endpoints included rehospitalizations and/or drug therapy modifications for worsening heart failure. Results from the normal sinus rhythm arm of MUSTIC provided strong evidence of benefit. The mean distance walked in 6 minutes was 23% greater with CRT than during the inactive pacing phase (P <0.001). Significant improvement was also seen in quality of life and NYHA functional class ranking. There were fewer hospitalizations during active resynchronization therapy. The atrial fibrillation group evaluated in MUSTIC demonstrated similar improvements, although the magnitude of benefit was slightly less.

Multicenter InSync Randomized Clinical Evaluation

MIRACLE was the first prospective, randomized, double-blind, parallel-controlled clinical trial designed to evaluate the merits of CRT and to further elucidate potential mechanisms of action of CRT.[25,26] Primary endpoints were NYHA class, quality of life score (using the Minnesota Living with Heart Failure questionnaire), and 6-minute hall walk distance. Secondary endpoints included assessments of a composite clinical response, cardiopulmonary exercise performance, neurohormone and cytokine levels, QRS duration, cardiac structure and function (as determined by echocardiography), and a variety of measures of worsening heart failure and combined morbidity and mortality.

The MIRACLE trial was conducted between 1998 and 2000. Four hundred and fifty-three patients with moderate to severe symptoms of heart failure associated with a left ventricular ejection fraction ≤35% and QRS duration of at least 130 msec were randomized (double-blind) to cardiac resynchronization (n = 228) or to a control group (n = 225) for 6 months, while conventional therapy for heart failure was maintained.[26] Compared with the control group, patients randomized to CRT demonstrated a significant improvement in quality of life score (–18 vs. –9 points, P = 0.001), 6-minute walk distance (+39 vs. +10 m, P = 0.005), NYHA functional class ranking (–1 vs. 0 class, P <0.001), treadmill exercise time (+81 vs. +19 seconds, P = 0.001), peak VO$_2$ (+1.1 vs. +0.1 mL/kg/min, P <0.01), and left ventricular ejection fraction (LVEF) (+4.6% vs. –0.2%, P <0.001). Patients randomized to CRT demonstrated a highly significant improvement in a composite clinical heart failure response endpoint, compared to control subjects, suggesting an overall improvement in heart failure clinical status. In addition, when compared with the control group, fewer patients in the CRT group required hospitalization (8% vs. 15%) or intravenous medications (7% and 15%) for the treatment of worsening heart failure (both P <0.05). In the resynchronization group, the 50% reduction in hospitalization was accompanied by a significant reduction in length of stay, resulting in a 77% decrease in total days hospitalized over 6 months compared to the control group. The major limitation of the therapy was due to unsuccessful implantation of the device in 8% of patients. The results of this trial led to the U.S. FDA approval of the InSync system in August 2001, the first approved CRT system in America, allowing the introduction of CRT into clinical practice.

The MIRACLE trial also provided persuasive evidence supporting the occurrence of reverse left ventricular remodeling with chronic CRT. In the MIRACLE trial, serial Doppler echocardiograms were obtained at baseline 3, and 6 months in a subset of 323 patients.[26,33] Cardiac resynchronization therapy for 6 months was associated with reduced end-diastolic and end-systolic volumes (both P <0.001), reduced left ventricular mass (P <0.01), increased ejection fraction (P <0.001), reduced mitral regurgitant blood flow (P <0.001), and improved myocardial performance index (P <0.001) as compared with control (Fig. 14-1). These effects are similar

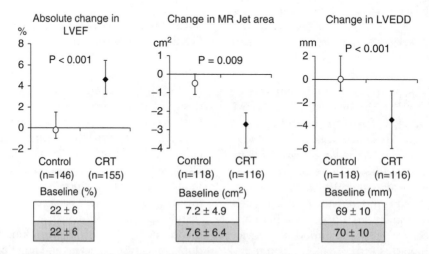

Figure 14-1   Effects of cardiac resynchronization therapy on cardiac structure and function from the MIRACLE trial. Pair median changes from baseline at 6 months are shown. Error bars represent 95% confidence intervals. CRT—cardiac resynchronization therapy; LVEDD—left ventricular end diastolic dimension; LVEF—left ventricular ejection fraction; MR—mitral regurgitation. (From reference 26, with permission.)

to those seen with β-blockade in heart failure but were seen in MIRACLE in patients already receiving β-blocker therapy.

Multicenter InSync-ICD Randomized Clinical Evaluation

The MIRACLE ICD study was designed to be almost identical to the MIRACLE trial. MIRACLE ICD was a prospective, multicenter, randomized, double-blind, parallel-controlled clinical trial intended to assess the safety and efficacy of a combined CRT-ICD system in patients with dilated cardiomyopathy (LVEF ≤35%, left ventricular end diastolic dimension [LVEDD] ≥55 mm), NYHA Class III or IV heart failure, ventricular dyssynchrony (QRS ≥130 msec), and an indication for an ICD. Primary and secondary efficacy measures were essentially the same as those evaluated in the MIRACLE trial, but also included measures of ICD function (including the efficacy of antitachycardia therapy with biventricular pacing).

Of 369 patients receiving devices and randomized, 182 were controls (ICD active, CRT inactive) and 187 were in the resynchronization group (ICD active, CRT active). At 6 months, patients assigned to active CRT had a greater improvement in median quality of life score (−17.5 vs. −11.0, P = 0.02) and functional class (−1 vs. 0 class, P = 0.007) than controls, but were no different than controls in the change in distance walked in 6 minutes (55 m vs. 53 m, P = 0.36).[27] Peak oxygen consumption increased by 1.1 mL/kg/min in the resynchronization group versus 0.1 mL/kg/min in controls (P = 0.04), while treadmill exercise duration increased by 56 seconds in the CRT group and decreased by 11 seconds in controls (P = 0.0006). The magnitude of improvement was comparable to that seen in the MIRACLE trial, suggesting that heart failure patients with an ICD indication benefit as much from CRT as those patients without an indication for an ICD. The combined CRT-ICD device used in this study was approved by the FDA for use in NYHA Class III and IV systolic heart failure patients with ventricular dyssynchrony and an ICD indication in June 2002.

CONTAK CD

The CONTAK CD trial enrolled 581 symptomatic heart failure patients with ventricular dyssynchrony (QRS > 120 msec), and malignant ventricular tachyarrhythmias, who were all candidates for an ICD.[28] Following unsuccessful implant attempts and withdrawals, 490 patients were available for analysis. The study did not meet its primary endpoint of a reduction in disease progression, defined by a composite endpoint of heart failure hospitalization, all-cause mortality, and ventricular arrhythmia requiring defibrillator therapies, although the trends were in a direction favoring improved outcomes with CRT. However, the CONTAK CD trial did demonstrate statistically significant improvements in peak oxygen uptake and quality of life in the resynchronization group compared to control subjects, although quality of life was improved only in NYHA Class III and IV patients without right bundle branch block. Left ventricular dimensions were also reduced, and LVEFs increased, as seen in other trials of CRT. Importantly, the improvement seen in peak VO_2 with cardiac resynchronization was again comparable to that observed in the MIRACLE trial. Improvements in NYHA functional class were observed in NYHA Class III-IV patients. The CONTAK CD device was approved by the FDA for use in NYHA Class III and IV systolic heart failure patients with ventricular dyssynchrony and an ICD indication in May 2002.

Cardiac Resynchronization in Heart Failure Trial

The Cardiac Resynchronization in Heart Failure (CARE HF) trial was designed to evaluate the effects of resynchronization therapy without an ICD on morbidity and mortality in patients with NYHA Class III or IV heart failure and ventricular dyssynchrony.[29,30] Eight hundred and nineteen patients with LVEFs of 35% or less and ventricular dyssynchrony defined as a QRS duration ≥150 msec or a QRS duration between 120 msec and 150 msec with echocardiographic evidence of dyssynchrony were enrolled in this randomized, unblinded controlled trial and followed for an average of 29.4 months.[30] Four hundred and four patients were assigned to receive optimal medical therapy alone and 409 patients were randomized to optimal medical therapy plus resynchronization therapy alone. The risk of death from any cause or unplanned hospitalization for a major cardiac event, the primary endpoint analyzed as time to first event, was significantly reduced by 37% in the treatment group compared to control subjects (hazard ratio, 0.63; 95% confidence interval [CI], 0.51 to 0.77; P <0.001; Fig. 14-2). In the CRT group, 82 patients (20%) died during follow-up compared to 120 patients (30%) in the medical group, yielding a significant 36% reduction in all-cause mortality with resynchronization therapy (hazard ratio, 0.64; 95% CI, 0.48 to 0.85; P <0.002). Resynchronization therapy also significantly reduced the risk of unplanned hospitalization for a major cardiac event by 39%, all-cause mortality plus heart failure hospitalization by 46%, and heart failure hospitalization by 52%.

Comparison of Medical Therapy, Pacing, and Defibrillation in Heart Failure

Begun in early 2000, COMPANION was a multicenter, prospective, randomized controlled clinical trial designed to compare drug therapy alone to drug therapy in combination with cardiac resynchronization in patients with dilated cardiomyopathy, an IVCD, NYHA Class III or IV heart failure, and no indication for a device.[31,32] COMPANION randomized 1520 patients into one of three treatment groups in a 1:2:2 allocation: Group I (308 patients) received optimal medical care only, Group II (617 patients) received optimal medical care and the Guidant CONTAK TR (biventricular pulse generator), and Group III (595 patients) received optimal medical care and the CONTAK CD (combined heart failure/ bradycardia/tachycardia device). The primary endpoint of the COMPANION trial was a composite of all-cause mortality and all-cause hospitalization, measured as time to first event, beginning from time of randomization. Secondary endpoints

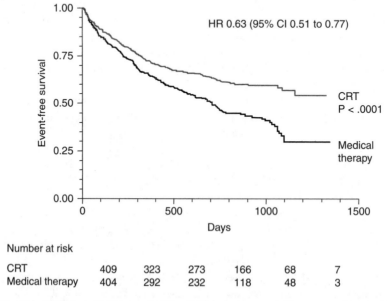

Figure 14-2   Kaplan-Meier estimates of risk of all-cause mortality or unplanned hospitalization for a major cardiac event in patients randomized to CRT compared to conventional medical therapy in the CARE-HF trial. CI—confidence interval; CRT—cardiac resynchronization therapy; HR—hazard ratio. (From reference 30, with permission.)

included all-cause mortality and a variety of measures of cardiovascular morbidity. When compared to optimal medical therapy alone, the combined endpoint of mortality or heart failure hospitalization was reduced by 35% for patients receiving CRT and 40% for patients receiving CRT-ICD (both P <0.001). For the mortality endpoint alone, CRT patients had a 24% risk reduction (P = 0.060) and CRT-ICD patients experienced a risk reduction of 36% (P <0.003), when compared to optimal medical therapy. COMPANION confirmed the results of earlier resynchronization therapy trials in improving symptoms, exercise tolerance, and quality of life for heart failure patients with ventricular dyssynchrony. In addition, COMPANION showed for the first time the impact of CRT-ICD in reducing all-cause mortality.

▶ LIMITATIONS OF CARDIAC RESYNCHRONIZATION THERAPY

The success rate for placement of a transvenous cardiac resynchronization system has ranged from about 88–92% in clinical trials. Thus, some patients undergoing an implant procedure will not receive a functioning system using this approach. Implant-related complications are similar to those seen with standard pacemakers and defibrillators, with the additional risk of dissection or perforation of the coronary sinus. This is a rare event but may lead to substantial morbidity and even mortality in heart failure patients.

Despite the results of randomized controlled CRT trials, some patients do not respond to this therapy. The nonresponder rate for cardiac resynchronization therapy appears to be about 25%, a rate that is similar to the nonresponder rate for heart failure drug therapies. A variety of factors have been proposed as contributing to the nonresponder rate associated with CRT including suboptimal left ventricular lead placement, suboptimal atrioventricular (AV) and interventricular (VV) timing, ventricular scar, and heart failure disease progression. One identifiable cause of poor response is loss of resynchronization. A specific programming sequence should be performed in

the clinic to determine capture thresholds and document that left ventricular capture is present. Lead dislodgement or a change in capture threshold may result in the loss of left ventricular pacing and thus the beneficial effects of CRT may also be lost. It is also possible that left ventricular lead placement and pacing thresholds are fine but resynchronization is lost for other reasons. For example, anything that frequently or consistently inhibits left ventricular stimulation can effectively inhibit CRT. If the AV interval is too long and the patient's intrinsic PR conduction inhibits biventricular pacing, deterioration may occur. The AV interval may have been programmed appropriately but accelerated intrinsic AV conduction could result in loss of effective biventricular pacing. This is commonly seen when atrial fibrillation occurs, resulting in a rapid ventricular response competing with biventricular pacing. Frequent premature ventricular contractions may also inhibit ventricular pacing output. While follow-up of the device itself and battery life are similar to that seen for contemporary dual-chamber pacemakers and defibrillators and generally managed by an implanting physician, heart failure specialists, general cardiologists, and primary care providers should possess the knowledge required to recognize the aforementioned limitations of resynchronization therapy and troubleshoot them.

▶ INDICATIONS FOR CARDIAC RESYNCHRONIZATION THERAPY IN HEART FAILURE PATIENTS

The 2005 ACC/AHA heart failure guideline proposes a Class I indication for CRT.[1] Patients with LVEF ≤35%, normal sinus rhythm, and NYHA functional Class III or ambulatory Class IV symptoms despite recommended optimal medical therapy and who have ventricular dyssynchrony should receive CRT, unless contraindicated. Currently, the guideline defines ventricular dyssynchrony as a QRS duration of at least 120 msec. However, echocardiography appears to be a promising way to define ventricular dyssynchrony in the future, so that a newer definition of ventricular dyssynchrony may one day prevail. This is being studied in the Predictors of Responsiveness to CRT (PROSPECT) trial.[34] Other ongoing trials of CRT are evaluating the usefulness of this therapy in NYHA Class I and II patients and in patients with narrow QRS durations but with echocardiographic evidence of ventricular dyssynchrony.

▶ SUDDEN CARDIAC DEATH IN HEART FAILURE

Patients with heart failure and left ventricular systolic dysfunction are at increased risk for sudden cardiac death (SCD).[35,36] Sudden cardiac death is the leading cause of mortality in patients with heart failure and occurs at a rate of six-to-nine times that is seen in the general population. A randomized controlled trial of β-blockade in heart failure demonstrated that patients with NYHA Class II or III symptoms die most frequently as a result of SCD.[37] This study estimated the proportion of total mortality attributable to SCD at 64% and 59% for NYHA Class II and III patients, respectively. In contrast, the major cause of death in Class IV patients was worsening heart failure.

Given this high incidence of SCD in heart failure, it was easy to hypothesize that an ICD used as prophylactic therapy would reduce total mortality by reducing the incidence of SCD. A series of recently completed and published studies have confirmed this notion.[38–43] These studies focused mainly on patients with coronary artery disease and left ventricular dysfunction and more recently on those patients with left ventricular systolic dysfunction of any cause.

▶ RANDOMIZED CONTROLLED TRIALS OF IMPLANTABLE CARDIOVERTER DEFIBRILLATORS IN HEART FAILURE

Several early studies including the Multicenter Automatic Defibrillator Implantation Trial (MADIT), the Coronary Artery Bypass Graft (CABG)-Patch trial, and the Multi-center Unsustained Tachycardia Trial (MUSTT) supported the benefit of prophylactic ICD implantation.[38–40] The landmark trials establishing a role for ICDs as primary prevention of mortality in heart failure patients are MADIT II, the Prophylactic Defibrillator Implantation in Patients with Nonischemic Dilated Cardiomyopathy (DEFINITE) trial, and the National Institutes of Health sponsored Sudden Cardiac Death-Heart Failure Trial (SCD-HeFT).[41–43]

Multicenter Automatic Defibrillator Implantation II Trial

MADIT II, a randomized controlled trial, was prospectively designed and powered to assess the survival benefit of ICDs in a population of post-MI patients with reduced ejection fractions (<30%). Importantly, this trial included no arrhythmic markers such as nonsustained or inducible ventricular tachycardia for inclusion. A total of 1232 patients were randomly assigned in a 3:2 ratio to receive an ICD (742 patients) or conventional medical therapy (490 patients). During an average follow-up of 20 months, the all-cause mortality rates were 19.8% in the conventional therapy arm and 14.2% in the ICD group (31% relative risk reduction, P = 0.016).[41] The effect of ICD therapy on survival was similar in subgroup analyses stratified according to age, gender, ejection fraction, NYHA class, and the QRS interval. Moreover, β-blocker utilization was 72% in these patients and was well balanced between the ICD and conventional therapy groups.

Of note, the majority of patients enrolled into MADIT II were classified in NYHA Class II or III. Class IV patients were excluded and the Class I cohort was relatively small. The average left ventricular ejection fraction was 23%. These findings suggest that heart failure patients with mild-to-moderate symptoms and moderate-to-severe reductions in LVEF may benefit the most from a prophylactic ICD. Moreover, in contrast to MADIT I, where the survival benefit of ICD therapy was seen early post-randomization, the survival benefit observed in MADIT II began approximately 9 months after the device was implanted. The authors suggested that this difference may be due to a lower-risk population enrolled in MADIT II, the absence of arrhythmia as risk stratification for entry, and/or the use of more aggressive medical treatment. Regardless of the explanation, this observation may be important when considering the timing of device placement in eligible patients.

Prophylactic Defibrillator Implantation in Patients with Nonischemic Dilated Cardiomyopathy Trial

While MADIT II enrolled exclusively post-MI patients with an ischemic cause of left ventricular systolic dysfunction and heart failure, the DEFINITE trial was the first randomized trial of primary prevention therapy with an ICD in nonischemic cardiomyopathy patients.[42] Such patients also exhibit high rates of SCD; however, until recently, there has been little consensus regarding the management of SCD risk in such patients. This may be due, in part, to limitations in objective risk assessment, in that no invasive or noninvasive testing procedure has been shown to accurately determine which nonischemic heart failure patient is likely to die suddenly. Also clouding the picture were older observations suggesting that the prophylactic administration of an antiarrhythmic agent, amiodarone, might prolong survival in nonischemic cardiomyopathy patients.[44]

The DEFINITE trial was a prospective evaluation of 458 patients with nonischemic dilated cardiomyopathy. Entry criteria included an ejection fraction of ≤35%, a history of symptomatic heart failure, and the presence of ambient arrhythmias defined as an episode of nonsustained ventricular tachycardia or at least 10 premature ventricular contractions per 24-hour period on continuous ambulatory electrocardiographic monitoring. Two hundred and twenty-nine patients were randomized to each arm of the study to receive either an ICD and standard medical therapy or standard medical therapy alone. Compliance with medical therapy was excellent and included an angiotensin-converting enzyme inhibitor (ACE-I) in 86% of the cohort and a β-blocker in 85%. The patients were followed for a mean of 29 ± 14.4 months with a primary endpoint of all-cause mortality.

There were 68 deaths reported in DEFINITE, 28 in the ICD group, and 40 in the standard therapy group. The implantation of an ICD yielded a nonsignificant 35% reduction in death from any cause (hazard ratio, 0.65; 95% CI, 0.4 to 1.06; P = 0.08) and significantly reduced the risk of sudden death by a remarkable 80% (hazard ratio, 0.20; 95% CI, 0.06 to 0.71; P = 0.006). In the subgroup of NYHA Class III patients, all-cause mortality was significantly decreased in the ICD arm (hazard ratio, 0.37, 95% CI 0.15 to 0.90; P = 0.02).

Although this study was underpowered and did not reach statistical significance with respect to the primary endpoint of all-cause mortality for the entire randomized cohort, the results demonstrated a strong trend toward a survival advantage for patients receiving an ICD. It is worth mentioning that the all-cause mortality reduction seen in DEFINITE was 35%, a value that is strikingly similar to the 31% relative risk reduction observed in the ischemic population studied in MADIT II. The statistical power of DEFINITE was affected by a low rate of SCD in both groups, which may be related to aggressive utilization of ACE-I and β-blockade in this trial.

Sudden Cardiac Death-Heart Failure Trial

The results of the SCD-HeFT trial, published in 2005, have had a substantial impact on current practice and reimbursement guidelines for ICDs.[43] This landmark randomized controlled trial enrolled 2521 patients from 148 mostly American centers between 1997 and 2001. Patients with NYHA Class II (70%) or III (30%) heart failure and reduced LVEF (≤35%; mean about 25%) of either ischemic or nonischemic etiology were eligible

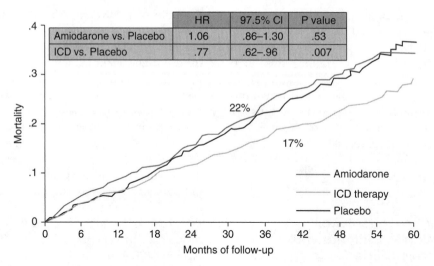

	HR	97.5% CI	P value
Amiodarone vs. Placebo	1.06	.86–1.30	.53
ICD vs. Placebo	.77	.62–.96	.007

Figure 14-3   Kaplan-Meier estimates of risk of all-cause mortality in patients randomized to an ICD compared to amiodarone compared to conventional medical therapy in the SCD-HeFT trial. CI—confidence interval; HR—hazard ratio; ICD—implantable cardioverter defibrillator. (From reference 43, with permission.)

for the study. SCD-HeFT was a three-arm trial, comparing treatment with an ICD to amiodarone and placebo. Specifically, SCD-HeFT addressed the following issues in heart failure treatment: (1) whether or not empirical amiodarone therapy saved lives in well-treated NYHA Class II and III heart failure patients with no arrhythmic indication for the drug and (2) whether or not a prophylactic ICD saved lives in such patients with heart failure from either an ischemic or nonischemic cause.

In SCD-HeFT, patients received standard heart failure therapy, if tolerated, which included an ACE-I or angiotensin receptor blocker (85%), β-blocker (69%), and aldosterone antagonists (19%), compatible with guidelines recommendations at the time the study was conducted. The median follow-up was 45.5 months. Importantly, the cohort was equally divided between ischemic and nonischemic causes of heart failure, allowing an important subgroup analysis of these cohorts to be done.

Mortality rates in the ICD, amiodarone, and placebo groups were 17.1%, 24%, and 22.3% at 3 years and 28.9%, 34.1%, and 35.9%, respectively, at 5 years. The ICD was associated with a statistically significant 23% reduction in all-cause

mortality compared to placebo (hazard ratio 0.77; 97.5% CI, 0.62 to 0.96, P = 0.007). Outcomes on amiodarone were not significantly different from placebo across all subgroups (hazard ratio 1.06; 97.5% CI, 0.86 to 1.30) (Fig. 14-3). Similar degrees of benefit were noted in patients with ischemic (21% mortality reduction) and nonischemic (27% mortality reduction) heart failure, thus confirming the findings of MADIT II and DEFINITE, respectively. The SCD-HeFT trial provides the most robust evidence to date supporting the prophylactic use of an ICD in patients with NYHA Class II and III systolic heart failure of virtually any cause.

▶ INDICATIONS FOR PROPHYLACTIC IMPLANTABLE CARDIOVERTER DEFIBRILLATOR IMPLANTATION IN HEART FAILURE PATIENTS

The 2005 ACC/AHA heart failure guideline endorses Class I indications for the use of an ICD as primary prevention of all-cause mortality in well-treated NYHA Class II and III patients with

LVEFs of less than or equal to 30% and either ischemic or nonischemic cardiomyopathy.[1] There is a Class IIa indication for such patients with ejection fractions of 31–35%. The reasoning behind these separate indications stems from the fact that MADIT II and SCD-HeFT used different ejection fraction criteria for enrollment. In any event, patients with moderate-to-severe left ventricular systolic dysfunction and NYHA Class II or III heart failure should receive an ICD, unless they have a poor chance of survival (<1 year) related to some comorbidity or a contraindication to the implantation or use of this device.

▶ LEVERAGING IMPLANTABLE DEVICES TO MONITOR HEART FAILURE

Implantable devices can provide substantial physiological information about heart failure patients. Such information may be useful in evaluating heart failure clinical status and/or in predicting episodes of heart failure decompensation. If these devices are reliable in the latter sense, the use of this information may improve heart failure outcomes by reducing the risk of worsening heart failure. For example, many implantable CRT and ICD devices can provide information on atrial heart rate and rhythm, ventricular heart rate and rhythm, patient activity level, heart rate variability (HRV), and in some cases, intrathoracic impedance, which has been proposed as a measure of lung "wetness."

Many implantable devices record an activity trend, providing an objective record of the number of hours per day that patients are physically active. The activity level may serve as a useful teaching and reinforcement tool to both the patient and family about the importance and level of activity. Since exercise intolerance is a manifestation of worsening heart failure, a decrease in patient activity level may provide one clue to disease progression or decompensation. This measurement may be viewed as complimentary to the patient history and, perhaps, more objective. In fact, patients may reduce their activity level without conscious recognition, until their heart failure becomes overtly decompensated. The objective measure of activity may have predictive value for worsening heart failure and is currently under investigation.

Heart rate variability reflects the balance between sympathetic and parasympathetic nervous system activity in the heart, with a decrease in HRV serving as a marker of increased sympathetic and decreased parasympathetic tone.[45] An analysis from Adamson et al. showed that HRV diminished in the days to weeks leading up to a hospitalization for worsening heart failure, suggesting that decreases in HRV may predict episodes of worsening heart failure.[46] This idea is biologically plausible, given our understanding of the changes in the neurohormonal milieu that occur as heart failure worsens. Specifically, sympathetic activation has been viewed as a hallmark of worsening heart failure, consistent with the findings of decreased HRV preceding decompensation.

Since most patients with decompensation exhibit pulmonary congestion due to an elevated left ventricular filling pressure, indirect measurement of lung water or direct measurement of left ventricular filling pressure or its surrogate may be useful in managing heart failure patients on an outpatient basis. Implantable devices can monitor fluid status by assessing changes in intrathoracic impedance. Electrical impedance can be determined between the ICD lead residing within the right ventricle and the device generator or "can." Using this approach, electrical impedance is measured across the lung, from the tip of the lead to the generator. The principle that is exploited is quite simple: water conducts electricity better than air, so increasing lung water is associated with a decrease in electrical impedance. Using this technique, electrical impedance may be assessed multiple times throughout the day and followed for changes over time. In a small study of 33 patients, intrathoracic impedance changes demonstrated the ability to predict hospitalizations for decompensated heart failure 10–14 days in advance of the event.[47] The challenge for clinicians is knowing how to react to this information, especially in the absence of signs or symptoms of congestion.

Thus, additional studies are underway to better understand the use and potential of this approach. Finally, a new generation of even more sophisticated implantable monitoring devices is under investigation. These devices allow continuous or intermittent assessment of hemodynamics, generally focused on the direct measurement or estimation of left-sided filling pressure.

▶ OTHER INVESTIGATIONAL IMPLANTABLE DEVICES FOR THE TREATMENT OF HEART FAILURE

Another electrical approach to heart failure currently under investigation has been called cardiac contractility modulation or CCM.[48] This investigational implantable device delivers an intermittent electrical impulse to the heart during the absolute refractory period of the ventricle. While the mechanism of action of CCM is incompletely understood, it may be thought of as a form of electrical conditioning of the heart whereby electrically medicated changes in myocyte calcium handling improve contractility. This improvement in contractility occurs in association with a reduction in myocardial oxygen consumption, suggesting improved efficiency of the heart.[49] This favorable relationship between myocardial contractility and work has been associated with improved outcomes for other heart failure therapies, such as CRT. A large-scale randomized controlled trial of CCM is underway. Other implantable heart failure devices are in preclinical and clinical evaluation. Among these are cardiac support devices (CSDs) that provide either passive or elastic ventricular restraint that may favorably affect functional status and remodeling. While these are surgically implanted devices, minimally invasive techniques have been developed for their deployment. An investigational ventricular partitioning device now under study attempts to replicate the effects of surgical ventricular restoration (SVR; discussed in Chap. 15) surgery, using a less invasive catheter-based approach to deployment. Nonimplantable devices are also being used or investigated for the treatment of heart failure. A discussion of these devices is beyond the scope of this chapter.

▶ SUMMARY

The device era for heart failure management is upon us, ushered in by the routine use of CRT and primary prevention ICDs. Specifically, CRT is intended for patients with ventricular dyssynchrony and moderate-to-severe heart failure. Substantial experience suggests that it is safe and effective, with patients demonstrating significant improvement in clinical symptoms, functional status, exercise capacity, and outcomes. The beneficial effects of CRT on ventricular structure and function have also been demonstrated. Prophylactic implantation of an ICD is also now of proven benefit in heart failure patients, specifically in those with NYHA Class II and III disease. Emerging implantable monitoring technologies may improve our ability to avoid episodes of heart failure decompensation. Other investigational devices may add incremental benefit to the treatment of heart failure, using novel approaches to improving cardiac structure, function, and/or energetics.

▶ REFERENCES

1. Hunt SA, Abraham WT, Chin MH, et al. ACC/AHA 2005 Guideline Update for the Diagnosis and Management of Chronic Heart Failure in the Adult: summary article. *Circulation*. 2005;112:1825–1852 and *J Am Coll Cardiol*. 2005;46:1116–1143.
2. Xiao HB, Brecker SJ, Gibson DG. Effects of abnormal activation on the time course of the left ventricular pressure pulse in dilated cardiomyopathy. *Br Heart J*. 1992;68:403–407.
3. Littmann L, Symanski JD. Hemodynamic implications of left bundle branch block. *J Electrocardiol*. 2000;33(Suppl):115–121.
4. Saxon LA, Kerwin WF, Cahalan MK, et al. Acute effects of intraoperative multisite ventricular pacing on left ventricular function and activation/ contraction sequence in patients with depressed

ventricular function. *J Cardiovasc Electrophysiol.* 1998;9:13–21.

5. Kerwin WF, Botvinick EH, O'Connell JW, et al. Ventricular contraction abnormalities in dilated cardiomyopathy: effect of biventricular pacing to correct interventricular dyssynchrony. *J Am Coll Cardiol.* 2000;35:1221–1227.

6. Farwell D, Patel NR, Hall A, et al. How many people with heart failure are appropriate for biventricular resynchronization? *Eur Heart J.* 2000;21:1246–1250.

7. Aaronson KD, Schwartz JS, Chen TM, et al. Development and prospective validation of a clinical index to predict survival in ambulatory patients referred for cardiac transplant evaluation. *Circulation.* 1997;95:2660–2667.

8. Xaio HB, Roy C, Fujimoto S, et al. Natural history of abnormal conduction and its relation to prognosis in patients with dilated cardiomyopathy. *Int J Cardiol.* 1996;53:163–170.

9. Unverferth DV, Magorien RD, Moeschberger ML, et al. Factors influencing the one-year mortality of dilated cardiomyopathy. *Am J Cardiol.* 1984;54:147–152.

10. Shamim W, Francis DP, Yousufuddin M, et al. Intraventricular conduction delay: a prognostic marker in chronic heart failure. *Int J Cardiol.* 1999;70:171–178.

11. Brophy JM, Deslauriers G, Rouleau JL. Long-term prognosis of patients presenting to the emergency room with decompensated congestive heart failure. *Can J Cardiol.* 1994;10:543–547.

12. Cazeau S, Ritter P, Bakdach S, et al. Four chamber pacing in dilated cardiomyopathy. *PACE.* 1994;17:1974–1979.

13. Foster AH, Gold MR, McLaughlin JS. Acute hemodynamic effects of atrio-biventricular pacing in humans. *Ann Thorac Surg.* 1995;59:294–300.

14. Cazeau S, Ritter P, Lazarus A, et al. Multisite pacing for end-stage heart failure: early experience. *Pacing Clin Electrophysiol.* 1996;19:1748–1757.

15. Blanc JJ, Etienne Y, Gilard M, et al. Evaluation of different ventricular pacing sites in patients with severe heart failure: results of an acute hemodynamic study. *Circulation.* 1997;96:3273–3277.

16. Leclercq C, Cazeau S, Le Breton H, et al. Acute hemodynamic effects of biventricular DDD pacing in patients with end-stage heart failure. *J Am Coll Cardiol.* 1998;32:1825–1831.

17. Kass DA, Chen CH, Curry C, et al. Improved left ventricular mechanics from acute VDD pacing in patients with dilated cardiomyopathy and ventricular conduction delay. *Circulation.* 1999; 99:1567–1573.

18. Gras D, Mabo P, Tang T, et al. Multisite pacing as a supplemental treatment of congestive heart failure: preliminary results of the Medtronic Inc. InSync Study. *Pacing Clin Electrophysiol.* 1998;21:2249–2255.

19. Auricchio A, Stellbrink C, Sack S, et al. The Pacing Therapies for Congestive Heart Failure (PATH-CHF) Study: rationale, design, and endpoints of a prospective randomized multicenter study. *Am J Cardiol.* 1999;83:130D–135D.

20. Auricchio A, Stellbrink C, Block M, et al, for the Pacing Therapies for Congestive Heart Failure Study Group. Effect of pacing chamber and atrioventricular delay on acute systolic function of paced patients with congestive heart failure. *Circulation.* 1999;99:2993–3001.

21. Auricchio A, Klein H, Spinelli J. Pacing for heart failure: selection of patients, techniques, and benefits. *Eu J Heart Fail.* 1999;1:275–279.

22. Gras D, Leclercq C, Tang A, et al. Cardiac resynchronization therapy in advanced heart failure the multicenter InSync clinical study. *Eur J Heart Fail.* 2002;4:311–320.

23. Cazeau S, Leclercq C, Lavergne T, et al, for the Multisite Stimulation in Cardiomyopathies (MUSTIC) Study Investigators. Effects of multisite biventricular pacing in patients with heart failure and intraventricular conduction delay. *N Engl J Med.* 2001;344:873–880.

24. Leclercq C, Walker S, Linde C, et al. Comparative effects of permanent biventricular and right-univentricular pacing in heart failure patients with chronic atrial fibrillation. *Eur Heart J.* 2002;23:1780–1787.

25. Abraham WT, on behalf of the Multicenter InSync Randomized Clinical Evaluation (MIRACLE) Investigators and Coordinators. Rationale and design of a randomized clinical trial to assess the safety and efficacy of cardiac resynchronization therapy in patients with advanced heart failure: the Multicenter InSync Randomized Clinical Evaluation (MIRACLE). *J Card Fail.* 2000; 6:369–380.

26. Abraham WT, Fisher WG, Smith AL, et al, for the Multicenter InSync Randomized Clinical Evaluation (MIRACLE) Investigators and Coordinators. Double-blind, randomized controlled trial of cardiac resynchronization in

chronic heart failure. *N Engl J Med*. 2002; 346:1845–1853.

27. Young JB, Abraham WT, Smith AL, et al. Safety and efficacy of combined cardiac resynchronization therapy and implantable cardioversion defibrillation in patients with advanced chronic heart failure. The Multicenter InSync ICD Randomized Clinical Evaluation (MIRACLE ICD) trial. *JAMA*. 2003;289:2685–2694.

28. Higgins SL, Hummel JD, Niazi IK, et al. Cardiac resynchronization therapy for the treatment of heart failure in patients with intraventricular conduction delay and malignant ventricular tachyarrhythmias. *J Am Coll Cardiol*. 2003; 42:1454–1459.

29. Cleland JGF, Daubert JC, Erdmann E, et al, on behalf of The CARE-HF study Steering Committee and Investigators. The CARE-HF study (CArdiac REsynchronisation in Heart Failure study): rationale, design and end-points. *Eur J Heart Fail*. 2001; 3:481–489.

30. Cleland JGF, Daubert JC, Erdmann E, et al, for the Cardiac Resynchronization—Heart Failure (CARE-HF) Study Investigators. The effect of cardiac resynchronization on morbidity and mortality in heart failure. *N Engl J Med*. 2005;352:1539–1549.

31. Bristow MR, Feldman AM, Saxon LA, for the COMPANION Steering Committee and COMPANION Clinical Investigators. Heart failure management using implantable devices for ventricular resynchronization: Comparison of Medical Therapy, Pacing, and Defibrillation in Chronic Heart Failure (COMPANION) trial. *J Card Fail*. 2000;6:276–285.

32. Bristow MR, Saxon LA, Boehmer J, et al. Cardiac-resynchronization therapy with or without an implantable defibrillator in advanced chronic heart failure. *N Engl J Med*. 2004;350:2140–2150.

33. St. John-Sutton MG, Plappert T, Abraham WT, et al. Effect of cardiac resynchronization therapy on left ventricular size and function in chronic heart failure. *Circulation*. 2003;107:1985–1990.

34. Yu CM, Abraham WT, Bax J, et al. Predictors of Response to Cardiac Resynchronization Therapy (PROSPECT) study design. *Am Heart J*. 2005;149: 600–605.

35. Uretsky B, Sheahan R. Primary prevention of sudden cardiac death in heart failure: will the solution be shocking? *J Am Coll Cardiol*. 1997;30:1589–1597.

36. Stevenson WG, Stevenson LW, Middlekauff HR, et al. Sudden death prevention in patients with advanced ventricular dysfunction. *Circulation*. 1993;88:2953–2961.

37. Effects of Metoprolol CR/XL in Chronic Heart Failure: Metoprolol CR/XL Randomised Intervention Trial in Congestive Heart Failure (MERIT-HF). *Lancet*. 1999;353:2001–2007.

38. Moss AJ, Hall WJ, Cannom DS, et al., for the Multicenter Automatic Defibrillator Implantation Trial Investigators. Improved survival with an implanted defibrillator in patients with coronary disease at high risk for ventricular arrhythmia. *N Engl J Med*. 1996;335:1933–1940.

39. Bigger JT. Prophylactic use of implanted cardiac defibrillators in patients at high risk for ventricular arrhythmia after coronary artery bypass graft surgery. *N Engl J Med*. 1997;337:1569–1575.

40. Buxton AE, Lee KL, Fisher JD, et al, for the Multicenter Unsustained Tachycardia Trial Investigators. A randomized study of the prevention of sudden death in patients with coronary artery disease. *N Engl J Med*. 1999;341:1882–1890.

41. Moss AJ, Zareba W, Hall J, et al, for the Multicenter Automatic Defibrillator Implantation Trial II Investigators. Prophylactic implantation of a defibrillator in patients with myocardial infarction and reduced ejection fraction. *N Engl J Med*. 2002;346:877–883.

42. Kadish A, Dyer A, Daubert JP, et al. Prophylactic defibrillator implantation in patients with nonischemic dilated cardiomyopathy. *N Engl J Med*. 2004;350:2151–2157.

43. Bardy GH, Lee KL, Mark DB, et al. Amiodarone or an implantable cardioverter-defibrillator for congestive heart failure. *N Engl J Med*. 2005; 352:225–237.

44. Doval HC, Nul DR, Grancelli HO, et al. Randomized trial of low-dose amiodarone in severe congestive heart failure. Grupo de Estudio de la Sobrevida en la Insuficiencia Cardiaca en Argentina (GESICA). *Lancet*. 1994;344:489–490.

45. Nolan J, Batin PD, Andrews R, et al. Prospective study of heart rate variability and mortality in chronic heart failure. *Circulation*. 1998;98:1510–1516.

46. Adamson P, Smith A, Abraham W, et al. Continuous autonomic assessment in patients with symptomatic heart failure. *Circulation*. 2004;2389–2394.

47. Yu CM, Wang L, Chau E, et al. Intrathoracic impedance monitoring in patients with heart failure. Correlation with fluid status and feasibility of early warning preceding hospitalization. *Circulation.* 2005;112:841–848.

48. Pappone C, Augello G, Rosanio S, et al. First human chronic experience with cardiac contractility modulation by nonexcitatory electrical currents for treating systolic heart failure: mid-term safety and efficacy results from a multicenter study. *J Cardiovasc Electrophysiol.* 2004;15:418–427.

49. Morita H, Suzuki G, Haddad W, et al. Cardiac contractility modulation with non-excitatory electric signals improves left ventricular function in dogs with chronic heart failure. *J Cardiac Failure.* 2003;9:69–75.

CHAPTER 15

Surgical Approaches to Heart Failure

ROBERT E. MICHLER, MD/MICHAEL ZEMBALA, MD/DANIEL J. GOLDSTEIN, MD

▶ INTRODUCTION

Despite tremendous advances in the medical management of HF, the gold standard for the treatment of end-stage HF remains cardiac transplantation. Several surgical alternatives for the treatment of HF are currently being investigated. Some approaches involve an extension of current conventional cardiac operations like mitral valve repair while others seek to induce changes in the geometry of the left ventricle to render it a more efficient pump. This chapter outlines surgical approaches to congestive HF in the most common clinical situations.

▶ CORONARY REVASCULARIZATION IN THE PATIENT WITH SEVERE LEFT VENTRICULAR DYSFUNCTION

Numerous studies over the last decade have demonstrated that left ventricular dysfunction secondary to myocardial stunning and hibernation can be a reversible phenomenon following coronary revascularization.[1,2] Therefore, it is believed that selection of patients who have coronary artery disease and left ventricular dysfunction for surgical revascularization be based on the presence of viable myocardium.[3-5] The implications of distinguishing viable from nonviable myocardium are important in determining which patients may benefit from coronary revascularization. A recent meta-analysis, which pooled 24 studies and some 3000 patients, suggested that viable myocardium may represent an unstable substrate leading to improvement in survival with revascularization.

The Coronary Artery Surgery Study (CASS) trial was the first clinical trial that assessed the impact of surgical coronary revascularization in patients with left ventricular dysfunction.[6] In comparing 420 medically treated and 231 surgically treated patients with left ventricular ejection fraction (LVEF) ≤35% in the nonrandomized registry cohort, Alderman et al. reported that coronary artery bypass graft (CABG) improved survival. The benefit was most apparent for patients with angina and LVEF ≤25%; medically treated patients in this cohort had a 43% 5-year survival while CABG recipients benefited from a 63% 5-year survival. Operative mortality in the CASS series was 6.9%. Clearly, much has changed in the medical and surgical treatment of advanced coronary disease since that time. The CASS trial was conducted prior to the routine use of angiotensin-converting enzyme (ACE) inhibitors, β-blockers, and statins. Advances in surgical management including routine use of internal mammary and other arterial conduits, improved cardioplegic solutions, and off-pump techniques, among others, have resulted in marked reductions in operative morbidity and mortality in increasingly ill patients. These radical changes

have lessened, if not obviated, the applicability of the results of the CASS and other early trials to current practice.

In an attempt to identify differential indications for CABG versus cardiac transplantation, Hausmann studied patients with end-stage ischemic cardiomyopathy and LVEF between 10% and 30% who underwent CABG. The 225 study patients had been referred as possible cardiac transplant candidates.[7] The major candidacy criterion for bypass grafting was ischemia diagnosed by myocardial thallium scintigraphy and echocardiography. The operative mortality was 7.1%, with an actuarial survival of 90.8% at 2 years, 87.6% at 4 years, and 78.9% at 6 years. During the same time period, 231 patients with end-stage coronary artery disease and a mean LVEF of 21% underwent orthotopic heart transplantation at the same institution. The operative mortality in the transplant group was 18.2%, and the actuarial survival at 6 years was 68.9%. Significant causes of early death in the transplant group were infection (40.5%) and early rejection (26.2%). Among their observations, the authors noted that an area of 20% or more of the total heart mass defined as viable by preoperative testing portends promising results after CABG. A summary of several reports depicting the results of conventional CABG in patients with severe left ventricular dysfunction is depicted in Table 15-1.

Off-pump revascularization has emerged as another option for the treatment of severe

▶ **Table 15-1** Summary of reports evaluating the results of surgical revascularization in patients with severe left ventricular dysfunction

Author	Year	n	EF range (%)	Operative mortality	Survival (%)
Pigott	1985	77	15–35	1.3	76 at 5 years
Kron	1989	39	10–20	2.6	83 at 3 years
Elefteriades	1997	125	10–30	5.2	71 at 5 years
Hausmann	1997	514	10–30	7.1	91 at 2 years
Mickleborough	2000	125	<20	4	72 at 5 years
Selim Isbir	2003	212	17–30	5.6	73 at 4 years
Nishi	2003	42	<30	2.4	83 at 5 years
Appoo	2004	430	<30	4.6	77 at 5 years

ischemic left ventricular dysfunction. Recent evidence indicates that some of the associated morbidities encountered with conventional arrested heart technique may be reduced with beating heart surgery.[8] Off-pump beating heart CABG is typically performed by total avoidance of cardiopulmonary bypass and minimization of aortic manipulation. Arom et al. compared 45 patients with LVEF <30% who underwent off-pump revascularization with 132 similarly impaired patients who underwent conventional grafting during the same time period.[9] The former benefited from reduced perioperative blood loss and perioperative myocardial injury. Operative mortality was lower in the off-pump group, but it did not reach statistical significance. Goldstein et al. reported on 100 consecutive patients with a mean ejection fraction (EF) of 26 ± 4% who underwent beating heart revascularization.[10] Patients received a mean of 3.5 grafts with 83% internal mammary artery use. Observed mortality was 3% with a predicted mortality of 5.3%. Observed-to-expected ratio was 0.56. Incidence of adverse events compared favorably with both that reported in the Society of Thoracic Surgeons Database for all CABG patients regardless of left ventricular function, and also to a concurrent CABG cohort. One-year survival was 85%. Freedom from cardiac readmission was 88% and freedom from angina was 83%. No patient required repeat percutaneous or surgical intervention. Further studies are necessary to define the indications for off-pump revascularization in this high-risk cohort of patients.

In the absence of confirmatory randomized data, it is generally accepted that in the presence of documented contractile reserve (myocardial viability) and graftable targets with good runoff, and in the absence of significant right ventricular dysfunction, pulmonary hypertension, and marked left ventricular dilation, patients with coronary artery disease and left ventricular dysfunction should be strongly considered for coronary revascularization rather than cardiac transplantation. As mentioned later (page 205 of this chapter), the comparative safety and efficacy of coronary revascularization plus optimal medical therapy versus optimal medical therapy alone is under evaluation in a large randomized controlled trial in patients with ischemic HF who are not considered sick enough for cardiac transplantation.

▶ AORTIC STENOSIS AND SEVERE LEFT VENTRICULAR DYSFUNCTION

The most common etiology of aortic stenosis (AS) is age-related degeneration of the aortic valve followed by a congenitally bicuspid valve and then rheumatic disease. Regardless of the etiology, the resulting left ventricular obstruction from chronic AS leads to chronic pressure overload of the left ventricle, leading to compensatory hypertrophy. Uncorrected AS eventually leads to systolic and diastolic dysfunction as the hypertrophied myocardium cannot compensate for the increased wall stress generated.

Aortic valve replacement (AVR) is possible in patients with severe AS and HF. In order to identify patients who may be better candidates for high-risk AVR, attempts have been made to stratify patients on the basis of presence or absence of reversible left ventricular dysfunction.[11] A recent study documented the use of dobutamine echocardiography to differentiate between those patients with severe AS, left ventricular dysfunction, a low transvalvular gradient, and irreversible myocardial damage from those with reversible myocardial dysfunction.[12] Dobutamine echocardiography is thus used to determine aortic valve area in two different flow states (baseline and stress), so that severe AS, which is fixed, can be distinguished from AS that is flow-dependent. Patients with flow-dependent AS will demonstrate a decrease in valve area with the increased flows caused by the enhanced inotropic-mediated contractile state. AVR is more likely to be beneficial in these patients, as the depressed contractility is due to increased afterload, also known as "afterload mismatch," and is, therefore, recoverable.

Only a few published series have been undertaken to examine the outcomes of patients with severe AS (valve area <0.75 cm²) and LVEF<35% or New York Heart Association (NYHA) Class IV symptoms who undergo AVR.[13] A report by Powell et al. described an operative mortality of 18%, with prior myocardial infarction being a risk factor for perioperative mortality. Based on the high operative mortality, the authors suggested avoiding AVR in these patients.[14]

Review of the published studies (Table 15-2) suggests high perioperative mortality (7–21%) but improved functional capacity in most survivors. Long-term survival was not recorded in most studies, but in those studies that did, 5-year survival was at least comparable to that achieved with cardiac transplantation. Based on these reports, the general consensus is that in patients with AS and severe left ventricular dysfunction in whom contractile reserve can be documented, AVR (1) can be performed with an acceptable operative mortality, (2) leads to symptomatic improvement in most survivors, and (3) confers a short- and long-term survival benefit in comparison to medical therapy.

► AORTIC REGURGITATION AND SEVERE LEFT VENTRICULAR DYSFUNCTION

Aortic regurgitation (AR) results from improper coaptation of the aortic valve leaflets leading to regurgitant blood flow into the left ventricle during diastole. The pathophysiology of AR involves *both* volume and pressure overload of the left ventricle. AR has numerous etiologies, including hypertension, calcific, degenerative and rheumatic disease, endocarditis, and aortic annular dilatation as a result of connective tissue disorders (such as Marfan syndrome), or even trauma. Chronic AR leads to left ventricular eccentric hypertrophy to compensate for the volume and pressure overload. With continued uncorrected AR, myocardial fibrosis eventually occurs, resulting either from subclinical ischemia secondary to increased wall stress and diminished diastolic coronary flow, and/or from stress-triggered myocyte apoptosis. Progressive fibrosis leads to irreversible cardiac dysfunction and severe HF symptomatology.

The natural history of patients with chronic AR and low EF (<35%) and/or NYHA Class III–IV symptoms treated medically is extremely poor.[15] Survival for medically treated severe AR at 5 years

► **Table 15-2** Summary of studies evaluating aortic valve replacement in patients with aortic stenosis and severe left ventricular dysfunction

Author	Year	n	Mean AVA* (cm²)	EF (%)	Operative mortality	Improved NYHA Class	Survival
Obadia	1995	112	0.4	NR*	7.1	Yes	78% at 5 yrs
Snopek	1996	11	NR†	38	9	Yes	NR
Connolly	1997	154	0.6	27	9	Yes	NR
Connolly	2000	52	0.7	26	21	Yes	NR
Monin	2001	45	0.7	35	18	Yes	NR
Pereira	2002	39	0.75	35	8	Yes	78% at 4 yrs
Rothenburger	2003	35	0.66	NR	NR	Yes	64% at 5 yrs
Tarantini	2003	52	<1.0‡	<35	8	Yes	NR
Vaquette	2005	155	0.35†	≤30	12	Yes	NR

*Aortic valve area
†Not recorded
‡Indexed aortic valve area (cm²/m²)

has been reported to be between 20% and 66%. Current guidelines for patients with AR recommend AVR best for symptomatic patients and for those asymptomatic patients who show signs of deteriorating left ventricular function or have an EF <35% or diastolic diameter approaching 75 mm or an end-systolic diameter approaching 55 mm. AVR is best tolerated and associated with acceptable morbidity and mortality in patients with preserved or slightly disturbed ventricular function. AVR is currently recommended in severe AR even when EF is depressed. Clearly defining the risks and benefits of AVR in this patient population would allow better allocation of treatment options, which include AVR, medical vasodilator therapy, and cardiac transplantation.[16]

Table 15-3 depicts the major clinical reports outlining the outcomes of AVR in patients with severe regurgitation and systolic dysfunction. The consensus from the available literature is that for patients with severe left ventricular dysfunction and chronic AR, even those with markedly dilated left ventricles, AVR can be performed with an acceptable operative mortality of approximately 8–15%. Long-term survival approaches 70% at 5 years, which is better than with no treatment or medical treatment alone, as inferred from natural history studies. However, no studies that directly compare medical therapy to AVR in this subgroup exist, and probably will not exist, as the prognosis of medical treatment alone for dilated cardiomyopathy secondary to AR is extremely poor.

▶ MITRAL VALVE SURGERY IN SEVERE LEFT VENTRICULAR DYSFUNCTION

It is well established that secondary or functional mitral regurgitation worsens both symptoms and prognosis in patients with left ventricular dysfunction of ischemic and nonischemic etiology. Volume overload resulting from mitral valve regurgitation leads to ventricular dilatation and dysfunction, which subsequently leads to further regurgitation through annular dilatation. Thus, a vicious downhill cycle is perpetuated whereby ventricular dilatation potentiates mitral regurgitation and mitral regurgitation potentiates ventricular dilatation. Despite maximal medical therapy, these patients face an extremely poor probability of survival unless they undergo cardiac transplantation.

In the majority of patients, the functional regurgitation produces a central jet, which is easily treated with reduction ring annuloplasty. Zealous supporters of either rigid or flexible annuloplasty rings exist and no convincing data exist to support one type over the other. There appears to be a growing consensus, however, that a complete rather than a partial (or posterior) ring should be used as recent data suggest improved freedom from recurrent regurgitation. Some authors suggest that the intertrigonal distance does, in fact, increase in the setting of cardiomyopathy. In the presence of leaflet pathology, more sophisticated repairs like triangular and

▶ **Table 15-3** Summary of clinical studies investigating the outcome of aortic valve replacement for patients with severe left ventricular dysfunction

Author	Year	n	EF (%)	Operative mortality	5-yr survival
Bonow	1985	50	37	0	63%
Acar	1996	46	<40	6.5	84%
Klodas	1997	128	NR*	7.8	72%
Chaliki	2002	43	35	14	72%
Rothenburger	2003	20	<30	NR	74%

*Not recorded

quadrangular resections, chordal shortening and transfers, and edge-to-edge (Alfieri) repairs have been successfully used to preserve the mitral apparatus and avoid the adverse effects of mitral prosthetic implantation.

Bolling et al., in 1995, were the first to report the early outcome of remodeling mitral annuloplasty with a flexible posterior ring in 16 patients with severe HF and mitral regurgitation.[17] Twelve of their patients had a nonischemic cardiomyopathy and the other 4 an ischemic cardiomyopathy. Functional capacity was improved in all patients, and mean LVEF rose from 16% to 25%, with reduction in regurgitation volume and left ventricular volume. The most impressive result of this study was that patients with severe left ventricular systolic dysfunction in whom LVEF was probably overestimated by the presence of severe mitral regurgitation were able to tolerate a major surgical procedure for correction of mitral regurgitation. This observation was instrumental in reversing the widely held opinion that corrective surgery should not be performed in patients with severe mitral regurgitation and an EF <30%. A summary of reports evaluating the outcomes of mitral valve repair in dilated cardiomyopathy are outlined in Table 15-4.

Rothenburger et al. recently reported a series of 31 patients with mitral regurgitation and EF <30% who underwent isolated repair or replacement with complete preservation of the subvalvar apparatus.[18] They reported comparable results between the two groups, with 1-, 2-, and 5-year survival rates of 91%, 84%, and 74%, respectively. Functional results were also equally good. Similarly, early available data from David et al. indicate that replacement of the mitral valve with preservation of the subvalvular structures can result in postoperative left ventricular systolic function that is comparable to that with valvular repair.[19] In situations where the native valve leaflet(s) is (are) excised, preservation of the subvalvular structures can be achieved by incorporating the chordal leaflet attachments between the annular suture line and the prosthetic cloth rim. In other situations where one or both valve leaflets are kept intact, this can be

achieved by incorporating the plicated leaflet structure with transannular sutures. In these latter instances, clinical and functional studies have suggested that preservation of the posterior leaflet is more important in maintaining left ventricular systolic function. Although preservation of the anterior leaflet is technically feasible, obstruction of the left ventricular outflow tract is possible if too much of the anterior leaflet structure is left intact. Such outcomes with chordae-preserving mitral valve replacement are certainly at odds with the previously reported superiority of repair over replacement in terms of left ventricular function and hemodynamics.

In conclusion, functional mitral regurgitation commonly occurs in patients with severe left ventricular dysfunction regardless of etiology. Presence of even mild regurgitation has been associated with poor long-term prognosis. Early and intermediate results with implantation of an undersized flexible ring in the mitral annulus suggest that correction of functional regurgitation results in partial reversal of left ventricular remodeling and in symptomatic improvement. Intermediate results are superior to medical treatment alone and comparable to cardiac transplantation. The long-term benefit of this procedure remains to be demonstrated, and only randomized trials comparing optimal medical management with mitral valve surgery will ascertain the potential benefits of surgically attained mitral competence on the long-term outcomes of patients with dilated cardiomyopathies.

▶ VENTRICULAR REMODELING THERAPIES

Several studies have documented that left ventricular volume is a sensitive prognostic parameter for both early and late mortal and morbid events after a myocardial infarction.[20–23] The paradigm of progressive left ventricular dilatation is grossly oversimplified but simply understood through Laplace's Law. Left ventricular wall stress/tension (δ) is proportional to the radius (r) and pressure (P) within the left ventricular

▶ **Table 15–4** Clinical series reporting mitral valve repair in the setting of dilated cardiomyopathy and severe left ventricular dysfunction

Author	Year	n	Symptoms/NYHA	EF	Study design	Operation	Op mortality	Survival
Chen	1998	81	III/IV	<30%	Retro[2]	MV Repair[4] CABG	11%	73% at 1 yr, 38% at 5 yrs
Bishay	2000	4	III/IV	<35%	Retro	MVR/Repl[5]	2.30%	89% at 1 yr, 72% at 3 yrs
Calafiore	2001	49	III/IV	<35%	Retro	MV Repair/Repl[5] CABG	4.10%	90% at 1 yr, 78% at 5 yrs
Bolling	2002	125	III/IV	<25%	Retro	MV Repair	5%	80% at 1yr, 70% at 2 yrs
Rothenberger	2002	31	III/IV	<30%	Retro	MV Repair/Repl	6.50%	91% at 1 yr, 77% at 5 yrs
Szalay	2003	30	NR[1]	<30%	Retro	MV Repair	6.60%	93% at 2 yrs
Gummert	2003	66	NR	<30%	Retro	MV Repair	6.10%	86% at 1 yr, 66% at 5 yrs
Kawaguchi	2003	66	III	<30%	Retro	NR	6.10%	86% at 1 yr, 56% at 5yrs
Bolling	2004	"over" 200	III/IV	mean 16%	Retro	MV Repair	5%	82% at l yr, 52% at 5 yrs
Haan	2004	727	NR	<30%	Retro STS[3]	NR	5.45%; 1.7% for repair	NR
Ghosh	2004	23	III/IV	<30%	Retro	MV Repair/Repl	8.70%	87% at 1 yr, 78% at 2 yrs
Calafiore	2004	91	III/IV	<35%	Retro	MV Repair/Repl[5] CABG	4.40%	78% at 5yrs
Ngaage	2004	43	81% III/IV	<30%	Retro	MV Repair[4] other valve	2.30%	84% at 1 yr, 33% at 5 yrs
De Bonis	2005	77	III/IV	<35%	Retro	MV Repair[5] CABG	3.80%	90% at 3 yrs
Wu	2005	126	NR	<30%	Retro	MV Repair	4.80%	NR

[1]Not recorded
[2]Retrospective review
[3]Retrospective review of Society of Thoracic Surgeons database
[4]Mitral valve repair
[5]Mitral valve repair or replacement

chamber and inversely proportional to left ventricular wall thickness (T), with average wall stress estimated by the following equation: $\delta = rP/(2)T$. Whether approaching the concept from the level of the individual myocyte (tension-length) or from the level of the left ventricular chamber (pressure-volume), increasing cardiac myocyte stress becomes an impediment to effective contraction. Therefore, a solution is to reduce left ventricular chamber radius/volume and thereby reduce myocardial wall stress.

Surgical ventricular reconstruction (SVR) is by far the most extensively studied and applied technique for reshaping the dilated left ventricle. Its goal is to reduce left ventricular volume and create a more geometrically optimal chamber by excluding scar in either akinetic or dyskinetic antero-apical and septal segments. Unlike partial posterior left ventriculectomy or the Batista[24] procedure, SVR attempts to directly address specific diseased areas of the left ventricle, most commonly the anterior apex. SVR reshapes the endoventricular contour by placing a patch, often at the level of a purse string suture that encircles the transition zone of myocardial asynergy (Fig. 15-1). The operation is accompanied by complete revascularization including a graft to the left anterior descending artery (to perfuse septal perforators and viable myocardium), and mitral valve repair or replacement as necessary. By grafting the left anterior descending artery, the high intraventricular septum is preserved, thereby enhancing postoperative circumferential shortening. The trade-off comes in the extent to which the longitudinal axis of the left ventricle can be reduced and is ultimately determined by the position of the new apex. In an attempt to avoid catastrophic postoperative restrictive ventricular physiology, Vincent Dor (who began performing the procedure in the early 1985) has recommended that ventricular sizing be routinely performed using a balloon sizer/shaper. Furthermore, it has been suggested that the purse string suture and patch be sutured at an oblique angle toward the aortic outflow tract while still excluding septal akinetic segments in order to prevent the creation of a "box-like" ventricle.

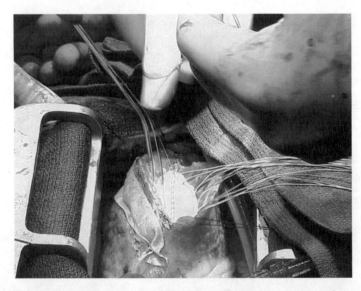

Figure 15-1 SVR procedure. The patient's head is toward the bottom of the figure. The anterior wall of the left ventricle has been opened down to the apex. A Dacron patch has been sutured to the septum and free wall of the left ventricle, effectively creating a more elliptical shape. The two edges of the left ventricle will be reapproximated in a final closure.

The validity of the SVR procedure was documented by the RESTORE group, an 11-center multinational group that evaluated the efficacy and durability of this procedure. In the most recent update from the group's registry, the outcome of 1198 postinfarction patients was reported.[25] Concomitant procedures included bypass grafting in 95%, mitral valve repair in 22%, and mitral valve replacement in 1%. Overall 30-day mortality was 5.3% and the need for perioperative mechanical support was uncommon (<9%). Global systolic function improved with an increase in EF from 29% ± 11% to 39% ± 12% and a reduction in left ventricular end-systolic volume index from 80 ± 51 mL/m² to 57% ± 34% mL/m². Overall 5-year survival was 69% ± 3%. Predictors of death were EF ≤30%, advanced NYHA class, age ≥75 years, and left ventricular end-systolic volume index ≥80 mL/m². Remarkably, 5-year freedom from rehospitalization for HF was 78% and 85% of patients who were in NYHA Class I or II.

While the RESTORE group's data are compelling, randomized evaluation of this procedure is absent, especially in comparison to coronary bypass surgery alone. To this end, the National Heart, Lung, and Blood Institute's (NHLBI) multicenter, international, randomized Surgical Treatment for Ischemic Heart Failure (STICH) trial began enrolling patients with HF and CAD in the spring of 2002.[26] The goal of this trial is to determine whether a benefit over medical therapy can be found for coronary revascularization in patients with multivessel coronary artery disease, LVEF ≤35%, HF, and no indication for bypass surgery (left main or unstable angina). In addition, STICH will examine whether any benefit from coronary bypass surgery can be enhanced by ventricular reconstruction surgery in patients with dilated ventricles. One major focus of the STICH trial will be to determine the long-term outcome and durability of SVR.

There is some evidence demonstrating further remodeling and left ventricular redilatation after SVR. Franco-Cereceda and colleagues noted that a cohort of patients who underwent SVR had indirect physiological evidence of progressive reductions in diastolic compliance.[27] This yet to be understood phenomenon may be attributed to (1) progression of left ventricular myocyte hypertrophy and fibrosis; (2) further progression of coronary artery disease; and/or (3) iatrogenic factors, namely, too aggressive a reduction in left ventricular volume at SVR, thereby creating a restrictive ventricular physiology that precludes adequate diastolic function.

It is likely, given the chronicity of disease prior to surgical therapy and the preexistence of remodeled remote myocardium, that, despite decreased systolic wall stress, there is not an adequate augmentation of diastolic elastance in some patients to allow for complete reversal or attenuation of continued left ventricular remodeling. The surgeon, though able to reduce left ventricular chamber size dramatically, does not reduce chamber volume back to normal values (normal left ventricular end-systolic volume index = 24 mL/m² vs. RESTORE group postprocedure = 69 mL/m²). It is not surprising that improved survival rates and less physiological derangements are seen in those patients with better preoperative function, less left ventricular dilatation, and shorter delay to surgical therapy. Therefore the intrinsic properties within the chronically remodeled myocardium limit the surgeon's ability to completely return chamber size (wall stress) to normal without risking too small a ventricle and compromised diastolic function.

One solution to the problem of chronicity is earlier identification of patients at risk for progressive dilatation and compromised function post myocardial infarction. Left ventricular dilatation generally follows global decreases in left ventricular function by up to several months and exercise challenge may be a predictor of those that will eventually develop left ventricular dilatation. If the promise of earlier intervention holds true, it may be possible to surgically exclude areas of asynergy prior to crossing the yet to be defined threshold of wall stress that inevitably leads to progressive and possibly irreversible ventricular remodeling, dilatation, and global left ventricular systolic dysfunction.

▶ VENTRICULAR ASSIST DEVICES

Ventricular assist devices (VADs) are blood pumps used to support the failing heart in critically ill patients with end-stage HF. Whether placed intracorporeally or paracorporeally, these pumps take over the function of the damaged left (or right) ventricle and restore more normal hemodynamics and end-organ perfusion.[28] Left ventricular assist devices, or LVADs, have been used in three clinical situations: (1) as bridge to transplantation in patients who are listed for transplantation but decompensate before a suitable donor heart becomes available, (2) as bridge to recovery in patients who are expected to recover left ventricular function (e.g., fulminant myocarditis), or (3) as permanent alternatives to transplantation in patients who are not considered to be candidates for transplantation.

Bridge to Transplantation

"Bridge to transplantation" is the most common indication for use of LVADs. Typical patients supported are those with large myocardial infarctions, those with myocarditis, and, most commonly, patients with chronic progressive end-stage HF.

It has been shown that patients bridged with an LVAD have excellent survival to transplantation and post-transplant survival equal to that seen with unsupported patients.[29] Furthermore, because most LVADs are wearable, patients can be discharged home to recover and rehabilitate and hence can undergo cardiac transplantation in a more stable condition.[30]

The usual clinical scenario is that of a patient listed for transplantation who deteriorates clinically requiring inotropic and/or balloon pump support. As results are markedly better when mechanical support is instituted early, HF physicians now alert their surgical colleagues of patients who are demonstrating more subtle signs of deterioration including worsening urine output, more marked hyponatremia, need for escalation of diuretics, and/or the need to institute inotropic support.

Several devices have received approval by the U.S. Food and Drug Administration (FDA) for use as a bridge to cardiac transplantation. These include the HeartMate VE (Thoratec Corporation), the Thoratec paracorporeal (PVAD) and intracorporeal (IVAD), and the Novacor LVAS (WorldHeart Corporation). Three second-generation axial flow pumps (DeBakey VAD, HeartMate II, and Jarvik Flowmaker) are undergoing clinical trials for bridging to transplantation in the United States. Characteristics of devices currently available or in clinical trials in the United States are outlined in Table 15-5. In experienced centers, successful bridging to transplantation occurs for 70–80% of VAD recipients.

Left Ventricular Assist Devices as a Destination Therapy (Alternative to Transplant, Lifetime Support)

The Randomized Evaluation of Mechanical Assistance for the Treatment of Congestive Heart failure (REMATCH) trial sought to compare maximum medical therapy to implantation of the Thoratec HeartMate device for a group of extremely ill patients with end-stage heart disease who, by any account, were the sickest patients ever enrolled in a randomized HF trial.[31] In this landmark NHLBI-supported trial, patients randomized to receive an LVAD benefited from improved survival and quality of life compared to the medically treated cohort. The trial highlighted the limitations associated with these large, pulsatile pumps including the high incidence of septic complications and their limited long-term reliability, thereby establishing benchmarks for the development of newer pump technologies. The positive results of this trial opened the doors to FDA and CMS approval and reimbursement of the Thoratec HeartMate XVE device as alternative to transplantation. Two second-generation miniaturized axial flow pumps (DeBakey VAD and HeartMate II) are currently undergoing randomized trials in the United States for the destination therapy indication.[32] Regardless of indication,

▶ **Table 15-5** Summary of clinical series reporting results of partial left ventriculectomy (Batista procedere) published in the last 7 years

Author	Year	n	Mean EF (%)	Operative mortality (%)	Survival	Comments
Lucchese	2000	44	22	NR*	38% at 1 year	High mortality, arrhythmias, and recurrent heart failure
Vural	2000	27	19	18.5	64% at 3 years	Improved functional status and EF
Moreira	2001	43	NR	21	58% at 1 year	Cardiac redilation in survivors
Franco-Cereceda	2001	62	16	NR	60% at 3 years	Early and late failures preclude widespread use
Etoch	2001	20	14	10	40% at 3 years	Recurrent heart failure
Chang	2001	17	21	41	NR	Recurrent heart failure
Gradinac	2001	38	NR	18	61% at 2 years	Improved functional capacity in survivors
Claus	2003	39	NR	NR	44% at 4 years	High mortality, no long-term improvement
Ascione[†]	2003	506	19	17	50–85% at 1 year 45–72% at 2 years	High early mortality, satisfactory late results
Bestetti	2004	14	17	28	29% at 1 year	PLV[‡] not an adequate treatment

*Not recorded
[†]Review of the literature
[‡]Partial left ventriculectomy

institution of mechanical support with a VAD(s) is associated with significant morbidity and mortality. This should not be unexpected as patients undergoing these procedures suffer from end-stage heart disease, are often supported with inotropic and pressor medications as well as intra-aortic balloon pumps, and carry other comorbidities associated with low-flow states.

The most common early complications of left VAD support are perioperative bleeding and right HF.[33] The former occurs in close to 60% of VAD recipients (regardless of type of device used) and is a result of a large operation often associated with prolonged extracorporeal circulation and hypothermia. In addition to the expected perioperative coagulopathy and platelet dysfunction induced by cardiopulmonary bypass, the propensity for bleeding is further increased by (1) routine use of anticoagulants, antiplatelet drugs, and broad-spectrum antibiotics among these patients with advanced cardiac disease; (2) the malnourished state of many of these patients; and (3) hepatic dysfunction associated with low-flow state and congestive hepatopathy from right HF.

Right HF occurs in approximately 30% of patients and is defined as the need for inotropic support for more than 2 weeks postoperatively or the need for institution of right heart support. The exact etiology of right HF following institution of LVAD support remains controversial. Late complications of VAD support vary among the different devices but involve issues of device-related infection and limited reliability.

▶ **HEART TRANSPLANTATION**

Orthotopic replacement of the failing heart with a donor allograft remains the gold standard therapy for the treatment of end-stage heart disease. Indeed, cardiac transplantation is associated with unrivaled late survival and quality of life resulting from improvements in immunosuppression and in the prevention and treatment suppress of infection.[34] Unfortunately, the number of donors has reached a plateau over the past few years, at a time when the number of potential recipients has continued to grow. This critical discrepancy mandates that patients be strictly evaluated for candidacy for transplantation. This typically occurs during a multidisciplinary session where all clinical, psychological, and sociological aspects of each patient are discussed. In most centers, the *minimum* requirements for consideration for transplantation include (1) a history of repeated hospitalization for congestive HF, (2) escalation in the intensity of medical therapy, and (3) a reproducible VO_{2max} of <14 mL/Kg/min. Unfortunately, many patients who meet the above criteria are excluded from transplantation because of the presence of *absolute* exclusionary criteria. These include (1) irreversible pulmonary hypertension (increased risk of right ventricular failure and death), and (2) active infection and malignancy. Several other *relative* contraindications exist and are weighed in when the final decision is made. These include advanced age (usually >65 years), presence of end-organ complication of diabetes, advanced restrictive or obstructive lung disease, advanced liver disease, renal insufficiency unrelated to low-flow state, significant peripheral vascular disease, morbid obesity, unstable social/family environment, demonstrable lack of compliance with medical/dietary therapy, active substance (alcohol, tobacco, or drug) abuse, and presence of a psychiatric disorder that would compromise adherence to medical therapy.

Patients on the waiting list are classified into one of three classes based on their clinical status, defined as follows: UNOS status 1A patients are those who have either been on mechanical circulatory support for <30 days, or have an intra-aortic balloon pump, or are on high-dose inotropic agents with continuous hemodynamic monitoring, or are expected to live <1 week. Status 1B is assigned to those patients who have been on mechanical circulatory support for >30 days or are on continuous low-dose inotropic support (without hemodynamic monitoring) on an inpatient or outpatient basis. UNOS status 2 includes all other active patients on the waiting list, namely those who are homebound and on no mechanical or inotropic support; and UNOS status 7 are patients who have been placed on the list because they satisfied the criteria for listing but who were inactivated because of some recent medical condition.

Once a suitable heart donor is identified and the organ is allocated, a timetable is set and organized to keep the transportation time and cold ischemia time of the procured organ to a minimum. Implantation occurs almost exclusively in the orthotopic position. In most centers, bicaval (as opposed to biatrial) technique is preferred as the latter is associated with a higher incidence of postoperative arrhythmias and tricuspid valve dysfunction.

Survival following transplantation has continued to improve. At present, 1-year survival approaches 85%, 5-year survival is approximately 75%, and 50% of adult recipients will be alive for 10 years.[35] Survival is best for patients (1) with congenital and dilated cardiomyopathies, (2) who are younger recipients, (3) who underwent transplantation since 1999, (4) with lower pulmonary vascular resistance, (5) who did not receive a VAD as a bridge to transplantation.

The most important dichotomous factors associated with 1-year mortality include congenital heart disease etiology, presence of temporary circulatory support, ventilator dependency, presence of renal failure requiring dialysis, hospitalization at the time of transplantation, donor history of cancer, a female recipient-to-male donor pairing, and cerebrovascular disease as the cause of donor death. Continuous factors associated with 1-year mortality include recipient age, recipient weight, donor age, donor/recipient weight ratio, transplant center volume, ischemia time and preoperative pulmonary artery diastolic pressure, bilirubin, and serum creatinine.

Functional status of transplant recipients is excellent on short- and long-term follow-up. Indeed, 80–85% of recipients have no activity limitations for up to 7 years following transplantation, and <5% require total assistance at any time. Cardiac transplant recipients benefit from freedom from rehospitalization that exceeds 70% for 7-year survivors.

Immunosuppressive strategies have evolved since the advent of cyclosporine in 1983. Approximately 46% of patients receive induction immunosuppression consisting of polyclonal globulin, OKT3, or interleukin-2R antagonist. Maintenance immunosuppression consists of a triple drug therapy that most often includes a calcineurin inhibitor (cyclosporine or tacrolimus), an antimetabolite (mycophenolate mofetil or azathioprine), and prednisone. In most centers, efforts are directed towards a progressive reduction of steroid therapy to minimal levels. Novel immunosuppressive agents including molecularly engineered humanized monoclonal antibodies are being evaluated in an effort to reduce the complications associated with the use of the traditional triple drug therapy.

The most common complications of transplantation include hypertension, renal dysfunction, hyperlipidemia, diabetes, and coronary artery vasculopathy. Malignancy is a well-recognized complication of prolonged immunosuppression and it is documented in 3%, 16%, and 26% of transplant recipients at 1, 5, and 8 years following transplantation. Cutaneous malignancies and lymphoma are by far the most commonly encountered. The latter often regresses with a reduction in immunosuppression.

Causes of death vary according to time after transplantation. The most common early (within 30 days) cause of death is primary allograft failure. Acute rejection, infection, coronary vasculopathy, and graft failure are the most commonly cited causes of death from 30 days to 3 years after transplantation. Malignancy and coronary vasculopathy are the predominant causes of death in long-term survivors.

▶ SUMMARY

Despite tremendous advances in the medical management of congestive HF, the gold standard for the treatment of end-stage congestive HF remains cardiac transplantation. The acknowledged critical limitation of sufficient suitable organ donors has resulted in the refinement and development of novel surgical alternatives for the treatment of congestive HF. These approaches include the extension of current conventional cardiac operations such as mitral valve repair to the failing ventricle, surgically reconstructing the size and shape of the failing left ventricle in order to render it a more efficient pump, and partial replacement of the ventricle with a mechanical device. One day the continued evolution of such therapies is likely to have a significant epidemiologic impact on patients suffering from end-stage HF.

▶ REFERENCES

1. Bolognese L, et al. Left ventricular remodeling after primary coronary angioplasty: patterns of left ventricular dilation and long-term prognostic implications. *Circulation*. 2002:106: 2351–2357.

2. Migrino RQ, et al. End-systolic volume index at 90 and 180 minutes into reperfusion therapy for acute myocardial infarction is a strong predictor of early and late mortality. *Circulation*. 1997;96: 116–121.

3. Sawada S, et al. Incremental value of myocardial viability for prediction of long-term prognosis in surgically revascularized patients with left ventricular dysfunction. *J Am Coll Cardiol*. 2003;17:42(12):2106–2108.

4. Kang WJ, et al. Prognostic value of rest (201)Tl-dypiridamole stress (99m)Tc-sestamibi gated SPECT for predicting patient-based clinical outcomes after bypass surgery in patients with left ventricular dysfunction. *J Nucl Med*. 2003; 44(11):1735–1740.

5. Pitt M, et al. Coronary artery surgery for ischemic heart failure: risks, benefits, and the importance of assessment of myocardial viability. *Prog Cardiovasc Dis*. 2001;43(5):373–386.

6. Killip T, et al. Coronary Artery Surgery Surgery Study (CASS): A randomized trial of coronary bypass surgery. Eight years follow up and survival in patients with reduced ejection fraction. *Circulation*. 1985;72:V102–V109.

7. Hausmann H, et al. Decision making in end stage coronary artery disease: revascularization or heart transplantation? *Ann Thor Surg*. 1997;64:1296–1302.

8. Cleveland JC, et al. Off pump coronary artery bypass grafting decreases risk adjusted mortality and morbidity. *Ann Thorac Surg*. 2001;72: 1282–1288.

9. Arom KV, et al. Is low ejection fraction safe for off pump coronary bypass operation? *Ann Thorac Surg*. 2000;70:1021–1025.

10. Goldstein DJ, et al. Multi-vessel off pump revascularization in patients with severe left ventricular dysfunction. *Eur J Cardiothorac Surg*. 2003;24:72–80.

11. deFilippi CR, et al. Usefulness of dobutamine echocardiography in distinguishing severe from non-severe valvular aortic stenosis in patients with depressed left ventricular function and low transvalvular gradients. *Am J Cardiol*. 1995;75: 191–194.

12. Monin JL, et al. Aortic stenosis with severe ventricular dysfunction and low transvalvular pressure gradients: risk stratification by low-dose dobutamine echocardiography *J Am Coll Cardiol*. 2001;37:2001–2107.

13. Pereira JJ, et al. Survival after aortic valve replacement for sefvere aortic stenosis with low transvalvular gradients and severe left ventricular dysfunction. *J Am Coll Cardiol*. 2002;39: 1356–1363.

14. Powell DE, et al. Aortic valve replacement in patients with aortic stenosis and severe left ventricular dysfunction. *Arch Intern Med*. 2000;160:1337–1341.

15. Dujardin KS, et al. Mortality and morbidity of aortic regurgitation in clinical practice: a germ follow up study. *Circulation*. 1999;99: 1851–1857.

16. Scheuble S, et al. Aortic insufficiency: defining the role of pharmacotherapy. *Am J Cardiovasc Drugs*. 2005;5(2):113–120.

17. Bolling S, et al. Early outcome of mitral valve reconstruction in patients with end stage cardiomyopathy. *J Thorac Cardiovasc Surg*. 1995;109:676–683.

18. Rothenburger M, et al. Mitral valve surgery in patients with poor left ventricular function. *Thorac Cardiovasc Surg*. 2002;6:351–354.

19. David TE, et al. Left ventricular function after mitral valve surgery. *J Heart Valve Dis*. 1995;4(Suppl2):S175–S180.

20. DiDonato M, et al. Akinetic versus dyskinetic postinfarction scar: relation to surgical outcome in patients undergoing endoventricular patch

plasty repair. *J Am Coll Cardiol.* 1997;29(7): 1569–1575.

21. Lee TH, et al. Impact of left ventricular cavity size on survival in advanced heart failure. *Am J Cardiol.* 1993;72:672–677.

22. Pfeffier MA, et al. Ventricular enlargement and reduced survival after myocardial infarction. *Circulation.* 1987;75(suppl IV):IV-93–IV-97.

23. White HD, et al. Left ventricular end-systolic volume as the major determinant of survival after recovery from myocardial infarction. *Circulation.* 1987;76:44–51.

24. Batista RJV, et al. Partial left ventriculectomy to improve LV function. *J Card Surg.* 1996;11:96–97.

25. Athanasuleas CL, et al. Surgical anterior ventricular endocardial restoration in the dilated remodeled ventricle after anterior MI. RESTORE group. *Am Coll Cardiol.* 2001;37(5): 1199–1209.

26. Doenst T, et al. To STICH or not to STICH. *J Thorac Cardiovasc Surg.* 2005;129:246–249.

27. Franco-Cereceda A, et al. Partial left ventriculectomy for dilated cardiomyopathy *J Thorac Cardiovasc Surg.* 2001:121:879–893.

28. Goldstein, DJ, et al. Medical progress: implantable left ventricular assist devices. *N Engl J Med.* 1998;339:1522–1533.

29. Morgan JA, et al. Does bridging to transplantation with a left ventricular assist device adversely affect posttransplantation survival: a comparative analysis of mechanical versus inotropic support. *J Thorac Cardiovasc Surg.* 2003;126(4):1188–1190.

30. Holman WL, et al. Treatment of end-stage heart disease with outpatient ventricular assist devices. *Ann Thorac Surg.* 2002;73(5):1489–1493.

31. Rose EA, et al. Long-term mechanical left ventricular assistance for end-stage heart failure. *N Engl J Med.* 2001;345(20):1435–1443.

32. Goldstein DJ, et al. Safety and feasibility, trial of the MicroMed DeBakey ventricular assist device as a bridge to transplantation. *J Am Coll Cardiol.* 2005;45(6):962–963.

33. Ochiai Y, et al. Predictors of severe right ventricular failure after implantable left ventricular assist device insertion: analysis of 245 patients. *Circulation.* 2002;106(12 Suppl): I198–I202.

34. Goldstein DJ, et al. Cardiac allotransplantation. In: Rose EA, Stevenson LW (eds): *Management of End Stage Heart Disease*, 1st ed. Philadelphia:PA; Lippincott-Raven, 1998, pp 177–185.

35. Massad M. Current trends in transplantation. *Cardiology.* 2004;101:79–92.

CHAPTER 16

When to Refer Patients for Heart Transplantation

MARYJANE FARR, MD/DONNA MANCINI, MD

▶ INTRODUCTION

Timely referral of patients for heart transplant evaluation requires a keen awareness of when medical management has begun to fail, and the identification of the development of irreversible end-organ damage from chronically reduced cardiac output. Unfortunately, many candidates come to the attention of transplant centers when they are at the end of their life. They are malnourished and typically dependent on inotropic medications and other modes of advanced cardiac support (e.g., intra-aortic balloon pump, mechanical ventilation). Though prior reports describe comparable survival of patients undergoing both elective and urgent transplantation, those patients undergoing urgent transplants have more prolonged recovery periods and more comorbidities including infections and renal failure from their decompensated state. Late referral also precludes the opportunity for patients and families to fully comprehend the short- and long-term care needed for transplantation to be successful.

Because donor organs remain scarce, only the sickest patients with minimal comorbidities are considered for transplantation. This chapter reviews the transplant evaluation process, which conditions are absolute and relative contraindications, and how patients are serially assessed for either delisting or upgrading to a more urgent status. The recent practice of alternate listing (use of less than perfect organs for older patients or patients with substantial comorbidities) will also be discussed.

▶ TRANSPLANT EVALUATION

Patients evaluated for transplant include those patients with New York Heart Association (NYHA) Class III–IV heart failure (HF) with severe left ventricular dysfunction, patients with refractory ischemia, or patients with incessant arrhythmias despite maximal medical or interventional therapies. Upon referral, a reassessment of cardiac function, ischemic burden, and medication tolerance is performed. If the patient is

ambulatory, functional status is assessed by measuring peak VO_2 (oxygen consumption) during cardiopulmonary exercise testing (CPEX) (Fig. 16-1). CPEX testing has emerged as an important prognostic tool to guide the selection of transplant candidates. The initial study demonstrating the utility of this technique was performed in the late 1980s at the University of Pennsylvania. All ambulatory patients referred for transplant evaluation underwent CPEX testing.[1] One hundred and sixteen patients were studied and divided into three groups on the basis of peak VO_2:

Group I: peak VO_2 <14 mL/kg/min and listed for transplant

Group II: peak VO_2 >14 mL/kg/min and transplant listing deferred

Group III: peak VO_2 <14 mL/kg/min, but not offered transplant listing because of a significant comorbidity

One-year survival was 94% in patients with preserved exercise capacity (VO_2 >14 mL/kg/min),

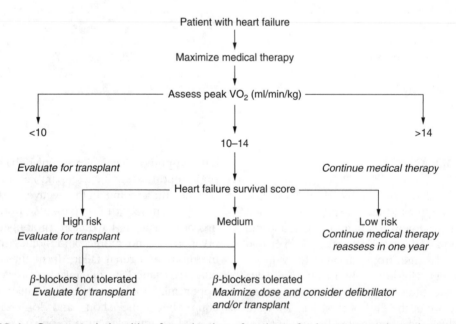

Figure 16-1   Suggested algorithm for selection of patients for heart transplantation, using peak exercise oxygen consumption (VO_2) and heart failure survival. (Butler J, Khadim G, Paul KM, et al. Selection of patients for heart transplantation in the current era of heart failure therapy. *J Am Coll Cardiol*. 2004;43:787–793.)

70% in patients with reduced VO_2 listed for transplant, and 47% in the group with VO_2 <14 mL/kg/min, but who were not offered transplantation. The 70% survival in Group II patients was artificially high as all urgent transplants were counted as censored observations. This study demonstrated that patients with VO_2 >14 mL/kg/min have a 1-year survival comparable to survival after transplant, indicating that transplant could be safely deferred. Patients with a VO_2 <14 mL/kg/min have a significantly worse survival and should be listed. From this, CPEX testing emerged as a key component of the transplant evaluation process.

Since the initial study, many investigators have attempted to improve the predictive value of this test by analyzing the VO_2 expressed as a percentage of predicted value and/or by adding ancillary data acquired during testing such as the anaerobic threshold, ventilatory response, and heart rate/blood pressure response. Peak exercise VO_2 is affected by age, gender, body weight, pulmonary function, muscle mass, and overall fitness. Patients included in the analysis of VO_2 data are those who have achieved maximal exercise testing with identification of ventilatory anaerobic threshold. Whether peak VO_2 normalized for predicted values better predicts mortality than absolute VO_2 is unclear.[2-4] As the majority of transplant candidates continue to be middle-aged men, absolute peak VO_2 is probably as effective a predictor as percent-predicted VO_2, though at the extremes of age the reverse may occur. Peak VO_2 does predict increased mortality in a continuous fashion, without a distinct cut-point, which abruptly increases risk.[5,6]

In the last 20 years, a few centers have used hemodynamic data measured at peak exercise with an invasive pulmonary catheter to guide triage decisions. Wilson and colleagues evaluated 64 patients referred for cardiac transplant using CPEX testing and simultaneous invasive hemodynamic monitoring.[7] Forty-four percent of patients with a normal cardiac response to exercise (as defined by the Higginbotham equation) had a peak VO_2 <14 mL/kg/min, while 33% of patients with a peak VO_2 >14 mL/kg/min had a severely impaired peak exercise cardiac output.[8] Wilson concluded that invasive hemodynamic information should be used in combination with VO_2 to determine transplant eligibility, and patients with a low VO_2 who demonstrate appropriate cardiac function at peak exercise may not benefit from organ replacement, as the etiology for the low VO_2 is a peripheral and not central cardiac mechanism.

Mancini and colleagues repeated Wilson's protocol to validate his conclusions, but found that peak VO_2 did correlate with peak cardiac output in their patients.[9] Although peak VO_2 and peak cardiac output were positively correlated, in multivariate analysis only left ventricular stroke work and stroke work index were shown to predict survival (stroke work is derived from measurements of mean arterial blood pressure, heart rate, pulmonary capillary wedge pressure, and cardiac output). The inability to predict survival using either VO_2 or cardiac output may have been due to small sample size (65 patients). Nevertheless, the addition of hemodynamic monitoring to CPEX adds a level of complexity that is difficult to routinely perform. At this time routine use of hemodynamic monitoring during exercise is not advocated.

More recently, ventilatory data during CPEX testing have emerged as a significant predictor of mortality in patients with HF. The ventilatory response to exercise, measured as the ratio of V_E to VCO_2, is increased in patients with HF. V_E/VCO_2, also called the ventilatory equivalent for carbon dioxide, expresses the amount of ventilation required to eliminate a given amount of CO_2 produced by metabolizing tissues. Because it is measured at the mouthpiece during expiration, it is strongly influenced by dead-space breathing. For some patients, an elevated V_E/VCO_2 ratio (normal $V_E/VCO_2 = 25$) reflects an increased stimulus to breathe off accumulating CO_2, whereas in others it may reflect abnormal breathing patterns secondary to overstimulation of peripheral ergoreceptors and/or pulmonary congestion. V_E/VCO_2 has emerged as a powerful prognostic indicator of survival in patients with HF. In one study, a V_E/VCO_2 slope >34 was associated with a higher NYHA functional class, a lower ejection fraction, lower peak VO_2, and lower survival rate at 18 months.[10] V_E/VCO_2 has not yet been evaluated in a large prospective cohort to more precisely define the sickest transplant candidates.

Although data derived from CPEX testing can yield powerful information, there are other, more routine clinical markers that have prognostic value. Aaronson and colleagues developed a statistical model to predict survival in ambulatory HF patients referred for transplant evaluation.[11] This model, called the Heart Failure Survival Score (HFSS), is a multivariable predictive index that was derived from data on 80 clinical characteristics of 268 ambulatory patients with advanced HF. The final model included the smallest number of noninvasive variables that could predict survival. The HFSS was later validated in a cohort of 223 patients with advanced HF. The final seven variables included different aspects of HF physiology: myocardial ischemia, resting heart rate, mean arterial blood pressure, ejection fraction, intraventricular conduction delay, peak VO_2, and serum sodium. The total HFSS was calculated by summing the individual variables, with each variable weighted slightly differently. A HFSS >8.09 correlated with a 1-year event-free survival of 93%, whereas a HFSS ≤8 was associated with a 1-year event-free survival significantly worse than that expected after transplant. Accordingly, patients without contraindications to transplant are listed if the HFSS is <8.

Current practice utilizes the VO_2 >14 mL/kg/min cutoff for deferring listing, with serial assessment every 6–18 months to monitor for deterioration. Some, but not all, centers also incorporate the HFSS into the evaluation. As for invasive hemodynamic data obtained at peak exercise, the debate continues over whether an invasive procedure provides prognostic information that is not already evident from noninvasive assessment. In cases where there is a marked dissociation of peak VO_2 and peak cardiac output (as obtained through invasive hemodynamic measurements, or at peak exercise with dobutamine stress-echo), there is a genuine concern that heart transplant may not markedly improve functional capacity. Thus,

there is continued interest in developing noninvasive strategies to assess cardiac output at peak exercise and correlate it with peak VO_2.

Finally, data regarding evaluation for heart transplant candidacy using peak VO_2 and the HFSS were derived in cohorts of patients before the "β-blocker era." Because β-blockers decrease heart rate, peak exercise capacity is generally not improved despite their positive impact on survival. The value of peak VO_2 in predicting survival in the β-blocker era has been examined. Most studies confirm the continued value of this variable, although with the improved survival with β-blockers, the cut-point for VO_2 is probably lower in the range of 10–12 mL/kg/min. For patients on β-blockers, the HFSS rather than peak VO_2 seems to predict more accurately who should be listed.[12,13]

▶ CANDIDATE SELECTION CRITERIA

Once it has been determined that a patient is ill enough for transplant listing and that all conventional strategies have been exhausted, the next part of the evaluation focuses on absolute and relative contraindications to successful transplantation. In the early years of transplant, a set of empirically derived contraindications were generated from experienced transplant programs.[14] These traditional exclusion criteria are listed in Table 16-1. The exclusion criteria list was formulated as a consensus among heart transplant experts who either through clinical experience or outcome analysis determined that the listed factors were significant obstacles to short- and/or long-term survival. Selection criteria continue to evolve as new therapies emerge for comorbidities, newer immunosuppressive therapies simplify posttransplant care, and more experience is gained.

Age

The age guideline for transplant varies between transplant centers. Age >65 years as an upper

▶ **Table 16-1** Traditional exclusion criteria

Age >65 years
Fixed pulmonary vascular resistance >6 Wood units
Peptic ulcer disease within 3 months
Pulmonary embolism within 3 months
Brittle diabetes mellitus or diabetes with significant end-organ damage
Symptomatic peripheral vascular disease (e.g., claudication, transient-ischemic attacks)
"Brittle" hypertension – requiring multidrug therapy
Significant obstructive pulmonary disease (FEV_1 <1 L/min)
Amyloidosis
HIV+ status
Morbid obesity (Body mass index >35)
Malignancy <2 years prior
Renal insufficiency (creatinine >2.5 mg/dL or creatinine clearance <50 mL/min)
Severe liver dysfunction (bilirubin >2.5 mg/dL or transaminases >2x normal)
Active alcohol or substance abuse
Untreated mental illness
Poor social support/psychosocial instability

Source: Mudge GH, Goldstein S, Addonizio LJ, et al. The 24th Bethesda Conference: cardiac transplantation. Task Force 3: recipient guidelines/prioritization. *J Am Coll Cardiol.* 1993;22:21–31.

limit of transplantability has been examined carefully, because of the increased incidence of HF as well as comorbidities in this age group.[15,16] An analysis of patients >65 years who underwent cardiac transplantation between 1992 and 2002 demonstrated similar 1- and 10-year actuarial survival rates when compared to a younger cohort matched for sex, HF etiology, United Network of Organ Sharing (UNOS) status at time of transplant, immunosuppressive regimen, and other pretransplant comorbidities, for example, hypertension and diabetes.[17] There were no differences in postoperative ICU or total length of stay, but there was an increase in posttransplant coronary artery disease in the older population. Survival posttransplantation of older patients in other single-center studies has been variable, with some investigators reporting an improved survival in older patients and other centers a comparable or worse survival (Fig. 16-2).

Pulmonary Hypertension

Severe, fixed pulmonary hypertension (>6 Wood units) remains a contraindication as the newly transplanted normal right ventricle (RV) cannot generate the pressure to overcome the resistance across the pulmonary bed with resultant RV dilatation and failure. Some degree of pulmonary hypertension is acceptable and can be managed perioperatively with vasodilation or with inhaled nitric oxide. The risk for worsening survival increases in a continuous fashion as the pulmonary vascular resistance increases.[18,19] Preoperatively patients with moderate-to-severe pulmonary hypertension are often placed on home milrinone infusion to allow some relaxation of pulmonary vascular resistance. Another strategy is to offer implantable mechanical assistance as a bridge to transplantation, for the purpose of unloading the left heart and thereby allowing some recovery/relaxation of the pulmonary circuit.

Recent Pulmonary Embolism

Pulmonary embolism often results in pulmonary infarct. In the setting of immunosuppressive therapy, this can develop into a pulmonary

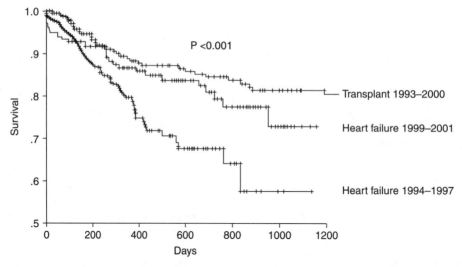

Figure 16-2   Cumulative survival for patients in the past era and current era demonstrates a significantly better survival for patients in the current era. After an initial higher mortality rate after transplantation, overall 1-year survival is comparable to medical therapy for patients in the current era and better than heart failure therapy in the past era. (Butler J, Khadim G, Paul KM, et al. Selection of patients for heart transplantation in the current era of heart failure therapy. *J Am Coll Cardiol*. 2004;43:787–793.)

abscess, which can be very difficult to eradicate posttransplant.[20] For this reason, most centers require a 3-month waiting period after a pulmonary embolism. Monitoring the resolution of lung damage by serial chest computerized tomography (CT) scans can sometimes shorten this delay to transplant.

Severe Chronic Obstructive Pulmonary Disease

Severe chronic obstructive pulmonary disease (COPD) remains a contraindication to transplant due to the high risk of ventilator dependence postoperatively. Also, patients are at risk for more frequent decompensation requiring mechanical ventilation during seasonal influenza and/or from pneumonia/bronchitis. Lastly, quality of life and functional status often remain limited secondary to chronic respiratory disease. Thus, transplantation of the heart makes no major impact on quality of life, although it may improve quantity.

Recent Peptic Ulcer Disease

Recent peptic ulcer disease is a temporary contraindication because gastric lesions can be colonized with cytomegalovirus (CMV) or candida, which can later cause systemic disease. Most centers wait 3 months after the occurrence of gastric ulcer before offering transplant.

Diabetes Mellitus

Over time there has been a liberalization of accepting patients with diabetes. Patients with "brittle" diabetes typically remain ineligible for transplantation. Many of these patients were diagnosed with juvenile diabetes and have been on insulin for many years. They often have multiorgan damage related to diabetes, including the etiology of their heart disease. The high doses of steroids initially required at the time of transplantation can cause severe hyperglycemia and ensuing metabolic disarray that can recur during episodes of rejection, which is largely treated with pulse steroids.

However, many patients with insulin-dependent diabetes have undergone successful cardiac transplantation even with evidence of mild-to-moderate end-organ damage. These patients must be very motivated to manage their own care in a meticulous fashion in order for transplant to be safe and successful. For patients with diabetes, similar posttransplant outcomes when compared to patients without diabetes have been described in some studies, but not in others.[21,22]

Human Immunodeficiency Virus Seropositivity

A limited number of patients with human immunodeficiency virus (HIV) disease have undergone cardiac transplantation in the United States. Individual cases suggest that outcomes are maximized when patients enter transplantation with a high CD4 count and undetectable viral load. As highly active antiretroviral therapy (HAART) markedly prolongs the lives of patients with HIV, referral of these patients for cardiac transplantation may become more common.

Amyloidosis

For most transplant centers, amyloidosis remains a contraindication to transplant. To be considered for transplant, amyloid deposition must be limited to the heart. However, recurrence of amyloid in the transplanted heart has been described as early as 4 months postoperatively, though some recipients have survived more than 4 years.[23-25] Thus transplant is possible, but low-term survival is unacceptably low particularly when using a scarce resource. Recently, a few centers have combined heart transplantation with autologous stem cell transplant in patients with isolated cardiac amyloidosis and have demonstrated improved survival.[26] In our center, we have offered combined heart stem cell transplant to 11 patients. None of the patients thus far have had recurrence of amyloidosis, with our longest follow-up being 3 years.

Psychosocial Instability

Psychosocial evaluation is an important aspect of the transplant evaluation. Active or recent alcohol and drug addiction continue to be a contraindication to transplantation. Additionally, patients must have a history of medical compliance as well as a family member or significant other who can assist with their health needs. For some patients, the rigors of transplantation may simply be too overwhelming to manage. Patients must also have a stable living situation. Patients who are noncompliant prior to transplant are unlikely to be successful recipients. The result is organ rejection and a lost opportunity for another listed candidate.

▶ WAITING LIST DEMOGRAPHICS

After the cardiac transplant evaluation is completed, the case is presented before a multidisciplinary transplant committee and a decision is made regarding listing. If the decision is made to proceed to transplant, the patient is then listed for transplant with the UNOS. The priority status of the patient is also determined and registered, along with the patient's blood type, age, weight, height, and need for crossmatch. When a donor is identified, regional procurement agencies match the organ to the recipient, based not only on the priority status, but also by time on the list and geographic location.

While each transplant candidate is considered individually for potential listing, candidacy algorithms are somewhat influenced by the number and summed characteristics of the patients already waiting. For example, patients with blood type O have prolonged wait times due to competition for organs while the wait for type AB patients can be just a few months. Body weight is a key variable in wait time, particularly for patients who do not resemble their "geographic" body type. Similarly, sensitized patients (frequently multiparous women or patients who have required multiple transfusions) will also have a more prolonged wait due to need to prospectively identify a negative crossmatch.

From 1992 to 2001, the mean waiting time on the list significantly increased with 46% of registrants now waiting >2 years. Patients are designated as Status 1A, 1B, or 2. Status 1A patients are considered to have <30 days to live, and by definition must be in an ICU, on one or two high-dose inotropic agents with an indwelling pulmonary catheter, or those patients requiring mechanical support (intra-aortic balloon pump, mechanical ventilator, or an assist device). Status 1B patients are stable on low-dose inotropic support or have a normal functioning ventricular assist device, either in the hospital or at home. Prior to 1998, Status 1 patients had not yet been divided into 1A and 1B categories.

▶ MANAGEMENT OF LISTED PATIENTS

It is sometimes the case that referral to a transplant center allows a "fresh look" at an individual patient. Medication regimens are altered, dietary teaching is reviewed, and often high-risk revascularization with ventricular assist device "backup" results in improvement in functional status. Patients may initially be listed, but if they demonstrate sustained, objective improvement in peak VO$_2$, they may be well enough to be delisted. This is appropriate, although not very common. In one study evaluating the outcomes of patients listed for ≥6 months on the waiting list demonstrated that <5% of patients become well enough to be delisted.[27] More often, Status 2 patients undergo serial reevaluation for subacute decompensation and development of new or worsening comorbidities, for example, progressive pulmonary hypertension. Patients who demonstrate poor compliance, that is, inability to keep appointments or follow recommendations, are often placed on probation and occasionally removed from the list.

We recently analyzed long-term follow-up data for sequential measurement of peak VO$_2$ and HFSS in 227 transplant candidates.[28] Survival to *reevaluation*, free from UNOS 1 transplant or left ventricular assist device (LVAD), was determined by the Kaplan-Meier method with censoring at UNOS 2 transplant. Survival differed by HFSS stratum (P <0.001) and by peak VO$_2$ stratum (P <0.001). Patients who deteriorated from low- to medium- or high-risk HFSS or peak VO$_2$ had worse survival than those who remained low risk (P <0.01 and P <0.001 respectively). Medium- or high-risk patients who improved to low risk tended to have higher survival than those who remained medium or high risk (P = 0.06 and P <0.16 respectively). Patients who improved to low risk had a 1-year survival of 72% for both HFSS and peak VO$_2$. However, patients who improved to low risk and were treated with β-blockers had a 1-year survival (89% for HFSS and 83% for peak VO$_2$) comparable to that post-transplant (84%). Both peak VO$_2$ and the HFSS can be successfully used for serial evaluation of HF mortality risk in ambulatory patients with advanced HF. Patients on the heart transplant waiting list should undergo serial evaluation to assess their continued need for transplantation. Patients who have been judged too well for transplantation should also be periodically reevaluated to determine if their HF has become severe enough to warrant placement on the transplant waiting list.

▶ ALTERNATE LISTING

Criteria for identifying a donor heart have been developed to maximize transplant outcome. The ideal donor organ comes from a patient <30 years old, who has suffered no chest wall contusion, with no prior medical conditions, no current infections, no history of substance abuse, and an anticipated ischemic time <2 hours (cross-clamp to implantation). Ideal donors are scarce, and for this reason, there has been a relaxation of criteria, particularly regarding age, with a more focused view on coronary artery disease, left ventricular hypertrophy, and risk factors for coronary artery disease. In these situations, angiogram or even dobutamine stress echo are performed prior to accepting the organ. Donor age was the first criteria to be relaxed in response to the donor shortage. Numerous studies have been done demonstrating that an aging heart without coronary artery disease does not appear to translate into worsened outcome for the recipient.[29–31]

The practice of alternate listing began when it was observed that many potential organs are refused. Some programs have created a "second list" whereby patients with high-risk situations (e.g., age >65 years, HIV+, amyloidosis), who would have been turned down for transplant in the past, can now be offered an alternate heart. These cases are more difficult to manage, because of the additional comorbidities, and pose novel questions related to how far a program should reach to consider either a high-risk donor or a high-risk recipient. Alternative listing first began in 1996 at UCLA, mostly expanding the age of the donor organ to patients who had minor exclusion criteria (e.g., diabetes mellitus).[32] The algorithm established was that a donor offer would be made to the targeted Status 1 patients, if declined then the organ would be offered to appropriate Status 2 patients. If still available, it would then be offered to a patient on the alternate list. These patients have the right to refuse the organ and can state their preferences in advance (e.g., some patients will refuse an organ from a donor with hepatitis C). It is important for referring cardiologists to recognize that aging patients or patients with comorbidities may still be eligible for transplantation, but that they may need to accept an alternate listing status.

Can a high-risk candidate who is transplanted with a high-risk organ have an optimal outcome? At UCLA, a recent study demonstrated worsened 90-day survival among transplant patient from the alternate list, compared to the standard list.[33] In our center, data on alternate list outcomes over the last 4 years indicate that there is no survival advantage to receiving a standard organ over an alternate organ.[34] There was no difference in 30- and 90-day survival, length of ICU stay, overall hospital stay, posttransplant circulatory support, or posttransplant continuous venovenous hemofiltration (CVVH). There was, however, a significant difference in intubation time and rate of sternal wound infection. Importantly, mortality postalternate heart transplantation was

primarily the result of infection and in no case was the result of primary graft failure. Interestingly, 22% of hearts used for the alternate list were acceptable for the standard list, but unmatchable. Thirty-two percent of alternate heart donors were categorized as such because of donor hepatitis B/C seropositivity. If outcome data from alternate listing continue to demonstrate that survival is comparable to standard listing, this may generate more interest in expanding the donor pool, as well as raise additional ethical questions regarding the definition of an "alternate" recipient.

▶ SUMMARY AND CONCLUSIONS

Cardiac transplantation has evolved into a highly successful strategy to offer a second chance to patients with end-stage HF. It is also a highly complex process of evaluation, monitoring, and ultimately matching the right organ with the right patient. It is important for referring cardiologists to clearly understand the process of transplant evaluation to identify more precisely which of their patients should be evaluated, and what their patients should expect when they come to a transplant center.

▶ REFERENCES

1. Mancini DM, Eisen H, Kussmaul W, et al. Value of peak exercise oxygen consumption for optimal timing of cardiac transplantation in ambulatory patients with heart failure. *Circulation*. 1991;83:778–786.

2. Aaronson K, Chen T, Mancini D. Demonstration of the continuous nature of peak VO2 for predicting survival in ambulatory patients evaluated for transplant. *J Heart Lung Transplant*. 1996;15:S66S.

3. Osada N, Chaitman BR, Miller LW, et al. Cardiopulmonary exercise testing identifies low risk patients with heart failure and severely impaired exercise capacity considered for heart transplantation. *J Am Coll Cardiol*. 1998;31: 577–582.

4. Stelken AM, Younis LT, Jennison SH, et al. Prognostic value of cardiopulmonary exercise testing using percent achieved of predicted peak oxygen uptake for patients with ischemic and dilated cardiomyopathy. *J Am Coll Cardiol.* 1996;27:345–352.

5. Aaronson K. Cardiopulmonary exercise testing identifies low risk patients with heart failure and severely impaired exercise capacity considered for heart transplantation. *J Am Coll Cardiol.* 1998;31:577–582.

6. Aaronson KD, Mancini DM. Is percentage of predicted maximal exercise oxygen consumption a better predictor of survival than peak exercise oxygen consumption for patients with severe heart failure? *J Heart Lung Transplant.* 1995;14:981–989.

7. Wilson J, Schwartz J, Sutton M, et al. Prognosis in severe heart failure: relation to hemodynamic measurements and ventricular ectopic activity. *J Am Coll Cardiol.* 1983;2:403–410.

8. Higginbotham MB, Morris KG, Williams RS, et al. Regulation of stroke volume during submaximal and maximal upright exercise in normal man. *Circ Res.* 1986;58:281–291.

9. Mancini D, Katz S, Donchez L, et al. Coupling of hemodynamic measurements with oxygen consumption during exercise does not improve risk stratification in patients with heart failure. *Circulation.* 1996;94:2492–2496.

10. Chua TP, Ponikowski P, Harrington D, et al. Clinical correlates and prognostic significance of the ventilatory response to exercise in chronic heart failure. *J Am Coll Cardiol.* 1997;29:1585–1590.

11. Aaronson K, Schwartz JS, Chen T, et al. Development and prospective validation of a clinical index to predict survival in ambulatory patients referred for cardiac transplant evaluation. *Circulation.* 1997;95:2660–2667.

12. Powhani A, Murali S, Mathier M, et al. Impact of beta-blocker therapy on functional capacity criteria for heart transplant listing. *J Heart Lung Transplant.* 2003;22:70–77.

13. Lund LH, Aaronson KD, Mancini DM. Predicting survival in ambulatory patients with severe heart failure on beta-blocker therapy. *Am J Cardiol.* 2003;92:1350–1354.

14. Mudge GH, Goldstein S, Addonizio LJ, et al. The 24th Bethesda Conference: cardiac transplantation. Task Force 3: recipient guidelines/prioritization. *J Am Coll Cardiol.* 1993;22:21–31.

15. Aronow WS. Epidemiology, pathophysiology, prognosis, and treatment of systolic and diastolic heart failure in elderly patients. *Heart Disease.* 5(4):279–294.

16. Bacchetta MD, Ko W, Gerardi LN, et al. Outcomes of cardiac surgery in nonagenarians: a 10-year experience. *Ann Thorac Surg.* 2003;75(4):1215–1220.

17. Morgan JA, John R, Weinberg AD, et al. Long-term results of cardiac transplantation in patients 65 years of age and older: a comparative analysis. *Ann Thorac Surg.* 2003;76:1982–1987.

18. Edwards BS, Rodeheffer RJ. Prognostic features in patients with congestive heart failure and selection criteria for cardiac transplantation. *Mayo Clin Proc.* 1992;67:485–492.

19. Kirklin JK, Naftel DC, Kirklin JW, et al. Pulmonary vascular resistance and the risk of heart transplantation. *J Heart Transplant.* 1988;7:331–335.

20. Young JN, Yazbeck J, Esposito G, et al. The influence of acute preoperative pulmonary infarction on the results of heart transplantation. *J Heart Transplant.* 1986;5(3):20–22.

21. Lang C, Beniaminovitz A, Edwards N, et al. Morbidity and mortality in diabetic patients following cardiac transplantation. *J Heart Lung Transplant.* 2003;22:244–249.

22. Shiba N, Chan MCY, Kwok BWK, et al. Analysis of survivors more than 10 years after heart transplantation in the cyclosporine era: Stanford experience. *J Heart Lung Transplant.* 2004;23:155–164.

23. Hosenpud JD, Demarco T, Frazier H, et al. Progression of systemic disease and reduced long-term survival in patients with cardiac amyloidosis undergoing heart transplantation: follow up results of a multi-center survey. *Circulation.* 1999;84(Suppl III):338–342.

24. Pelosi F, Cepehart J, Roberts WC. Effectiveness of cardiac transplantation for primary (AL) cardiac amyloidosis. *Am J Cardiol.* 1997;79:532–535.

25. Dubrey S, Simmn R, Skinner M, et al. Recurrence of primary (AL) amyloidosis in a transplanted heart with four-year survival. *Am J Cardiol.* 1995;76:739–741.

26. Mohty M, Albat B, Fegueux N, et al. Autologous peripheral blood stem cell transplantation for primary systemic amyloidosis. *Leukemia & Lymphoma.* 2001;41(1–2):221–223.

27. Aaronson KD, Mancini DM. Mortality remains high for outpatient transplant candidates with

prolonged (> months) waiting list time. *J Am Coll Cardiol.* 1999;33:1189–1195.

28. Lund LH, Aaronson KD, Mancini DM. Validation of peak exercise oxygen consumption and The Heart Failure Survival Score for serial risk stratification in advanced heart failure. (In press) 2005.

29. Chen JM, Rajasinghe HR, Sinha P, et al. Do donor characteristics really matter? Analysis of consecutive heart donors 1995–1999. *J Heart Lung Transplant.* 2002;21(5):608–610.

30. Tenderich G, Koerner MM, Stuettgen B, et al. Extended donor criteria: hemodynamic follow-up of heart transplant recipients receiving a cardiac allograft from donors ≥60 years of age. *Transplantation.* 1998;66(8):1109–1113.

31. Ibrahim M, Masters RG, Hendry PJ, et al. Determinants of hospital survival after cardiac transplantation. *Ann Thorac Surg.* 1995;59:604–608.

32. Laks H, Marelli D. *The Alternate Recipient List for Heart Transplantation: A Model for Expansion of the Donor Pool. Advances in Cardiac Surgery.* 1999, Vol 11, chapter 11:233–244.

33. Laks H, et al. Use of two recipient lists for adults requiring heart transplantation. *J Thorac Cardiovasc Surg.* 2003;125(1):49–59.

34. Chen JM, Russo MJ, Hammond KM, et al. Alternate waiting list strategies for heart transplantation maximize donor organ utilization. *Ann Thorac Surg.* 2005;80:224–228.

CHAPTER 17

Comorbidities and Heart Failure

HENRY KRUM, MBBS, PHD, FRACP/
RICHARD E. GILBERT, MBBS, PHD, FRACP

Many patients with chronic heart failure also have a range of comorbid conditions that both contribute to the etiology of the disease and may have a key role in its progression and response to therapy. This undoubtedly relates to heart failure being predominantly a disease of the elderly and driven by risk factors, which are important comorbid conditions in and of themselves.

▶ HYPERTENSION

Hypertension contributes pathogenetically to the development of systolic and diastolic heart failure. As well as being a major risk factor for ischemic heart disease, hypertension can also lead directly to the development of chronic heart failure by afterload-induced cardiac hypertrophy and impairment of diastolic function.[1,2] Early investigations of the characteristics of patients with chronic heart failure, such as the Framingham study, cited hypertension as the most frequent comorbidity.[3] However, in recent intervention trials, hypertension is cited less frequently as a comorbidity and the underlying etiology of chronic heart failure. About 15% of participants in Studies Of Left Ventricular Dysfunction trial (SOLVD) had diastolic blood pressure above 90 mm Hg on entry, but other studies have not reported on this issue.[4] It is likely that recent trials have underestimated the contribution of hypertension to the development and progression of chronic heart failure. Blood pressure falls as systolic chronic heart failure develops such that the contribution of hypertension to the failure syndrome may be underappreciated. Hypertension is also a major risk factor for ischemic heart disease, but with the ischemic contribution to heart failure listed as the primary cause, the underlying hypertension may be relegated to a secondary role and not acknowledged as a comorbidity. The effect of antihypertensive therapies in limiting the development of chronic heart failure in patients with essential hypertension supports a major contribution of this comorbidity to onset and progression of chronic heart failure.[5–8]

Intervention Studies

Placebo-controlled studies have examined the impact of antihypertensive therapy in the prevention of chronic heart failure amongst patients with elevated diastolic blood pressure and those with isolated systolic hypertension.[5–8] These studies have consistently demonstrated impressive reductions in the subsequent development of chronic heart failure amongst such patients.

Although the etiology of diastolic heart failure is incompletely understood, it is likely that hypertension is a major contributor. Therefore, a major goal of therapy in the hypertensive patient with diastolic heart failure should be the reduction of elevated blood pressure to target levels. Other key goals of therapy in this setting include avoidance

of fluid overload (whilst being vigilant for iatrogenic underperfusion), recognizing and treating ischemia and arrhythmia, and correcting underlying contributory valvular disease. A number of studies conducted primarily in patients with chronic heart failure and diastolic dysfunction are currently in progress or have recently reported their findings. These include the Irbesartan in Heart Failure with Preserved Systolic Function (I-PRESERVE) study with irbesartan, the Candesartan in Heart Failure: Assessment of Reduction in Mortality and Morbidity-Preserved (CHARM-Preserved) study with candesartan cilexetil, Study of the Effects of Nebivolol Intervention on Outcomes and Hospitalization in Seniors with Heart Failure (SENIORS) with nebivolol, and the Perindopril for Elderly People with Chronic Heart Failure (PEP-CHF) study with perindopril.[9–11] These studies enrolled patients with hypertension as a major comorbid factor, such as in the CHARM-Preserved study where 64% of the study population had preexisting or concomitant hypertension at baseline.

▶ ISCHEMIC HEART DISEASE

Coronary artery disease features prominently as an etiological factor in chronic heart failure patients.[12] As with hypertension, it is also likely that the contribution of ischemia to chronic heart failure is underreported.[13] Many patients enrolled in chronic heart failure trials may have ischemia but do not have a high level of documentation of this comorbidity. Furthermore, patients with *active* ischemia are often excluded from entry into these trials.

Coronary artery disease may lead to heart failure through a variety of mechanisms. Most dramatically, extensive myocardial necrosis will result in pump failure. Infarction of smaller areas may lead to regional contractile dysfunction and adverse remodeling with myocyte hypertrophy, apoptosis, and extracellular matrix deposition. In addition, transient reversible ischemia may occur with episodic dysfunction even in the presence of "normal" resting ventricular function.[14]

Thus, patients with myocardial ischemia may have hibernating (but potentially viable) myocardium.[15,16] Ventricular function may therefore be improved by myocardial revascularization in this setting.[17,18] In the CHRISTMAS study, over 50% of ischemic chronic heart failure patients had evidence of hibernation affecting two or more segments on echocardiography.[19]

However, this has not as yet been tested in a rigorous manner. Revascularization in such patients may result not only in improved ventricular function but also in long-term symptomatic and prognostic benefits.[20,21]

Many of the pathogenetic factors that contribute to endothelial dysfunction and atherosclerosis (and thus ischemia) are also involved in the ongoing progression of chronic heart failure.[22] These factors include activation of the renin-angiotensin-aldosterone, sympathetic, and endothelin systems.[23] Therefore, a component of the beneficial effects of neurohormonal antagonists in the management of chronic heart failure may occur on the basis of improvements in underlying ischemia. For example, angiotensin-converting enzyme (ACE) inhibitors improve coronary endothelial function (Trial on Reversing Endothelial Function [TREND]) and reduce development of chronic heart failure in patients at high risk of cardiovascular disease (Heart Outcomes Prevention Evaluation [HOPE]).[24,25] Similarly, the SOLVD and Survival and Ventricular Enlargement (SAVE) studies (in patients with systolic ventricular dysfunction) demonstrated both reductions in ischemic events and heart failure hospitalizations.[26,27] In the Carvedilol Postinfarction Survival Control in Left Ventricular Dysfunction (CAPRICORN) trial, patients with postmyocardial infarction (MI) ventricular systolic dysfunction derived benefit from the β-blocker carvedilol, both in terms of subsequent ischemic endpoints and chronic heart failure-related events.[28]

Several analyses have examined differences in responses to pharmacological therapies between ischemic and nonischemic etiologies of heart failure. In some studies, such as the Congestive Heart Failure Survival Trial of Antiarrhythmic Therapy (CHF-STAT) (amiodarone), the Prospective Randomized Amlodipine Survival Evaluation (PRAISE I) (amlodipine), and an early β-blocker study, the magnitude of the benefit appeared to be greater amongst patients with a nonischemic etiology.[29–31] In contrast, however, other trials have not reported substantial differences in clinical response between these etiologies (Cardiac Insufficiency Bisoprolol Study II [CIBIS-II], Carvedilol Prospective Randomized Cumulative Survival trial [COPERNICUS], Randomized Aldactone Evaluation Study trial [RALES], Evaluation of Losartan in the Elderly [ELITE II], and Valsartan Heart Failure Trial [Val-HeFT]).[32–36]

▶ DIABETES MELLITUS

Diabetes is a frequent and important, but commonly overlooked, comorbidity in patients with chronic heart failure. Subjects with diabetes are not only at higher risk of developing chronic heart failure but also have worse symptoms for their level of systolic function and a higher mortality compared with their nondiabetic counterparts.[37–39]

The Framingham study first reported an overrepresentation of diabetic patients amongst chronic heart failure patients, such that 14% of men and 26% of women with chronic heart failure were noted to have concomitant diabetes.[40] In a further report from Framingham, in which 5209 middle-aged community dwellers were followed prospectively for 10 years, diabetes was associated with a twofold increase in chronic heart failure in men and a fivefold increase in chronic heart failure in women.[41] Moreover, this increased risk of chronic heart failure persisted after adjustment for other potential confounders such as known coronary artery disease, age, blood pressure, and cholesterol.

Community-based studies in the elderly have also reported that diabetes was an independent risk factor for the development of chronic heart failure with relative risks of 1.7–2.9.[42–44] In the U.K. Prospective Diabetes Study (UKPDS), the development of chronic heart failure was examined over a 10-year period in almost

4000 community-based, middle-aged type 2 diabetic patients.[45,46] In these subjects, the absolute risk of hospitalization for chronic heart failure was 3–8.1 per 1000 patient years, depending on the assigned treatment group. This risk can be compared with those of nonfatal MI, nonfatal stroke, and renal failure at 7.5–9.5, 4–8.9, and 0.6–2.3 per 1000 patient years, respectively, in the same study.

Three major factors contribute to the high prevalence of chronic heart failure in diabetes: hypertension, coronary artery disease, and diabetic cardiomyopathy. Patients with diabetes characteristically develop premature atherosclerotic coronary artery disease, which is often widespread, asymptomatic, and presents late.[46] Indeed, patients with diabetes are two to three times more likely to develop chronic heart failure following MI, and diabetic women are at particularly high risk.[47] Hypertension, another risk factor for the development of chronic heart failure, is present in 71–93% of patients with type 2 diabetes.[48] Both experimental and clinical studies have provided evidence for the existence of a diabetic cardiomyopathy, independent of large vessel disease.[39,49,50] The clinical manifestations of this cardiomyopathy are poorly understood, with asymptomatic diastolic dysfunction a common finding on echocardiographic investigation in diabetic patients.[49] The role of autonomic dysfunction, endothelial dysfunction and abnormal energy metabolism, and the development of chronic heart failure in the diabetic patient is less well understood.[51]

The presence of chronic heart failure as a comorbidity should be taken into consideration in the choice of drugs used for the treatment of diabetes. In particular, metformin is contraindicated in the presence of chronic heart failure. Similarly, the thiazolidinediones should be avoided in patients with New York Heart Association (NYHA) III–IV disease and used with caution in patients with less severe chronic heart failure.

Intervention Studies

In the UKPDS, intensive blood glucose control did not significantly reduce the likelihood of macrovascular disease.[46] However, this study also examined the risk of complications at different levels of glycemia. In this prospective, observational component of UKPDS, a continuous relationship between glycemic exposure and the development of chronic heart failure was noted with no threshold of risk, such that for each 1% (absolute) reduction in hemoglobin A1c, there was an associated 16% decrease in hospitalization for heart failure.[52] Similar findings have also been recently reported in a large cohort study from the United States.[53]

The UKPDS additionally examined the effect of blood pressure control on the development of chronic heart failure in the diabetic patient. Tight blood pressure control was associated with a 56% reduction in the risk of chronic heart failure.[45] As with glycemia, the incidence of chronic heart failure was significantly associated with systolic blood pressure, such that a 10 mm Hg decrease in systolic blood pressure was accompanied by a 12% decrease in chronic heart failure, also with no apparent threshold of risk.[54] A number of other intervention trials using angiotensin receptor blockers have also shown a reduction in the development of chronic heart failure in high-risk patients, apparently independent of blood pressure.[55] Such studies, which included those in patients with diabetes, hypertension, and left ventricular hypertrophy (Losartan Intervention for Endpoint Reduction [LIFE]) and in patients with diabetic nephropathy (Irbesartan in Diabetic Nephropathy Trial [IDNT] and (Reduction in End Points in Noninsulin-Dependent Diabetes Mellitus with the Angiotensin II Antagonist Losartan [RENAAL]) highlight the importance of blocking the renin-angiotensin system in the prevention as well as in the treatment of heart failure in diabetes.[56–58]

Diabetes is a noted comorbidity in between 10% and >30% of participants in clinical trials in chronic heart failure.[59] Despite its limitations, analysis of the diabetic subgroup within these trials has provided significant insight into the relationship between chronic heart failure and diabetes and provided information on a range of pharmacological interventions including ACE inhibitors, angiotensin receptor blockers, and β-blockers. For instance, in SOLVD, diabetes was associated with increased mortality, but only in patients with ischemic cardiomyopathy (RR 1.37, CI: 1.21–1.55, P <0.0001) and not in those with a nonischemic cardiac dysfunction (RR 0.98).[60] Fortunately, patients with diabetes and ischemic cardiomyopathy do respond to therapeutic intervention, particularly following acute MI.[61]

Diabetes, particularly in the presence of chronic heart failure, has traditionally been viewed as a contraindication to the use of β-blocking agents. Nevertheless, β-blockers have been consistently shown to improve prognosis and reduce hospital admissions for systolic chronic heart failure when added to background ACE inhibitor and diuretic therapy. Furthermore, the major chronic heart failure-β-blocker trials have shown similar benefit in the diabetic subgroup such that this class of drug should be strongly considered in treating the diabetic patients with chronic heart failure.[62,63]

In Val-HeFT, the addition of the angiotensin receptor blocker valsartan, significantly reduced morbidity and mortality in patients with NYHA Class II–IV chronic heart failure, reporting a consistent beneficial effect among predefined subgroups of patients, including those with diabetes.[36]

Although patients with diabetes were not excluded in RALES, no subgroup analysis is mentioned.[34] However, patients with diabetes, in whom hyporeninemic hypoaldosteronism is common, may be at particularly high risk of developing hyperkalemia when an aldosterone antagonist is added to baseline ACE inhibitor therapy and vigilant monitoring of serum potassium is recommended.

▶ CARDIAC ARRHYTHMIAS

Many factors contribute to the frequent development of arrhythmias in chronic heart failure, including ischemia and infarction, electrophysiological abnormalities, myocardial hypertrophy, and the activation of various neurohormonal systems.[64] Furthermore, alterations in electrolyte status as well as the proarrhythmic effect of many antiarrhythmic heart failure drug therapies may also contribute.

Ventricular Arrhythmias

Ventricular arrhythmias in patients with chronic heart failure range from benign (asymptomatic premature ventricular contractions [PVC]) to fatal (ventricular fibrillation), with "sudden" death estimated to account for approximately half of all deaths amongst chronic heart failure patients.[65] In patients with advanced chronic heart failure, 11% had a prior cardiac arrest plus ventricular tachycardia and an additional 3.4% had a history of ventricular fibrillation.[65]

The management of ventricular arrhythmias in patients with established chronic heart failure is controversial. While amiodarone is the preferred antiarrhythmic in chronic heart failure patients with severe, symptomatic, and sustained ventricular tachycardia, large-scale trials do not support its prophylactic use in patients with nonsustained asymptomatic arrhythmias.[29,64] The antiarrhythmic properties of β-blockers, together with reductions in sudden death with these agents would suggest benefit in reducing lethal arrhythmias.[32,33,65]

Implantable cardioverter defibrillators (ICDs) have proven beneficial in patients with a high risk of sudden death, for example, those with impaired ventricular function, life-threatening ventricular arrhythmias, or survivors of sudden death.[66–68] As some of the studies contributing to the ICD database used electrophysiological entry criteria, for example, the Multicenter Automatic Defibrillator Implantation Trial (MADIT), this approach may also be indicated in selecting chronic heart failure patients for ICD.[66] Recently, the MADIT II trial has been terminated because of the benefit of ICDs (compared to standard medical therapy) in patients >1 month post-MI with a left ventricular ejection fraction (LVEF) ≤30% and ≥10 ventricular extrasystoles/hour on Holter monitoring.[69] As many ischemic chronic heart failure patients would fit this category, there are major potential cost implications to these observations, despite the relatively small absolute risk reduction observed.

Furthermore, amiodarone has been found to be inferior to ICD in reducing mortality in patients with systolic chronic heart failure of NYHA Class II–III severity.[70]

Atrial Fibrillation

Atrial fibrillation (AF) is a common concomitant morbidity with chronic heart failure, present in up to a third of all patients enrolled in major intervention trials. While AF is often a consequence of the many etiological factors contributing to chronic heart failure, it may (very rarely) lead to its development, particularly if the ventricular response is not adequately controlled. β-Blockers are frequently used (in conjunction with digoxin) to control ventricular response. Nonetheless, there is some controversy regarding their impact on outcome in patients with AF in the setting of chronic heart failure. In particular, in a subgroup analysis of the CIBIS-II trial of bisoprolol, there was no apparent benefit for active therapy amongst patients with AF, contrasting with the findings for the entire study cohort.[71] However, this heterogeneity in response was not observed in other chronic heart failure β-blocker trials such as with carvedilol.[72]

While there is no evidence that restoring sinus rhythm is superior to controlling the ventricular response in patients with chronic heart failure and AF, both electrical cardioversion and amiodarone, either alone or in combination, are often used.[73] The use of other antiarrhythmics is limited by their negative inotropic and proarrhythmic effects, although dofetilide improved AF reversion rates, without increasing mortality, in patients with chronic heart failure.[74]

Anticoagulation with warfarin should be standard therapy for heart failure patients with concomitant AF, unless contraindicated.[63] Far more controversial is the use of thromboprophylaxis in patients with ventricular dysfunction and normal sinus rhythm (see below).

▶ THROMBOEMBOLISM

There is evidence that chronic heart failure is associated with an increased risk of thromboembolism (e.g., because of the frequent presence of thrombi within akinetic segments of failing ventricle and an increased propensity to develop AF). The SOLVD trial clearly demonstrated an increase in the incidence in stroke (mainly thromboembolic) with decreasing ventricular function.[75] However, retrospective analyses of studies of antithrombotic therapy in chronic heart failure have yielded conflicting results.

There is an urgent need for prospective studies of anticoagulation in chronic heart failure patients in sinus rhythm, using agents such as warfarin. An early pilot trial, the Warfarin/Aspirin Study in Heart Failure (WASH) study, compared groups taking aspirin, warfarin, and no anticoagulation.[76] There was no significant difference between groups within this small study, although there was a tendency towards an increase in hospitalization in the aspirin group. This may be due to adverse interactions between aspirin and ACE inhibitor, offsetting the beneficial effects of the latter.

The Warfarin and Antiplatelet Therapy in Chronic Heart Failure (WATCH) trial compared open-label warfarin with blinded antiplatelet therapy (either aspirin or clopidogrel) in patients with NYHA Class II–IV symptoms and an LVEF of <30%.[77] The primary endpoint was a composite of all-cause mortality, nonfatal MI, and nonfatal stroke. Unfortunately, the study was truncated before full recruitment had been achieved and, consequently, was underpowered to explore planned primary or secondary endpoints. Nevertheless, hospitalization for heart failure seemed again to be increased in aspirin-treated patients.[77]

The precise role of inhibitors of adenosine diphosphate (ADP), of activation of platelets (e.g., clopidogrel), and of warfarin in prophylaxis of thromboembolism in chronic heart failure remain uncertain. Similarly, the role of newer agents, such as direct thrombin inhibitors, has not yet been prospectively studied in this condition.

▶ OTHER IMPORTANT COMORBID CONDITIONS

Respiratory Disorders and Sleep Apnea

The interaction between chronic heart failure and concomitant respiratory disease is an important one. Many patients with heart failure are commonly misdiagnosed as having airflow obstruction based on overlapping symptomatology (and vice versa). Careful consideration with regard to the possibility that both cardiac and respiratory disease may coexist is critical to the optimal evaluation and thus management of these patients.

β-Blockers are considered to be contraindicated in the chronic heart failure patient with airflow obstruction. In practice, because of the overwhelming benefits of these agents in systolic heart failure, patients with fixed or limited airway reversibility are often given these agents with surprisingly good tolerability.[78] It is not clear whether β-1 selective agents offer advantages in this regard compared to nonselective agents such as carvedilol.[79]

Sleep apnea may be both a cause and consequence of chronic heart failure. Central sleep apnea with Cheyne-Stokes respirations during sleep affects about 40% of patients with chronic heart failure.[80] Obstructive sleep apnea also frequently coexists and may also contribute to disease progression.[81] Trials of continuous positive airway pressure (CPAP) in such patients have, in the short term, improved autonomic dysfunction and increased LVEF.[82,83]

Cognitive Dysfunction and Dementia

There is clear-cut evidence that cognitive dysfunction coexists with heart failure.[84,85] Chronic heart failure is associated with low cardiac output, which may further compromise cerebral blood flow in a patient with borderline perfusion of their cerebrum. In addition, chronic heart failure is largely driven by vascular disease (at least in Western societies) and cerebrovascular disease is an important contributor to multi-infarct dementia.

Measures of cognitive function have rarely been studied in heart failure trials, unlike recent hypertension trials such as the Systolic Hypertension in Europe (SYST-EUR) trial and the Study on Cognition and Prognosis in the Elderly (SCOPE).[8,86] Given the consistent reporting of impaired cognitive function in cross-sectional studies of patients with heart failure, perhaps this should be considered as an end point for future trials of heart failure pharmacotherapy.

Hyperlipidemia

Despite the classical perception of the chronic heart failure patient as being cachectic with low-plasma cholesterol levels, hyperlipidemia in fact coexists with chronic heart failure in a significant percent of patients. In chronic heart failure intervention trials, up to 26% of patients were classified as being hyperlipidemic on entry.[87] Of particular interest is whether HMG-CoA reductase inhibitor (statin) therapy may be beneficial in patients with established chronic heart failure. This has never been formally tested in prospective trials, because trials of lipid-lowering therapy have generally excluded patients with significant left ventricular systolic dysfunction.[88–90] Furthermore, there is concern regarding these agents lowering ubiquinone (coenzyme Q10) levels, which may be important in maintenance of myocardial function in chronic heart failure.[91,92] In addition, maintenance of circulating lipoproteins may be necessary to lower elevated circulating levels of proinflammatory cytokines, which may adversely impact on disease progression.[93–95]

Nevertheless, as statins beneficially impact coronary artery disease progression, this may translate into long-term benefits in patients with chronic heart failure of an ischemic etiology. Indeed, post hoc, retrospective analyses of major lipid-lowering trials support statin therapy as being of benefit for chronic heart failure. In the Scandianavian Simvastatin Survival Study (4S) trial, simvastatin decreased the rate of development of chronic heart failure following MI as well as the mortality of patients who developed chronic heart failure during the course of the study.[96]

The impact of statin therapy in patients with established chronic heart failure has been retrospectively assessed in nonrandomized, subset analyses within major chronic heart failure intervention trials. In the Evaluation of Losartan in the Elderly (ELITE) II study, there was a significantly lower mortality in patients receiving statins (10.6%) compared to those who were not (17.6%).[97]

In this regard, antiapoptotic, endothelial progenitor cell stimulatory, and vascular endothelial growth factor-stimulatory effects, antagonism of proinflammatory cytokines, and antifibrotic effects of statins may contribute to improvement in myocardial function directly and independent of effects on coronary artery disease.[98–102] This hypothesis has been supported by animal studies in which a statin improved parameters of ventricular function and reduced pathological fibrosis in the absence of changes in plasma cholesterol.[103] Furthermore, some but not all remodeling studies have suggested improvement in systolic ventricular function with statin therapy.[104–107]

Chronic Anemia

Anemia is common in chronic heart failure, with a mean hemoglobin of 12 g/dL amongst such patients.[108] The likelihood of anemia in patients with chronic heart failure correlates with disease severity.[109]

Small-scale studies of administration of subcutaneous erythropoietin and intravenous iron to patients with chronic heart failure and mild anemia have been shown to produce improvement in patients' overall clinical status and ventricular function.[109,110] A large-scale study to examine the effect of anemia correction with erythropoietin on clinical outcomes has commenced (Reduction of Events with Darbepoetin alfa in Heart Failure [RED-HF]).

Despite the above considerations, the importance of identifying and correcting mild anemia is generally under-recognized within this patient cohort.

Renal Failure

The close relationship between cardiovascular and renal function in normal physiology is also apparent in the setting of disease, where renal dysfunction may develop secondary to cardiac disease or vice versa. As a consequence of accelerated atherosclerotic coronary artery disease, concomitant hypertension, and fluid retention, patients with primary renal disease are at high risk of developing heart failure.[111] Alternatively, patients with heart failure often have evidence of kidney dysfunction in the absence of intrinsic renal disease.[112] The observed reduction in glomerular filtration rate in chronic heart failure is a consequence of diminished cardiac output, with decreased renal perfusion and intrarenal vasoconstriction accompanied by sodium and water retention.[111] Indeed, given this relationship between renal function and cardiac output, it is perhaps not surprising that renal dysfunction is not only an adverse prognostic marker but is a stronger predictor of poor outcome in heart failure than NYHA functional class.[112,113]

Blockade of the renin-angiotensin system is a cornerstone of both chronic heart failure therapy and renoprotective treatment in patients with both diabetic and nondiabetic kidney disease.[58,114] However, as the renal vasoconstriction that develops in the setting of reduced cardiac output is angiotensin II-dependent, treatment with an ACE inhibitor or angiotensin receptor blocker frequently leads to a (usually clinically unimportant) increase in the serum creatinine.

Arthritis and Gout

Patients with chronic heart failure tend to be elderly, and therefore other noncardiovascular conditions of the elderly will frequently coexist.

Arthritis is one such condition, with antiarthritic therapy impacting on heart failure status. Both nonsteroidal anti-inflammatory drugs (NSAIDs) as well as the cyclo-oxygenase (COX)-2 selective inhibitors are frequently prescribed to patients with arthritis, and are associated with potentially significant cardiovascular adverse effects in the setting of the patient with chronic heart failure.[115,116] Sodium and water retention with these agents may adversely impact on volume status in part because of activation of vasodilator prostaglandins (PGs) such as PGE_2 and PGI_{2i} in the heart failure setting.[117,118]

The role of the PG-inhibitor aspirin in attenuating the beneficial effects of renin-angiotensin blockade in chronic heart failure is highly controversial.[119,120]

Concern has also been expressed that certain COX-2 inhibitors may be prothrombotic, clearly an unfavorable effect in chronic heart failure patients, particularly those with an ischemic etiology.[121]

Tumor necrosis factor (TNF) blockade, now an established therapy for rheumatoid arthritis and other autoimmune conditions, has been studied in patients with established chronic heart failure.[122] Blockade of this cytokine as a potential therapy for chronic heart failure is based on its multifaceted contribution to progression of this disease.[123] However, both the TNF receptor fusion protein, etanercept, and the monoclonal antibody, infliximab, did not result in beneficial outcomes in this setting.[124,125]

Gout is a common comorbid association in patients with heart failure. Heart failure patients have elevated levels of plasma urate and these levels confer adverse prognostic significance. However, a recent trial of xanthine oxidase inhibition in patients with heart failure did not demonstrate benefits on clinical outcomes.[126]

Gout is also common in heart failure patients because many of the treatments used in the management of this condition are associated with elevations in plasma urate, for example, diuretic therapies.

Treatment of gout in the patient with heart failure is made somewhat more complex by the contraindication to use of NSAIDs and COX-2 inhibitors, as above. Similarly, steroids are also best avoided in the management of this complication in the heart failure patient. Colchicine is the preferred treatment option in the acute management of this condition, with allopurinol recommended for recurrent attacks as chronic therapy if required.

Malignant Disease

Cancer chemotherapy, particularly with anthracycline derivatives, may lead to the development of CHF; the risk is directly related to cumulative anthracycline dosage.[127] Preexistent impairment of left ventricular (LV) systolic function represents a relative contraindication to aggressive chemotherapy with such agents.

Alkylating agents such as cyclophosphamide, ifosfamide, cisplatin, carmustine, busulfan, chloromethane, and mitomycin have also been associated with cardiotoxicity. Trastuzumab is an antibody therapy directed against the human epidermal growth factor receptor-2 (HER2), which increases survival in patients with metastatic breast cancer and is under evaluation in the adjuvant setting. It may cause a decrease in LVEF in a minority of patients via uncertain mechanisms.[128] The incidence of this adverse effect is increased if trastuzumab is given in conjunction with paclitaxel or anthracyclines. It differs from anthracycline cardiotoxicity in that it is not cumulative dose-dependent and often improves after withdrawal of treatment.

▶ CONCLUSIONS

Chronic heart failure is a complex disease with progression and response to therapy influenced by a number of important demographic factors and comorbid conditions. These demographic and comorbid factors may have a considerable impact on progression of chronic heart failure as well as guiding therapeutic decision-making for this condition.

► REFERENCES

1. Topol EJ, Traill TA, Fortuin NJ. Hypertensive hypertrophic cardiomyopathy of the elderly. *N Engl J Med*. 1985;312:277–283.

2. Bonow RO, Udelson JE. Left ventricular diastolic dysfunction as a cause of congestive heart failure: mechanisms and management. *Ann Intern Med*. 1992;117:502–510.

3. Levy D, Larson MG, Vasan RS, et al. The progression from hypertension to congestive heart failure. *JAMA*. 1996;275:1557–1562.

4. Kostis JB. The effect of enalapril on mortal and morbid events in patients with hypertension and left ventricular dysfunction. *Am J Hypertens*. 1995;8:909–914.

5. Kostis JB, Davis BR, Cutler J, et al. Prevention of heart failure by antihypertensive drug treatment in older persons with isolated systolic hypertension. SHEP Cooperative Research Group. *JAMA*. 1997;278:212–216.

6. MRC Working Party Medical Research Council: Trial of treatment in older adults: principal results. *BMJ*. 1992;304:405–412.

7. Dahlof B, Lindholm LH, Hansson L, et al. Morbidity and mortality in the Swedish Trial in Old Patients with Hypertension (STOP-Hypertension). *Lancet*. 1991;338:1281–1285.

8. Staessen JA, Fagard R, Thijs L, et al. Randomised double-blind comparison of placebo and active treatment for older patients with isolated systolic hypertension. The Systolic Hypertension in Europe (Syst-Eur) Trial Investigators. *Lancet*. September 13, 1997;350(9080):757–764.

9. Yusuf S, Pfeffer MA, Swedberg K; CHARM Investigators and Committees. Effects of candesartan in patients with chronic heart failure and preserved left-ventricular ejection fraction: the CHARM-Preserved Trial. *Lancet*. 2003;362:777–781.

10. Flather MD, Shibata MC, Coats AJ; SENIORS Investigators. Randomized trial to determine the effect of nebivolol on mortality and cardiovascular hospital admission in elderly patients with heart failure (SENIORS). *Eur Heart J*. 2005;26:215–225.

11. Cleland JG, Tendera M, Adamus J; The PEP investigators. Perindopril for elderly people with chronic heart failure: the PEP-CHF study. *Eur J Heart Fail*. 1999;1:211–217.

12. Sutton GC. Epidemiologic aspects of heart failure. *Am Heart J*. 1990;120:1538–1540.

13. Gheorghiade M, Bonow RO. Chronic heart failure in the United States: a manifestation of coronary artery disease. *Circulation*. 1998;97:282–289.

14. Vasan RS, Benjamin EJ, Levy D. Prevalence, clinical features and prognosis of diastolic heart failure: an epidemiologic perspective. *J Am Coll Cardiol*. 1995;26:1565–1574.

15. Braunwald E, Rutherford JD. Reversible ischemic left ventricular dysfunction: evidence for the "hibernating myocardium". *J Am Coll Cardiol*. 1986;8:1467–1470.

16. Rahimtoola SH. From coronary artery disease to heart failure: role of the hibernating myocardium. *Am J Cardiol*. 1995;75:16E–22E.

17. Elefteriades JA, Tolis G Jr, Levi E, et al. Coronary artery bypass grafting in severe left ventricular dysfunction: excellent survival with improved ejection fraction and functional state. *J Am Coll Cardiol*. 1993;22:1411–1417.

18. Ragosta M, Beller GA, Watson DD, et al. Quantitative planar rest-redistribution 201Tl imaging in detection of myocardial viability and prediction of improvement in left ventricular function after coronary bypass surgery in patients with severely depressed left ventricular function. *Circulation*. 1993;87:1630–1641.

19. Cleland JG, Pennell DJ, Ray SG, et al; Carvedilol hibernating reversible ischaemia trial: marker of success investigators. Myocardial viability as a determinant of the ejection fraction response to carvedilol in patients with heart failure (CHRISTMAS trial): randomised controlled trial. *Lancet*. 2003;362:14–21.

20. Eitzman D, al-Aouar Z, Kanter HL, et al. Clinical outcome of patients with advanced coronary artery disease after viability studies with positron emission tomography. *J Am Coll Cardiol*. 1992;20:559–565.

21. Di Carli MF, Asgarzadie F, Schelbert HR, et al. Quantitative relation between myocardial viability and improvement in heart failure symptoms after revascularization in patients with ischemic cardiomyopathy. *Circulation*. 1995; 92:3436–3444.

22. Harrison DG. Endothelial dysfunction in atherosclerosis. *Basic Res Cardiol*. 1994;89:87–102.

23. Lüscher TF, Boulanger CM, Dohi Y, et al. Endothelium-derived contracting factors. *Hypertension*. 1992;19:117–130.

24. Mancini GB, Henry GC, Macaya C, et al. Angiotensin-converting enzyme inhibition with quinapril improves endothelial vasomotor dysfunction in patients with coronary artery disease. The TREND (Trial on Reversing ENdothelial Dysfunction) Study. *Circulation.* 1996;94: 258–265.

25. Yusuf S, Sleight P, Pogue J, et al. Effects of an angiotensin-converting-enzyme inhibitor, ramipril, on cardiovascular events in high-risk patients. The Heart Outcomes Prevention Evaluation Study Investigators. *N Engl J Med.* 2000;342:145–153.

26. The SOLVD Investigators. Effect of enalapril on survival in patients with reduced left ventricular ejection fractions and congestive heart failure. *N Engl J Med.* 1991;325:293–302.

27. Pfeffer MA, Braunwald E, Moye LA, et al. Effect of captopril on mortality and morbidity in patients with left ventricular dysfunction after myocardial infarction. Results of the survival and ventricular enlargement trial. The SAVE Investigators. *N Engl J Med.* 1992;327:669–677.

28. Dargie HJ. Effect of carvedilol on outcome after myocardial infarction in patients with left-ventricular dysfunction: the CAPRICORN randomised trial. *Lancet.* 2001;357:1385–1390.

29. Singh SN, Fletcher RD, Fisher SG, et al. Amiodarone in patients with congestive heart failure and asymptomatic ventricular arrhythmia: Survival Trial of Antiarrhythmic Therapy in Congestive Heart Failure. *N Engl J Med.* 1995;333:77–82.

30. Packer M, O'Connor CM, Ghali JK, et al. Effect of amlodipine on morbidity and mortality in severe chronic heart failure. Prospective Randomized Amlodipine Survival Evaluation Study Group. *N Engl J Med.* 1996;335:1107–1114.

31. Woodley SL, Gilbert EM, Anderson JL, et al. Beta-blockade with bucindolol in heart failure caused by ischemic versus idiopathic dilated cardiomyopathy. *Circulation.* 1991;84:2426–2441.

32. CIBIS II investigators and committees. The cardiac insufficiency bisoprolol study II (CIBIS II): a randomised trial. *Lancet.* 1999;353:9–13.

33. Packer M, Coats AJ, Fowler MB, et al. Effect of carvedilol on survival in severe chronic heart failure. *N Engl J Med.* 2001;344:1651–1658.

34. Pitt B, Zannad F, Remme WJ, et al. The effect of spironolactone on morbidity and mortality in patients with severe heart failure Randomized Aldactone Evaluation Study Investigators. *N Engl J Med.* 1999;341:709–717.

35. Pitt B, Poole-Wilson PA, Segal R, et al. Effect of losartan compared with captopril on mortality in patients with symptomatic heart failure: randomised trial—the Losartan Heart Failure Survival Study ELITE II. *Lancet.* 2000;355:1582–1587.

36. Cohn JN, Tognoni G. A randomized trial of the angiotensin-receptor blocker valsartan in chronic heart failure. *N Engl J Med.* 2001;345:1667–1675.

37. Stone PH, Muller JE, Hartwell T, et al. The effect of diabetes mellitus on prognosis and serial left ventricular function after acute myocardial infarction: contribution of both coronary disease and diastolic left ventricular dysfunction to the adverse prognosis. The MILIS Study Group. *J Am Coll Cardiol.* 1989;14(1):49–57.

38. Gustafsson I, Hildebrandt P, Seibaek M, et al. Long-term prognosis of diabetic patients with myocardial infarction: relation to antidiabetic treatment regimen. The TRACE Study Group. *Eur Heart J.* 2000;21(23):1937–1943.

39. Gustafsson I, Hildebrandt P. Early failure of the diabetic heart. *Diabetes Care.* 2001;24(1):3–4.

40. McKee PA, Castelli WP, McNamara PM, et al. The natural history of congestive heart failure: the Framingham study. *N Engl J Med.* 1971;285(26):1441–1446.

41. Kannel WB, Hjortland M, Castelli WP. Role of diabetes in congestive heart failure: the Framingham study. *Am J Cardiol.* 1974;34(1):29–34.

42. Chen YT, Vaccarino V, Williams CS, et al. Risk factors for heart failure in the elderly: a prospective community-based study. *Am J Med.* 1999;106(6):605–612.

43. Chae CU, Pfeffer MA, Glynn RJ, et al. Increased pulse pressure and risk of heart failure in the elderly. *JAMA.* 1999;281(7):634–639.

44. He J, Ogden LG, Bazzano LA, et al. Risk factors for congestive heart failure in US men and women: NHANES I epidemiologic follow-up study. *Arch Intern Med.* 2001;161(7):996–1002.

45. UKPDS Group. Tight blood pressure control and risk of macrovascular and microvascular complications in type 2 diabetes: UKPDS 38. *BMJ.* 1998;317(7160):703–713.

46. UKPDS Group. Intensive blood-glucose control with sulphonylureas or insulin compared with conventional treatment and risk of complications in patients with type 2 diabetes (UKPDS 33). *Lancet.* 1998;352(9131):837–853.

47. Grundy SM, Benjamin IJ, Burke GL, et al. Diabetes and cardiovascular disease: a statement for healthcare professionals from the American Heart Association. *Circulation*. 1999;100(10):1134–1146.

48. Tarnow L, Rossing P, Gall MA, et al. Prevalence of arterial hypertension in diabetic patients before and after the JNC-V. *Diabetes Care*. 1994;17(11):1247–1251.

49. Poirier P, Bogaty P, Garneau C, et al. Diastolic dysfunction in normotensive men with well-controlled type 2 diabetes: importance of manoeuvres in echocardiographic screening for preclinical diabetic cardiomyopathy. *Diabetes Care*. 2001;24(1):5–10.

50. Bell DS. Diabetic cardiomyopathy: a unique entity or a complication of coronary artery disease? *Diabetes Care*. 1995;18(5):708–714.

51. Standl E, Schnell O. A new look at the heart in diabetes mellitus: from ailing to failing. *Diabetologia*. 2000;43(12):1455–1469.

52. Stratton IM, Adler AI, Neil HA, et al. Association of glycaemia with macrovascular and microvascular complications of type 2 diabetes (UKPDS 35): prospective observational study. *BMJ*. 2000;321(7258):405–412.

53. Iribarren C, Karter AJ, Go AS, et al. Glycemic control and heart failure among adult patients with diabetes. *Circulation*. 2001;103(22):2668–2673.

54. Adler AI, Stratton IM, Neil HA, et al. Association of systolic blood pressure with macrovascular and microvascular complications of type 2 diabetes (UKPDS 36): prospective observational study [see comments]. *BMJ*. 2000;321(7258):412–419.

55. Heart Outcomes Prevention Evaluation Study Investigators. Effects of ramipril on cardiovascular and microvascular outcomes in people with diabetes mellitus: results of the HOPE study and MICRO-HOPE substudy. *Lancet*. 2000;355(9200):253–259.

56. Dahlof B, Devereux RB, Kjeldsen SE; LIFE Study Group. Cardiovascular morbidity and mortality in the Losartan Intervention For Endpoint reduction in hypertension study (LIFE): a randomised trial against atenolol. *Lancet*. 2002;359:995–1003.

57. Brenner BM, Cooper ME, de Zeeuw D, et al. Effects of losartan on renal and cardiovascular outcomes in patients with type 2 diabetes and nephropathy. *N Engl J Med*. 2001;345 (12): 861–869.

58. Lewis EJ, Hunsicker LG, Clarke WR, et al. Renoprotective effect of the angiotensin-receptor antagonist irbesartan in patients with nephropathy due to type 2 diabetes. *N Engl J Med*. 2001;345(12):851–860.

59. Krum H, Gilbert RE. Demographics and concomitant disorders in heart failure. *Lancet*. 2003;362:147–158.

60. Dries DL, Sweitzer NK, Drazner MH, et al. Prognostic impact of diabetes mellitus in patients with heart failure according to the etiology of left ventricular systolic dysfunction. *J Am Coll Cardiol*. 2001;38(2):421–428.

61. Gustafsson I, Torp-Pedersen C, Kober L, et al. Effect of the angiotensin-converting enzyme inhibitor trandolapril on mortality and morbidity in diabetic patients with left ventricular dysfunction after acute myocardial infarction. Trace Study Group. *J Am Coll Cardiol*. 1999;34(1):83–89.

62. Haas SJ, Vos T, Gilbert RE, et al. Are beta-blockers as efficacious in patients with diabetes mellitus as in patients without diabetes mellitus who have chronic heart failure? A meta-analysis of large-scale clinical trials. *Am Heart J*. 2003;146:848–853.

63. Swedberg K, Cleland J, Dargie H; Task Force for the Diagnosis and Treatment of Chronic Heart Failure of the European Society of Cardiology. Guidelines for the diagnosis and treatment of chronic heart failure: executive summary (update 2005): The Task Force for the Diagnosis and Treatment of Chronic Heart Failure of the European Society of Cardiology. *Eur Heart J*. 2005;26:1115–1140.

64. Stevenson WG, Sweeney MO. Pharmacologic and nonpharmacologic treatment of ventricular arrhythmias in heart failure. *Curr Opin Cardiol*. 1997;12:242–250.

65. Stevenson WG, Middlekauff HR, Saxon LA. Ventricular arrhythmias in heart failure. Zipes DP, Jaife J eds. In: *Cardiac Electrophysiology: From Cell to Bedside*. 1995;848–863.

66. Moss AJ, Hall WJ, Cannom DS, et al. Improved survival with an implanted defibrillator in patients with coronary disease at high risk for ventricular arrhythmia. Multicenter Automatic Defibrillator Implantation Trial Investigators. *N Engl J Med*. 1996;335:1933–1940.

67. Buxton AE, Lee KL, Fisher JD, Multicenter Unsustained Tachycardia Trial Investigators.

A randomized study of the prevention of sudden death in patients with coronary artery disease. *N Engl J Med*. 1999;341:1882–1890.

68. The Antiarrhythmics versus Implantable Defibrillators (AVID) Investigators. A comparison of antiarrhythmic-drug therapy with implantable defibrillators in patients resuscitated from near-fatal ventricular arrhythmias. *N Engl J Med* 1997;337:1576–83.

69. Moss AJ, Zareba W, Hall WJ, et al. Prophylactic implantation of a defibrillator in patients with myocardial infarction and reduced ejection fraction. *N Engl J Med*. March 21 2002; 346(12):877–883.

70. Bardy GH, Lee KL, Mark DB; Sudden Cardiac Death in Heart Failure Trial (SCD-HeFT) Investigators. Amiodarone or an implantable cardioverter-defibrillator for congestive heart failure. *N Engl J Med*. 2005;352:225–237.

71. Lechat P, Hulot JS, Escolano S, et al. Heart rate and cardiac rhythm relationships with bisoprolol benefit in chronic heart failure in CIBIS II Trial. *Circulation*. 2001;103:1428–1433.

72. Joglar JA, Acusta AP, Shusterman NH, et al. Effect of carvedilol on survival and hemodynamics in patients with atrial fibrillation and left ventricular dysfunction: retrospective analysis of the US Carvedilol Heart Failure Trials Program. *Am Heart J*. 2001;142:498–501.

73. Wyse DG, Waldo AL, DiMarco JP; Atrial Fibrillation Follow-up Investigation of Rhythm Management (AFFIRM) Investigators. A comparison of rate control and rhythm control in patients with atrial fibrillation. *N Engl J Med*. 2002;347:1825–1833.

74. Moller M, Torp-Pedersen CT, Kober L. Dofetilide in patients with congestive heart failure and left ventricular dysfunction: safety aspects and effect on atrial fibrillation. The Danish Investigators of Arrhythmia and Mortality on (DIAMOND) Study Group. *Congest Heart Fail*. 2001;7:146–150.

75. Loh E, Sutton MS, Wun CC, et al. Ventricular dysfunction and the risk of stroke after myocardial infarction. *N Engl J Med*. 1997;336:251–257.

76. Cleland JG, Findlay I, Jafri S, et al. The Warfarin/Aspirin Study in Heart failure (WASH): a randomized trial comparing antithrombotic strategies for patients with heart failure. *Am Heart J*. July 2004;148(1):157–164.

77. Thatai D, Ahooja V, Pullicino PM. Pharmacological prevention of thromboembolism in patients with left ventricular dysfunction. *Am J Cardiovasc Drugs*. 2006;6:41–49.

78. Krum H, Ninio D, MacDonald P. Baseline predictors of tolerability to carvedilol in patients with chronic heart failure. *Heart*. December 2000;84(6):615–619.

79. Salpeter SS, Ormiston T, Salpeter E, et al. Cardioselective beta-blockers for chronic obstructive pulmonary disease. *Cochrane Database Syst Rev*. 2002;(2):CD003566.

80. Andreas S. Central sleep apnea and chronic heart failure. *Sleep*. 2000;23:S220–S223.

81. Tremel F, Pepin JL, Veale D, et al. High prevalence and persistence of sleep apnoea in patients referred for acute left ventricular failure and medically treated over 2 months. *Eur Heart J*. 1999;20:1201–1209.

82. Tkacova R, Dajani HR, Rankin F, et al. Continuous positive airway pressure improves nocturnal baroreflex sensitivity of patients with heart failure and obstructive sleep apnea. *J Hypertens*. 2000;18:1257–1262.

83. Naughton MT. Impact of treatment of sleep apnoea on left ventricular function in congestive heart failure. *Thorax*. 1998;53:S37–S40.

84. Scall RR, Petrucci RJ, Brozena SC, et al. Cognitive function in patients with symptomatic dilated cardiomyopathy before and after cardiac transplantation. *J Am Coll Cardiol*. 1989;14:1666–1672.

85. Cacciatore F, Abete P, Ferrara N, et al. Congestive heart failure and cognitive impairment in the elderly. *Arch Gerontol Geriatr*. 1995;20:63–68.

86. Skoog I, Lithell H, Hansson L; SCOPE Study Group. Effect of baseline cognitive function and antihypertensive treatment on cognitive and cardiovascular outcomes: Study on COgnition and Prognosis in the Elderly (SCOPE). *Am J Hypertens*. 2005;18:1052–1059.

87. Krum H, McMurray JJ. Statins and chronic heart failure: do we need a large-scale outcome trial? *J Am Coll Cardiol*. 2002;39:1567–1573.

88. Scandinavian Simvastatin Survival Study Group. Randomised trial of cholesterol lowering in 4444 patients with coronary heart disease: the Scandinavian Simvastatin Survival Study (4S). *Lancet*. 1994;344:1383–1389.

89. Sacks FM, Pfeffer MA, Moye LA, et al. The effect of pravastatin on coronary events after myocardial infarction in patients with average

cholesterol levels. Cholesterol and Recurrent Events Trial investigators. *N Engl J Med.* 1996; 335:1001–1009.

90. The Long-Term Intervention with Pravastatin in Ischaemic Disease (LIPID) Study Group. Prevention of cardiovascular events and death with pravastatin in patients with coronary heart disease and a broad range of initial cholesterol levels. *N Engl J Med.* 1998;339:1349–1357.

91. Mortensen SA, Leth A, Agner E, et al. Dose-related decrease of serum coenzyme Q10 during treatment with HMG-CoA reductase inhibitors. *Mol Aspects Med.* 1997;18(Suppl):S137–S144.

92. McMurray J, Chopra M, Abdullah I, et al. Evidence of oxidative stress in chronic heart failure in humans. *Eur Heart J.* 1993;14:1493–1498.

93. Rauchhaus M, Coats AJ, Anker SD. The endotoxin-lipoprotein hypothesis. *Lancet.* 2000; 356:930–933.

94. Rauchhaus M, Doehner W, Francis DP, et al. Plasma cytokine parameters and mortality in patients with chronic heart failure. *Circulation.* 2000;102:3060–3067.

95. Niebauer J, Volk HD, Kemp M, et al. Endotoxin and immune activation in chronic heart failure: a prospective cohort study. *Lancet.* 1999;353: 1838–1842.

96. Kjekshus J, Pedersen TR, Olsson AG, et al. The effects of simvastatin on the incidence of heart failure in patients with coronary heart disease. *J Card Fail.* 1997;3:249–254.

97. Segal R, Pitt B, Poole Wilson P, et al. Effects of HMG-CoA reductase inhibitors (statins) in patients with heart failure. *Eur J Heart Failure.* 2000;2(Suppl.2):96. (abstract)

98. Kaneider NC, Reinisch CM, Dunzendorfer S, et al. Induction of apoptosis and inhibition of migration of inflammatory and vascular wall cells by cerivastatin. *Atherosclerosis.* 2001;158:23–33.

99. Dimmeler S, Aicher A, Vasa M, et al. HMG-CoA reductase inhibitors (statins) increase endothelial progenitor cells via the PI 3-kinase/Akt pathway. *J Clin Invest.* 2001;108:391–397.

100. Kureishi Y, Luo Z, Shiojima I, et al. The HMG-CoA reductase inhibitor simvastatin activates the protein kinase Akt and promotes angiogenesis in normocholesterolemic animals. *Nat Med.* 2000;6:1004–1010.

101. Rosnenson RS, Tangney CC, Casey LC. Inhibition of proinflammatory cytokine production by pravastatin. *Lancet.* 1999;353:983–984.

102. Martin J, Denver R, Bailey M, et al. In vitro inhibitory effects of atorvastatin on cardiac fibroblasts: implications for ventricular remodelling. *Clin Exp Pharmacol Physiol.* 2005;32:697–701.

103. Bauersachs J, Galuppo P, Fraccarollo D, et al. Improvement of left ventricular remodeling and function by hydroxymethylglutaryl coenzyme a reductase inhibition with cerivastatin in rats with heart failure after myocardial infarction. *Circulation.* 2001;104:982–985.

104. Node K, Fujita M, Kitakaze M, et al. Short-term statin therapy improves cardiac function and symptoms in patients with idiopathic dilated cardiomyopathy. *Circulation.* 2003;108:839–843.

105. Sola S, Mir MQ, Lerakis S, et al. Atorvastatin improves left ventricular systolic function and serum markers of inflammation in nonischemic heart failure. *J Am Coll Cardiol.* 2006;47:332–337.

106. Bleske BE, Nicklas JM, Bard RL, et al. Neutral effect on markers of heart failure, inflammation, endothelial activation and function, and vagal tone after high-dose HMG-CoA reductase inhibition in non-diabetic patients with non-ischemic cardiomyopathy and average low-density lipoprotein level. *J Am Coll Cardiol.* 2006;47:338–341.

107. Krum H, Tonkin A, for the UNIVERSE Investigators. Effect of high-dose HMG CoA reductase inhibitor therapy on ventricular remodelling, pro-inflammatory cytokines and neurohormonal parameters in patients with chronic systolic heart failure: The UNIVERSE study. *J Am Coll Cardiol.* 2006;Suppl. (abstract)

108. Haber HL, Leavy JA, Kessler PD, et al. The erythrocyte sedimentation rate in congestive heart failure. *N Engl J Med.* 1991;324:353–358.

109. Silverberg DS, Wexler D, Blum M, et al. The use of subcutaneous erythropoietin and intravenous iron for the treatment of the anemia of severe, resistant congestive heart failure improves cardiac and renal function and functional cardiac class, and markedly reduces hospitalizations. *J Am Coll Cardiol.* 2000;35:1737–1744.

110. Silverberg DS, Wexler D, Sheps D, et al. The effect of correction of mild anemia in severe, resistant congestive heart failure using subcutaneous erythropoietin and intravenous iron: a randomized controlled study. *J Am Coll Cardiol.* 2001;37:1775–1780.

111. Ruilope LM, van Veldhuisen DJ, Ritz E, et al. Renal function: the Cinderella of cardiovascular

risk profile. *J Am Coll Cardiol.* 2001;38(7): 1782–1787.

112. Hillege HL, Girbes AR, de Kam PJ, et al. Renal function, neurohormonal activation, and survival in patients with chronic heart failure. *Circulation.* 2000;102(2):203–210.

113. Dries DL, Exner DV, Domanski MJ, et al. The prognostic implications of renal insufficiency in asymptomatic and symptomatic patients with left ventricular systolic dysfunction. *J Am Coll Cardiol.* 2000;35(3):681–689.

114. The GISEN Group (Gruppo Italiano di Studi Epidemiologici in Nefrologia). Randomised placebo-controlled trial of effect of ramipril on decline in glomerular filtration rate and risk of terminal renal failure in proteinuric, non-diabetic nephropathy. *Lancet.* 1997;349:1857–1863.

115. Page J, Henry D. Consumption of NSAIDs and the development of congestive heart failure in elderly patients: an underrecognized public health problem. *Arch Intern Med.* 2000;160: 777–784.

116. Feenstra J, Grobbee DE, Mosterd A, et al. Adverse cardiovascular effects of NSAIDs in patients with congestive heart failure. *Drug Saf.* 1997;17:166–180.

117. Harris CJ, Brater DC. Renal effects of cyclooxygenase-2 selective inhibitors. *Curr Opin Nephrol Hypertens.* 2001;10:603–610.

118. Katz SD. The role of endothelin-derived vasoactive substances in the pathology of exercise intolerance in patients with congestive heart failure. *Prog Cardiovasc Dis.* July–August 1995;38(1):23–50.

119. Cleland JGF. Anticoagulant and antiplatelet therapy in heart failure. *Curr Opin Cardiol.* 1997;12:276–287.

120. Teo KK, Yusuf S, Pfeffer M, et al. Effects of long-term treatment with angiotensin-converting enzyme inhibitors in the presence or absence of aspirin: a systematic review. *Lancet.* 2002; 360:1037–1043.

121. McAdam BF, Catella-Lawson F, Mardini IA, et al. Systemic biosynthesis of prostacyclin by cyclooxygenase (COX)-2: the human pharmacology of a selective inhibitor of COX-2. *Proc Natl Acad Sci USA.* 1999;96:272–277.

122. Pisetsky DS, St Clair EW. Progress in the treatment of rheumatoid arthritis. *JAMA.* 2001;286:2787–2790.

123. Shan K, Kurrelmeyer K, Seta Y, et al. The role of cytokines in disease progression in heart failure. *Curr Opin Cardiol.* 1997;12:218–223.

124. Mann DL, McMurray JJ, Packer M, et al. Targeted anticytokine therapy in patients with chronic heart failure: results of the Randomized Etanercept Worldwide Evaluation (RENEWAL). *Circulation.* 2004;109:1594–1602.

125. Chung ES, Packer M, Lo KH; Anti-TNF Therapy Against Congestive Heart Failure Investigators. Randomized, double-blind, placebo-controlled, pilot trial of infliximab, a chimeric monoclonal antibody to tumor necrosis factor-alpha, in patients with moderate-to-severe heart failure: results of the anti-TNF Therapy Against Congestive Heart Failure (ATTACH) trial. *Circulation.* 2003;107:3133–140.

126. Stiles S. Oxypurinol fails to improve HF outcomes in phase 2 trial. *www.theheart.org.* August 18, 2005.

127. Wouters KA, Kremer LC, Miller TL, et al. Protecting against anthracycline-induced myocardial damage: a review of the most promising strategies. *Br J Haematol.* 2005; 131:561–578.

128. Youssef G, Links M. The prevention and management of cardiovascular complications of chemotherapy in patients with cancer. *Am J Cardiovasc Drugs.* 2005;5:233–243.

CHAPTER 18

Disease Management Overview

ROBIN J. TRUPP, MSN, APRN, BC, CCRN, CCRC

▶ INTRODUCTION

Due to its tremendous clinical and financial impact, managing chronic diseases has become a focus for health-care policymakers and researchers. More than 100 million Americans have a chronic disease, and half of the health-care dollars in the United States are being spent on individuals with chronic illnesses.[1,2] These expenditures double when chronic disease produces limitations in physical activity.[1] As a chronic condition associated with marked physical debilitation and multiple comorbidities, heart failure (HF) ranks high on the list of chronic diseases in terms of prevalence, morbidity and

mortality, and financial costs in the United States and worldwide.[1] An increase in the aging population combined with aggressive treatment for and improved survival from acute coronary syndromes has contributed to the dramatic growth in the number of individuals with HF, where HF is expected to reach 10 million cases in the United States alone.

Managing HF is challenging for both health-care providers and patients. The United States has been criticized for providing health care on an episodic, acute illness basis and for the absence of a systematic approach to managing chronic disease. Rightfully so, since the majority of health-care dollars spent on HF result from inpatient care during hospitalization.[2] Over the past decade, many pharmacologic and nonpharmacologic treatment strategies have been evaluated in multicenter clinical trials. The good news is that many of these strategies work, giving those with HF an improved prognosis with reduced morbidity and mortality and improved quality of life.[3-6] The bad news is that these strategies have dramatically changed HF care over the past decade, making it quite complex as multiple medications, including medications that were previously contraindicated, and biomedical devices are now integral aspects of care.

Based upon the overwhelming evidence and the desire to improve treatment and the quality of care, the American College of Cardiology/American Heart Association published *Guidelines for the Evaluation and Management of Chronic Heart Failure in the Adult* in 2001.[6] These guidelines were subsequently updated in 2005.[7] Yet even with explicit recommendations for practice, gaps exist between best evidence and clinical practice in implementation of the guidelines. Rapid advances in biomedicine, the tendency to overlook information not used routinely, and learning new information concurrent with relearning forgotten information all contribute to nonadherence. Studies suggest that 30–40% of patients are not receiving care based upon current scientific evidence and that as much as 25% of the care provided to patients with chronic HF is either unnecessary or is potentially harmful.[8,9] One approach to bridging the gap between proven therapies and clinical practice has been the development of disease management (DM) programs.

▶ HISTORICAL PERSPECTIVES

As health-care costs continue to soar, everyone seems to be looking for new ways to reduce expenditures while improving patient outcomes and satisfaction. The first programs considered to be DM were introduced by the pharmaceutical industry as a tactic to increase pharmaceutical profits.[10] The largest pharmaceutical benefits management (PBM) firms, which process pharmacy claims for employers and health maintenance organizations (HMOs), and negotiate purchasing agreements with pharmaceutical manufacturers, were purchased by pharmaceutical companies in 1993 and 1994.[10] On average, patients with a single chronic condition see more than 3 physicians and fill 6 prescriptions annually, while individuals with 5 or more comorbidities have 15 physician visits and fill over 50 prescriptions per year.[11] By offering services to assist with managing patients with chronic diseases and/or programs designed to improve patient adherence to medications regimens, PBMs can directly effect drug sales. Thus, through systematic approaches making them providers of care for patients with chronic diseases, pharmaceutical manufacturers influence billions of dollars in revenue from HMOs while also expanding their industry's volume and profits.[10]

Other strategies geared toward reducing health-care expenditures have been developed. Critical pathways, guidelines, and care maps attempt to standardize care for individuals hospitalized with a particular disease or condition. These approaches are very effective in reducing length of stay and limiting inpatient resource utilization, but do little to address postdischarge needs or to prevent rehospitalization. For these reasons, more comprehensive approaches, such as DM, have been accepted by health-care institutions and organizations. "Disease management" is used as an umbrella term. The phrase "disease management" means different things to different people, has diverse operationalizations, and encompasses a wide range of concepts. Unfortunately there are no universal standards for DM programs. According to the Disease Management Association of America (DMAA), a voluntary organization formed in 1999 to promote a more scientific approach to measuring success of DM programs, full-service DM programs have six essential components (Table 18-1). Those with fewer components are considered DM support services and far outnumber the full-service programs available.[12] DMAA

▶ **Table 18-1** Essential components of disease management*

* Processes to identify the population of interest
* Evidence-based practice guidelines
* Collaborative practice models to include physician and support-service providers
* Patient self-management education
* Process and outcomes measurement, evaluation, and management
* Routine reporting mechanisms, including feedback loops

*Note: Full-service disease management programs must include all six components. Programs consisting of fewer components are disease management support services.
Source: Adapted from Disease Management Association of America.

defines DM as "a system of coordinated healthcare interventions and communications for populations with conditions in which patient self-care efforts are significant."[12] Since initial programs focused on reducing expenditures, managed care organizations were early adopters of DM due to the financial attractiveness. However, "true" DM is far more than fiscal in nature. For clarity purposes, the remainder of this chapter will utilize the DMAA definition.

DM programs are population-based approaches concentrating on costly chronic diseases, such as asthma, diabetes, or HF. Even though termed "disease" management, these programs intently focus on managing "patients" and use patient-centered outcomes as measures of success. Because of the significant accomplishments seen in improving outcomes, DM is being increasingly endorsed by policymakers and third-party payers. However, caution must be used when interpreting the findings in many of the articles published on DM. Flaws in the research design and/or data analysis, the lack of guidelines for evaluation, and inconsistencies in reviewing of such articles leave questions about the veracity in reported findings.[13-15] This may be one reason the National Committee for Quality Assurance in the United States announced plans in June 2000 to certify DM programs, using criteria based on effectiveness in quality, accreditation, and health improvement.[16]

Successful DM programs engage in collaborative practice with a multidisciplinary approach,

utilizing a health-care team with specialized education and training for that specific chronic condition. Traditional members include physicians, advanced practice nurses (APN), nurses, pharmacists, dietitians, and social workers, to name a few. Membership can be extended on a routine or ad hoc basis to palliative care clinicians, exercise specialists, home care nurses, clergy, psychologists, or others deemed essential. A prerequisite for any program is advanced education in the management of the disease for all team members. Using this approach, care is coordinated throughout the continuum of illness, throughout all providers of care, and throughout the health-care system.

To optimize collaboration, it is imperative that team members respect the unique skills and knowledge base of all members and encourage active involvement by all. Members have a clear vision of their responsibilities in order to achieve the common goals, which are beneficial to both the team and the patient. Examples of common goals include a reduction of the severity of symptoms and the impact of that disease. By working together, care can be extended across the natural course of the illness.

Collaboration between medicine and nursing is integral to success in DM, as physicians and APNs develop a partnership to manage the complex clinical issues associated with chronic illness. While the plan of care is typically established by the physician, the APN typically provides the majority of care and clinical management.

Importantly, this approach bestows the patient with increased access to the APN for both routine and urgent care. The APN works semiautonomously to accomplish medication optimization, symptom management skills, education to the patient and family, and communication between patient, family, and other caregivers. Routine processes of episodic care, with heavy emphasis on the use of hospitals and emergency departments, are broken as patients are instructed to contact the APN with concerns or changes in symptoms. Through proactive surveillance and early intervention, hospitalizations may be avoided, thereby both reducing health-care expenditures and increasing quality of life.[17,18]

DM endorses and employs evidence-based medicine, based upon the most current science, and cost-effective technology to deliver individualized care to those with specific chronic diseases. Many successful DM programs participate in clinical research, offering patients access to participate in investigations of novel medications or other therapies. Thus, DM is multifaceted and incorporates a variety of strategies and interventions to manage chronic illness. Individual programs determine the actual interventions that are used and how they are operationalized. For the vast majority of programs, patient education, lifestyle modifications to reduce further injury, outpatient monitoring, and self-care management strategies are important aspects of care.

Accurately defining quality care is problematic as well. In *The Quality Chasm* report, the Institute of Medicine outlined key recommendations to improve the quality of health care in the United States, focusing on health-care delivery and dimensions of health-care performance.[19] In this report, the patient's experience within the health-care system is fundamental to quality. Thus, the value of work, delivery systems, organizations, and policies is judged only by their ability to alleviate suffering, reduce disability, and improve the health of patients.[19]

Since its inception, DM has been interested in clinical and economic outcomes. While clinical outcomes are important and necessary measurements of success, patients ultimately judge their own health within the context of daily living. Thus comprehensive DM programs routinely evaluate changes in physical limitations and the impact of chronic disease on patients' lives. This is accomplished through either general or disease-specific health questionnaires, appraisal of physical performance, or standardized surveys. This information can, and should, be used to make individualized treatment decisions.

Financial and quality initiatives at local and federal levels have encouraged the employment of DM. Most recently the Medicare Prescription Drug, Improvement and Modernization Act of 2003 contains three sections that establish DM initiatives and provides the Center for Medicare and Medicaid Services (CMS) the authority to contract directly with DM companies and others qualified to manage chronic illness.[20] If deemed successful after a 3-year pilot, CMS may begin nationwide implementation of chronic care programs. Several insurers are also offering enhanced reimbursement for demonstrated quality care in episodic care (i.e., acute MI) or DM care (i.e., diabetes).[21] Linking reimbursement to achieving high-quality outcomes may be an effective strategy to improve adherence to evidence-based clinical practice guidelines and for healthier patients.

DM programs can be either "home grown," purchased from a variety of DM vendors, or a partnership with another institution that has already an existing DM program. Many vendors and individuals are also available as consultants to institutions interested in initiating or enhancing existing DM programs. If a choice is made to outsource DM, good decision-making and data interpretation must be involved to interpret the successes reported by that vendor and to understand exactly what is being purchased. If it sounds too good to be true, it most likely is.

▶ MODELS OF CARE IN DISEASE MANAGEMENT

Just as there is no universal definition of DM, there are no universal models for DM. As previously discussed, there is also great variety in the interventions utilized by DM programs. A variety of classification schemes have been suggested to facilitate comparison between programs, but there is no single system recognized at this time.[22,23] Following are some guiding principles in DM, adapted from AADM:[12]

- Health care should be delivered in the least intensive manner in the least intense environment possible.
- Treatment must focus on the whole individual with goals of preserving independence, function, comfort, and quality of life.
- Education on the chronic disease and symptom management, including when to seek intervention, should be provided to the patient and family.
- Any decisions about changes in care must be driven by quality data and should involve the patient and family.

▶ GOALS OF DISEASE MANAGEMENT PROGRAMS

Most patients with chronic disease are not well educated on managing their own diseases. Office visits with health-care providers are short and provide inadequate time for addressing chronic conditions or establishing clearly defined plans of care. The end result is a passive, ill-informed patient receiving episodic care, driven primarily by exacerbations rather than a proactive, comprehensive approach.

Goals for DM programs include integration of care, efficient processes for delivery of care, comprehensive care, and care based on best practice, as identified by the best clinical evidence available. This translates to a better educated patient, with improved access to contemporary care that is both resourceful and cost-effective.

▶ OUTCOME MEASUREMENTS

Documenting outcomes for the care provided is an expectation of all health-care disciplines. However, this documentation is more than simply collecting data and requires planning and the selection of valid and reliable instruments that are both sensitive and specific for the desired outcome. Measured outcomes can be clinical endpoints, such as exercise capacity, complication rates, or appropriate medication use, or indicative of resource utilization, such as length of stay, hospitalization rates, or office visits. Increasingly studies are reporting measures of satisfaction, encompassing patient and/or physician satisfaction as well as variables such as depression or caregiver burden (Table 18-2).

▶ **Table 18-2** Examples of outcome and process measurements for disease management programs

Quality	Satisfaction	Financial
Adherence to guidelines	Patient satisfaction	Resource use
Complication rates	Physician satisfaction	Hospitalization rates
Clinical assessment measures (i.e., blood pressure, weight)	Functional status/exercise capacity (i.e., stress test, 6-minute walk)	Readmission rates
Pharmacy utilization		Length of stay
Mortality rates	Quality of life	Emergency department visits
Disease-specific measures (i.e., ACE inhibitor use, glycosylated hemoglobin levels)	Caregiver burden	Outpatient visits and testing
Assessment of LVEF		
Laboratory values		

ACE—angiotensin-converting enzyme; LVEF—left ventricular ejection fraction

► HEART FAILURE DISEASE MANAGEMENT

Managing HF is challenging and requires the integration of inpatient and outpatient care. The goals of DM are to reduce symptoms and to improve morbidity, mortality, and quality of life in HF. Although guidelines are available to guide and direct the management of patients with HF or at risk for its development, the vast majority of clinicians managing the condition have fallen short of the standards.[9,18,24,25]

Numerous challenges are associated with managing HF. First, it is a complex disease requiring substantial resources for care. It is difficult for clinicians to keep abreast of the latest research findings, and adherence to published guidelines remains less than ideal. Many patients with HF are not prescribed medications proven to improve morbidity and mortality or are not prescribed evidence-based medications at doses deemed effective in clinical trials.[26,27] In addition, most patients have multiple comorbidities, making their care and management more complicated. Common comorbidities include hypertension, coronary artery disease, atrial fibrillation, renal insufficiency, sleep disorders, dyslipidemia, and diabetes.[28] Evidence suggests that many patients with HF are undiagnosed, and thus receive no treatment until advanced disease has developed, thereby missing any opportunities to slow or halt disease progression are lost.[29]

As previously discussed, the majority of health-care dollars in HF are spent during hospitalization. Postdischarge, these patients have readmission rates between 36% and 75% and increased mortality rates.[30] Age, gender, coronary artery disease, diabetes, and nonadherence to the medical regimen are risk factors for readmission.[31] All of these issues contribute favorably to and support the importance of DM in HF.

The American Heart Association's Expert Panel recommends the following principles for the development, implementation, and evaluation of DM initiatives:[20]

- The main goal should be to improve the quality of care and patient outcomes.
- Evidence-based, consensus-driven guidelines should be the basis of care and should be used to increase adherence to the most current evidence.
- DM programs should be within integrated and comprehensive systems. The patient-provider relationship is central.
- DM programs should be developed for all populations and should include under-served or vulnerable populations.
- Organizations involved in DM should be aware of and address potential conflicts of interest.

► MODELS OF HEART FAILURE DISEASE MANAGEMENT

The literature is filled with articles describing HF programs and their impact on outcomes. However, because of the diversity in the data measured and reported, it is difficult to discern exactly what intervention was most influential or to replicate the results. It is also difficult to compare programs due to the diversity of interventions used. Riegel and LePetri propose a classification system that can be used for comparison, based upon the provider(s) of the DM intervention: multidisciplinary models, case management models, and clinic models.[23] These models are discussed in greater detail below.

Multidisciplinary Models of Care

As previously described, this model involves multiple dedicated health-care clinicians, each approaching the patient from a unique perspective. The first prospective study of a multidisciplinary HF DM program was conducted by Rich et al. in 1993.[32] Using interventions that involved intensive education, medication adherence, discharge planning, and enhanced follow-up care, Rich reported significant reductions in HF hospitalizations that were evident 1 year later.

It is important to note that no two DM programs are identical. Similarities seen in the literature include characteristics of transitioning from hospital to home, individualized education and reinforcement, telephone monitoring, promoting self-care abilities, and the role of the nurse.[33–36] Nurses play a critical role as liaisons between the patient and the physician, through telephone monitoring, triage, and advice to patients. Because most HF DM utilize APNs, patients have increased access to care either through frequent follow-up, through the ability to be seen on an emergent basis, or through walk-in appointments. These programs emphasize the role of medications in treating HF and routinely review prescription and over-the-counter drugs to simplify and optimize regimens, utilize treatment protocols to manage changes in symptoms and/or weight, have established education plans for patients and families to enhance self-care, are involved in the discharge process to ease the transition from hospital to home care, and provide routine monitoring and access to care for outpatients. Reported successes include marked reductions in HF hospitalizations and shorter length of stay, higher ACE inhibitor and β-blocker utilization, and improved quality of life and functional capacity.[37,38]

Case Management Models

In this model, patients receive intense monitoring after hospital discharge. This monitoring may occur via the telephone or home visits, or remotely via electronic scales within the home. Case managers are typically nurses, but may be social workers, pharmacists, or physicians.[23] This model provides frequent, individualized education focusing on dietary sodium, medication adherence, and symptom monitoring. Case managers coordinate communication with the health-care clinicians about issues, concerns, or physical examination findings. Decreases in hospitalizations, length of stay, costs, and clinic and emergency department visits have been reported.[37,39] In fact, a recent article reported that a home-based

model may be most effective for fragile, elderly, or physically impaired patients who cannot travel to clinic appointments.[40]

Clinic Models of Care

Clinic models for DM in HF are outpatient clinics that are directed by HF specialists who are usually, although not always, cardiologists. Intense follow-up by physicians or APNs provides the basis of care, where emphasis is placed on treating modifiable causes of HF and optimization of medications. Education and reinforcement are major components of care. Flexible diuretic regimens allowing patients to adjust their doses based on daily weights originated in clinic models.[33,41] As with the others, reductions in all-cause and HF hospitalizations and emergency department visits are reported in the literature.[33,41]

► ESSENTIALS OF HEART FAILURE DISEASE MANAGEMENT

Adherence to prescribed medical regimens, including both pharmacologic and nonpharmacologic interventions, significantly impacts both the short- and long-term management of HF. Such treatment strategies have been well proven to slow disease progression, reduce hospital admissions, and improve overall symptom control.[42] However, despite the importance of these interventions, numerous barriers to adherence exist. Barriers may include lack of understanding of perceived benefit, lifestyle modifications, absence of social support, powerlessness, financial concerns, and time constraints. These barriers complicate patients' ability and willingness to adhere to the prescribed medical regimen. In addition, in the haste to shorten length of stay and reduce health-care expenditures, clinicians may simply treat the symptoms and fail to identify nonmedical causes for the decompensation. By taking the time to do a thorough assessment to identify barriers and then target problem areas, clinicians can better utilize the time spent with each patient, leading to a more individual-ized treatment plan and enhanced adherence.

Worsening Signs and Symptoms

Despite advanced warning signs and symptoms of decompensation, many patients either fail to recognize or fail to react. For example, Friedman and Griffin reported 90% of patients hospitalized due to decompensation experi-enced dyspnea 3 days prior to hospitalization.[44] Additionally 35% reported edema and 33% had cough 1 week prior to admission.[45] A survey by Carlson and Riegel revealed that most patients had experienced multiple symptoms of worsen-ing HF in the previous year, yet their knowledge of the importance of these signs and symptoms was poor.[46] Even though patients who had lived with HF for years were more likely to use appro-priate self-care strategies than newly diagnosed patients, they were uncomfortable in evaluating the effectiveness of their own actions.[46] Thus when patients fail to recognize or acknowledge worsening signs and symptoms, clinicians lose the chance to intervene and potentially avert hospitalization. Therefore, educating patients and their families on both the signs and symp-toms associated with worsening HF and what actions to take provides an excellent opportu-nity to reduce hospitalizations and ultimately reduce health-care expenditures. Establishing self-efficacy, or belief in the ability to control HF, is essential for patients to participate in their own care and better manage their disease.

Patients experiencing decompensated HF exhibit a constellation of signs and symptoms, including increased dyspnea and/or fatigue, weight gain, orthopnea, and paroxysmal noctur-nal dyspnea (PND). Essential aspects of educa-tion are presented in Table 18-3. Patients need simple advice on what changes in symptoms are important and clear endpoints that should prompt them to seek help. Whenever special equipment is involved, instruction on proper use and when to seek help are required. For example, daily weights require that the patient owns a scale, that the scale has numbers that can be read by the patient with a stable base large enough for them to stand on, and that the weights be obtained at approximately the same time each day. Education on when to call with weight changes is determined by the clinician and should be provided in written format and then reinforced frequently. In all cases, patients and families should be diligent in monitoring physical signs and symptoms. Establishing plans for notifying health-care providers of any changes are the logical next step and should include the identification of emergency contact numbers for doing so.

"Which program is best?" "What interven-tions are most effective?" Unfortunately those questions cannot be answered at this time, as no one trial has evaluated single models or inter-ventions against each other. In a meta-analysis of 33 randomized clinical trials of DM in HF, Roccaforte et al conclude that all produced simi-lar effects on outcomes and that the choice for a specific program should be driven by the resources available, patient population, and health-care system.[47]

▶ FUTURE IMPLICATIONS

Well-designed studies, employing long-term out-comes and a control group, are needed to evalu-ate the impact of patient management strategies in HF. Because of the variety of DM programs and interventions, a classification system for comparison between programs should be devel-oped.[48] As the evidence supporting HF DM con-tinues to mount, steps must be taken to identify those at risk for developing HF followed by aggressive treatment. Improving clinician adher-ence to the evidence-based treatment guidelines is also an important issue that must be addressed. Research in this area should answer some ques-tions as to why clinicians fail to follow clinical practice guidelines. In doing so, insight may be gained that will direct future work in enhancing adherence and ultimately improving outcomes for individuals with chronic HF.

▶ **Table 18-3** Fundamentals of heart failure patient education

Daily weights every day of your life.
- Use the same scale at the same time of the day wearing comparable clothing.
- Weigh first thing in the morning after going to the bathroom.
- Notify your health-care provider if you gain 3 or more pounds overnight or 5 pounds over 3 days *or* if you lose weight and experience dizziness upon standing up.

Maintain a low-sodium diet to help avoid fluid retention.
- A dietary intake of 2000 mg/day of sodium is recommended.
- Ask for written materials to help you make healthier choices.
- Salt is everywhere. Learn to read labels.

Be conscious of fluid intake.
- Do not drink 8 glasses of water per day if taking a diuretic (water pill). This defeats the purpose of that medication.
- Drink small sips when thirsty or when taking medications.
- Do not carry liquids with you.
- Fluid comes in a variety of formats: soup, Jello, ice, watermelon.

Be as active as possible.
- Engage in physical activity at least three to four times per week.
- Appropriate activities include activities like walking or biking.

Avoid any form of heavy lifting or isometric exercises.
(Isometric exercises are those in which a force is applied to a resistant object, such as pushing against a brick wall.)
- Treatment of heart failure is directed at reducing the workload in your heart, not straining it. Do not lift anything heavier than 10 pounds.

Notify your health-care provider of changes in your symptoms or weight.
- This includes weight gain of 3 or more pounds overnight or 5 pounds over 3 days, increased fatigue or shortness of breath, dizziness, or fever, to name a few.
- Your physician or nurse will give you additional, specific information to follow.
- Keep their emergency number available in case of need.

▶ **SUMMARY**

DM in HF is very effective in reducing the associated morbidity and mortality, halting or reversing the natural course of the condition, improving quality of life, and reducing overall health-care expenditures. Development of multifaceted programs that stress primary prevention through lifestyle modifications for risk reduction, early aggressive treatment using evidence-based approaches, and enhancing patient self-care may proactively diminish the staggering burden of HF on individuals, families, health-care systems, and society.

▶ **REFERENCES**

1. Clarke JL, Nash DB. The effectiveness of heart failure disease management: initial findings from a comprehensive program. *Disease Management.* 2002;4:215–223.

2. Hoffman C, Rice D, Sung. Persons with chronic conditions: their prevalence and costs. *JAMA.* 1996;276:1473–1479.

3. Dzau VJ. Mechanism of action of angiotensin-converting enzyme (ACE) inhibitors in hypertension and heart failure: role of plasma versus tissue ACE. *Drugs.* 1990;39(suppl 2):11–16.

4. Scow DT, Smith EG, Shaughnessy AF. Combination therapy with ACE inhibitors and

angiotensin-receptor blockers in heart failure. Available at: *www.aafp.org/afp/20031101/1795.html*. Accessed January 18, 2005.

5. Swedberg K, Kjekshus J, Snapinn S. Long-term survival in severe heart failure in patients treated with enalapril: Ten-year follow-up of CONSENSUS. *Eur Heart J.* 1999;20:136–139.

6. Hunt SA, Baker DW, Chin MH, et al. ACC/AHA guidelines for the diagnosis and treatment of chronic heart failure in the adult. *J Am Coll Cardiol.* December 2001;1–56.

7. Hunt SA, Abraham WT, Chin MH, et al. ACC/AHA 2005 Guideline update for the diagnosis and management of chronic heart failure in the adult - summary article. *Circulation.* 2005; 112:1825–1852 and *J Am Coll Cardiol.* 2005;46: 1116–1143.

8. Grol J, Grimshaw J. From best evidence to best practice: effective implementation of change in patients' care. *Lancet.* October 11, 2003;362: 1225–1230.

9. Fonarow GC, on behalf of the Steering Committee. The Acute Decompensated Heart Failure Registry (ADHERE): opportunities to improve care of patients hospitalized with acute decompensated heart failure. *Reviews in Cardiovascular Medicine.* 4(suppl 7):S21–S30.

10. Bodenheimer T. Disease management: promises and pitfalls. *NEJM.* 1999;340:1202–1205.

11. Chronic conditions: Making the case for ongoing care. Robert Wood Johnson Foundation, Available at http://www.rwjf.org/Research/Research Detail.jsp?1A = 142&id = 1502

12. Disease Management Association of America. Available at: *http://www.dmaa.org/dm_definition.asp*. Retrieved October 15, 2005.

13. Linden A, Roberts N. A user's guide to the disease management literature: recommendations for reporting and assessing program outcomes. *Am J Managed Care.* 2005;11:113–120.

14. Linden A, Adams J, Roberts N. Evaluating disease management program effectiveness: an introduction to time series analysis. *Disease Management.* 2003;6:234–245.

15. Linden A, Adams J, Roberts N. Using an empirical method for establishing clinical outcome targets in disease management programs. *Disease Management.* 2004;7:93–101.

16. NCQA News. NCQA announces intention to certify disease management programs. Available at: *http://www.ncqa.org/Pages/communication/news/disease_management.html*. Retrieved December 1, 2005.

17. Smith B, Forkner E, Zaslow B, et al. Disease management produces limited quality-of-life improvements in patients with congestive heart failure: evidence from a randomized trial in community-dwelling patients. *Am J Managed Care.* 2005;11:701–713.

18. Institute of Medicine. *Crossing the Quality Chasm: A New Health System for the 21st Century.* Washington, DC: National Academy Press, 2001.

19. Berwick DM. A user's manual for the IOM's "Quality Chasm" report. *Health Aff.* 2001;21(3): 80–90.

20. Faxon DP, Schwamm LH, Pasternak RC, et al. Improving quality of care through disease management: principles and recommendations from the American Heart Association's expert panel on disease management. *Circulation.* 2003;109: 2651–2654.

21. Mukherjee D, Eagle KA. Improving quality of cardiovascular care in the real world: how can we remove the barriers? *Am J Managed Care.* 2004;15(7):471–472.

22. Moser DK. Expert management of heart failure: optimal health care delivery programs. *Annu Rev Nurs Res.* 2000;18:91–106.

23. Riegel B, LePetri B. Heart Failure Disease Management Models. In: *Improving Outcomes in Heart Failure.* Moser DK, Reigel B, eds. Gaithersburg, MD, Aspen Publishers: 2001.

24. Fonarow GC, on behalf of the Steering Committee. The Acute Decompensated Heart Failure Registry (ADHERE): opportunities to improve care of patients hospitalized with acute decompensated heart failure. *Rev Cardiovasc Med.* 2003;4 (suppl 7):S21–S30.

25. Lee DS, Tu JV, Juurlink DN, et al. Risk-treatment mismatch in the pharmacotherapy of heart failure. *JAMA.* 2005;294:1240–1247.

26. Echemann M, Zannad F, Briancon S, et al. Determinants of angiotensin-converting enzyme inhibitor prescription in severe heart failure with left ventricular systolic dysfunction. *Am Heart J.* 2000;139:624–631.

27. Roe CM, Motheral BR, Teitelbaum F, et al. Angiotensin-converting enzyme inhibitor compliance and dosing among patients with heart failure. *Am Heart J.* 1999;138:818–825.

28. Berenson RA, Horvath J. Confronting the barriers to chronic care management in Medicaid.

Health Aff. January–June 2003:(suppl):W3-37–53.

29. Akosah KO, Moncher K, Schaper A, et al. Chronic heart failure in the community: missed diagnosis and missed opportunities. *J Card Fail.* 2001;7:232–238.

30. McDermott MM, Feinglass J, Lee PI, et al. Systolic function, readmission rates, and survival among consecutively hospitalized patients with congest heart failure. *Am Heart J.* 1997;134: 728–736.

31. Whellan DJ, Gattis WA, Gaulden L, et al. Disease management of congestive heart failure. *Am J Manag Care.* 1999;5(4):499–507.

32. Rich MW, Vinson JM, Sperry JC, et al. Prevention of readmissions in elderly patient with CHF: results of a prospective, randomized pilot study. *J Gen Intern Med.* 1993;8:585–590.

33. Fonarow GC, Stevenson LW, Walden JA, et al. Impact of a comprehensive heart failure management program on hospital readmissions and functional status of patients with advanced heart failure. *J Am Coll Cardiol.* 1997;30:725–732.

34. Holst DP, Kaye K. Richardson M, et al. Improved outcomes from a comprehensive management system for heart failure. *Eur J Heart Fail.* 2001;3: 619–625.

35. Hershberger R, Ni H, Nauman DJ, et al. Prospective evaluation of an outpatient heart failure management program. *J Card Fail.* 2001;7:64–74.

36. Clarke JL, Nash DD. The effectiveness of heart failure disease management: initial findings from a comprehensive program. *Disease Management.* 2002;5(4):215–774.

37. Whellan D, et al. Metaanalysis and review of heart failure disease management randomized controlled clinical studies. *Am Heart J.* 2005; 149(4):722–729.

38. McAlister FA, Stewart S, Ferrua S, et al. Multidisciplinary strategies for the management of heart failure patients at high risk for admission: a systematic review of randomized trials. *J Am Coll Cardiol.* 2004;44(4):810–819.

39. Riegel B, Carlson B, Unger A, et al. Effect of a computer-driven nurse case management telephone intervention on resource use in chronic heart failure patients. Amsterdam, Holland: European Society of Cardiology. 2000.

40. Ekman J, Swedberg K. Home-based management of patients with chronic heart failure – focus on content not just form! *Eur Heart J.* 2002;23:1323.

41. Kornowski R, Zeeli D, Averbuch M, et al. Intensive home-care surveillance prevents hospitalization and improves morbidity rates among elderly patients with severe congestive heart failure. *Am Heart J.* 1996;129:762–766.

42. Smith LE, Fabbri SA, Pai R, et al. Symptomatic improvement and reduced hospitalization for patients attending a cardiomyopathy clinic. *Clin Cardiol.* 1997;20:949–954.

43. Compliance or concordance: is there a difference? *Drugs & Therapy Perspectives.* 1999;13(1): 11–12.

44. Friedman M, Griffin JA. Relationship of physical symptoms and physical functioning to depression in patients with heart failure. *Heart & Lung.* 2001;30(2):98–104.

45. Vinson J. *Am Geriatr Soc.* Early readmission of elderly patients with congestive heart failure. 1990;38:1290–1295.

46. Carlson B, Riegel B. Self-care abilities of patients with heart failure. *Heart & Lung.* 2001;30(5): 351–359.

47. Roccaforte R, Demers C, Baldassarre F, et al. Effectiveness of comprehensive disease management programmes in improving clinical outcomes in heart failure patients: a meta-analysis. *Eur J Heart Failure.* 2005;7:1133–1144.

48. Whellan DJ, Cohen EJ, Matchar DB, et al. "Disease management in healthcare organizations" Results of in-depth interviews with disease management decision makers. *Am J Managed Care.* 2002;8:633–641.

CHAPTER 19

How to Develop a Heart Failure Management Pathway

Jennifer Farroni, RN, MSN, CNP/David Feldman, MD, PhD/
Sara Paul, RN, MSN, FNP

Despite advances in pharmaceuticals and technology, heart failure (HF) continues to be a large health-related economic burden. Numerous programs and systems have been implemented over the years in an attempt to decrease the cost and length of hospital stay involved in the care of patients with HF. Disease-based guidelines have helped to incorporate evidence-based practices into the care of HF patients. An instrument that has been put into practice to improve efficiency in using those guidelines is clinical-based pathways that define and organize the processes involved in patient care management.[1-5]

▶ CLINICAL MANAGEMENT PATHWAYS

Practice guidelines originated in the 1950s and were used by the industry to coordinate project development in a timely manner.[6] The medical field began using clinical management pathways in the 1980s when nurses developed them to structure patient care processes within a designated timeframe.[7] This was in response to the government's prospective payment system of diagnostic related grouping (DRG), which was implemented in 1983. With DRGs, payment for hospitalization is limited to a predetermined length of stay (LOS) based on the patient's diagnosis. This has led to an increased emphasis on containing costs in health care without sacrificing the quality of patient care.[8] HF disease management programs, multidisciplinary clinics, case management, observation units, patient telemanagement, and clinical pathways are multiple strategies that have been developed in attempts to reduce HF costs.[9]

Clinical management pathways, also known as critical pathways, caremaps, and integrated care pathways, are designed to be used in conjunction with the present standard of care as a tool to decrease variation in outcomes and maintain care within a specified LOS. They facilitate clinical interventions by guiding the patient's hospitalization through a sequence of steps toward a desired outcome. Clinical pathways are generally applied to high-volume diagnoses or procedures and those with longer LOS and mortality, such as HF, myocardial infarction, coronary artery bypass grafting, hip surgery, or vascular surgery. These procedures tend to have a predictable course of events during the hospitalization and marked variation in care.[10] Pathways are designed to be integrated management plans that improve clinical outcomes, resource usage, coordination and quality of care, and discharge process. With the use of clinical pathways, clinical performance variation is decreased and hospital LOS and related costs are reduced.[8,11,12] The content of clinical pathways designates the major interventions and patient outcomes, and is based on expert guidelines, current standards, and published clinical trials.[13]

► CLINICAL PATHWAY DEVELOPMENT

Clinical pathway development has historically been initiated by nursing, but in many institutions this led to lack of physician commitment.[10] Incorporating a multidisciplinary team to evaluate current practice and collect clinical data for development of the clinical pathway is the best way to begin the process and encourage involvement from nonnursing disciplines (Fig. 19-1).[14] Traditionally, a physician leader or "champion" heads the committee, contributing leadership and clinical expertise. The team may consist of physicians (cardiologists, emergency room physicians, internists), nurses, nurse practitioners, administrators, quality improvement (QI) committee members, case managers, and members from social services, nutrition, cardiac rehabilitation, respiratory therapy, and pharmacy.

A retrospective chart review of financial data, LOS, readmission data, mortality, and direct costs for HF admissions will more than likely illuminate the need for a clinical pathway to guide inpatient HF management within a designated timeframe. A literature review of current data on HF pathways and standards of care for HF provides the groundwork for developing a template. Clinical goals must be defined before developing the clinical pathway. The committee should set objectives and goals to include clinical outcomes measurement, Joint Commission on Accreditation of Healthcare Organizations (JCAHO) compliance, patient satisfaction, and clinical pathway monitoring.[11] The goals must be translated into elements of care in a sequence of events and expected patient progress over a designated timeframe.[12] To accomplish this, frequent team meetings are required. The format for a clinical pathway may range from a simple checklist to detailed steps for the process of care. Standardized admission and discharge orders may coincide with the pathway and provide a solid foundation to support the interventions on the pathway (App. 19-A).

Prior to implementation of the pathway, educational in-services on content of the pathway and QI concepts are provided to those involved with the care of HF patients. The physician leader presents the pathway to appropriate physicians at medical grand rounds and/or through memos. An HF nurse or advanced practice nurse in-services the inpatient staff, and patients receive a copy of their own pathway. The nursing staff provides education on the pathway to the patient and their family. Pathways should identify an accountable person to ensure that clinical outcomes are met in a timely fashion.[15]

Multidisciplinary roles within the pathway must be clearly defined as to those responsible for documenting information, analyzing data, and educating the patient and family. Variances are the patient outcomes or staff actions that do not meet the expectation of the pathway or do not occur within the designated timeframe. These variances should be tracked throughout the process of using and developing the pathway, in order to define areas that need improvement. Piloting of the pathway is necessary for analysis,

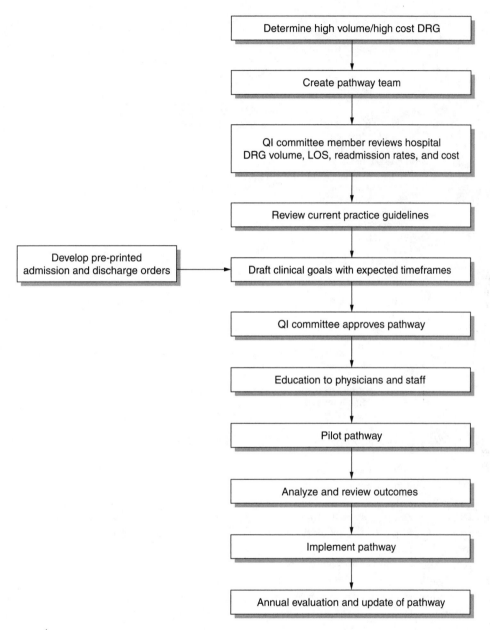

Figure 19–1 Clinical pathway development.

addressing staff concerns, and making revisions prior to final implementation.[7]

The categories of a HF clinical pathway usually include clinical outcomes, patient teaching, discharge planning, consults, treatments, diagnostic tests/procedures, medications, nutrition, and

activity (App. 19-B). The average LOS of an HF pathway is based on the DRG LOS. Preferably, the LOS of the clinical pathway is below that of the DRG in order to maximize cost benefits.

HF patient education is initiated during the hospitalization and patient teaching is performed

Dx: Congestive heart failure

Vital signs q 4 hours

Notify on-call provider if: SBP > 150 or < 90; DBP > 100 or < 40

Resp rate > 30 or increased SOB

Temp > 101.5

Chest pain

O_2 sat. < 90%

Urine output < 240ml/8 hrs.

Activity: Bedrest with BRP, advance per clinical pathway

Telemetry monitor

IV hep lock with flush per protocol

I & O q 8 hrs.

Weight on admission and qam

ECG on admission and STAT if chest pain occurs

PA & lateral CXR on admission

Cardiac fitness diet: _____ 2 gm Na _____ 3 gm Na

Other dietary requirements: _____

Fluid restriction: 2000 ml per day

Pulse oximetry spot check on admission, continuous if O_2 sat. < 90%

Echo if EF unknown or if not assessed in last 6 months

O_2 2L/NC prn or if O_2 sat. <90% on room air

Labs: CBC with diff, chem profile, Mg, BNP, PT/INR if on anticoagulant,

CK/CKMB, digoxin level, thyroid panel, liver function panel

QAM chem profile & Mg, fasting lipid profile x 1

Meds: ACE inhibitor/ARB _____

Beta-blocker _____

Spironolactone Y/N dose _____

Digoxin Y/N dose _____

IV furosemide dose _____

Other meds _____

Appendix 19-A   Standardized heart failure admission orders.

by the HF nurses. Printed educational materials are given to the patient and their family, and other audiovisual learning tools may be used, such as videotapes, heart models, or computer web-based programs. A longer, more detailed education session for the patient and family may take place in the outpatient setting. Consults along the pathway are specific to the patient's needs, but may include cardiac rehabilitation, nutrition, and smoking cessation. Diagnostic tests are specified as to when they should be performed during the hospitalization. HF medications may be listed on the pathway as outlined in national guidelines for HF care. Dietary guidelines and activity level advance as appropriate along the pathway.

Comprehensive hospital-specific performance and benchmarking reports about processes and outcomes of care are gathered by the QI committee and presented to the team on a quarterly basis.[13] A chart audit may also be used as part of the QI process to ensure that HF patient care adheres to the clinical pathway.[16] Identification of variances and evaluation of clinical indicators can lead to improvement in the process of managing patient care (Table 19-1). The pathway content is updated by yearly evaluation of patient variances and LOS, as well as reviewing current clinical practice for the specific diagnosis or procedure.

▶ BARRIERS TO CLINICAL PATHWAYS

Some health-care professionals feel that clinical pathways are time-consuming and "cookbook medicine," applicable to only the "ideal," not the complex patient. One large barrier to using a

Admission date	Phase 1 - Admission (Day 1)	Phase 2 - Treatment (Days 2–3)	Phase 3 - Discharge (Day 4)
Expected outcomes	Patient stabilized with improvement in SOB Diuresis started	Continued weight loss, improved respiratory status, vital signs, and electrolytes stable	Patient discharged in stable condition and on appropriate medications. Patient has all the necessary prescriptions. Follow-up appointment made
Diagnostic studies	History and physical Bloodwork: CBC, chem profile, Mg, BNP, PT/INR (if on coumadin) Cardiac enzymes if known ischemic cardiomyopathy, angina, or ECG changes 12 Lead EKG, CXR, pulse oximetry (spot check; continuous if O_2 sat <90%) ECHO with doppler flow studies if initial presentation or EF not measured in last 6 months Thyroid function studies if patient >65 yrs, atrial fib present, or other s/s hypo or hyperthyroidism Schedule cardiac cath, stress thallium or biopsy if indicated	Electrolytes and Mg^{++} at least q 3 days Continue diagnostics not completed in Phase 1 Repeat CXR if continued respiratory distress or otherwise indicated DC pulse oximetry if O_2 sat >90%	Electrolytes and Mg if not performed with in last 2 days DC pulse oximetry
Treatments	Telemetry, O_2 if needed, hep lock, I and O, daily weight, VS per unit routine, daily orthostatic BP Assess need for cardioversion if atrial fib present	Telemetry, wean O_2, hep lock, I and O, daily weight, VS per unit routine, daily orthostatic BP	DC telemetry, hep lock, and O_2

Appendix 19-B Congestive heart failure inpatient clinical management pathway.

Medications	• IV Diuretics • ACE Inhibitor or ARB (titrate to maintain SBP 90–100 without orthostatic hypotension) • β-blocker unless contraindicated • Aspirin if appropriate • If angina, may add nitrates • IV vasodilators or inotropes if severe pulmonary edema, symptomatic hypotension, or inadequate progress with conventional methods within first 48 hours of admission • Anticoagulation: SQ heparin if bedridden; full anticoagulation only if atrial fib, embolic event, or mural thrombus noted on echo • Aldosterone antagonist (consider for LV sys dysfunction in pts on standard therapy; pts should have normal serum K^+ and adequate renal function) • Assess need for statin therapy • Treat ventricular arrhythmias only if sustained or symptomatic • Potassium supplement if hypokalemic	Convert to oral medications Assess need for continued inotropes Continue to optimize vasodilators, diuretics, anti-anginals, beta blocker Assess need for K^+ or Mg^{++} replacement	Diuretic KCl/Mg replacement ACE inhibitor, ARB, or hydralazine/nitrates β-blocker Aldosterone blocker if appropriate Digoxin if appropriate Aspirin if CAD Statin therapy Patient given all discharge prescriptions
Nutrition	Cardiac fitness diet 2 gm Na^+ ___ 3gm Na^+ ___ Other ___ Fluid restriction 1000–1500 cc/day if serum Na < 125	Cardiac fitness diet 2 gm Na^+ ___ 3 gm Na^+ ___ Other ___ Discontinue fluid restriction if serum Na>125	Cardiac fitness diet Other ___
Activity	BR with BRP/ambulate if tolerated	Up OOB, ambulate in halls	Up ad lib Refer to cardiac rehab if appropriate
Education	Orient to unit routines Assess knowledge base/educational needs	Consult Cardiac Rehab nurse Consult Dietician for dietary teaching Institute teaching protocol for CHF, provide patient with teaching materials, patient & family view CHF video, provide medication cards, discuss purpose & side effects of medications Consult CHF nurse practitioner clinic	*Per CHF teaching protocol:* • Reinforce medication, diet, activity teaching • Address sexuality • What to report to CHF Nurse Practitioner or M.D.: weight gain, edema, orthopnea, paroxysmal dyspnea, exercise intolerance or frequent dry hacking cough • Daily weight • Importance of compliance!!

Appendix 19-B *(Continued)*

Discharge planning	Assess need for social services and/or home health referral if indicated	Continue to assess home care needs	*Discharge criteria:* Stable vital signs BP controlled without symptoms Weight close to baseline Minimal edema Respiratory status at baseline Able to perform ADLs without dyspnea or angina Verbalizes understanding of diet, activity & medication regimen Laboratory values acceptable Follow-up (including lab tests) scheduled Home arrangements made if necessary

Document each variance:

Date	Hospital day activities	Pt's progress corresponds to critical path? Yes/No	Describe variance	Signature

Appendix 19-B (*Continued*)

▶ **Table 19-1** Process and outcome indicators to evaluate heart failure clinical pathway

Process indicators	Criterion	Measure
Daily weight	Patients weighed daily	100% daily weight documented in chart
LV function assessed	Current LVEF documented on chart; measured within past 6 months	100% of patients have documented LVEF
Smoking cessation counseling	Advice or counseling given to all patients with history of smoking	100% of smokers receive counseling
Patient education	Written instructions/patient educational materials given to patients before discharge	100% of patients receive instruction/education
Follow-up appointments	Follow-up appointments made for HF clinic and/or primary care	All patients able to verbalize date and time of appointments
Outcome indicators	**Criterion**	**Measure**
Length of stay	Adheres to clinical management pathway	Discharged within DRG timeframe
Medications at discharge	Prescriptions written for ACE inhibitor or ARB, β-blocker, appropriate diuretic dose, aldosterone blocker if appropriate, anticoagulation if needed, other medicines	100% of patients discharged on appropriate HF therapy unless documented contraindication Prescriptions given to patients for at least 1-month supply
Readmission	Readmission >31 days postdischarge	Significant decrease in readmission days

ACE—angiotensin-converting enzyme; ARB—angiotensin receptor blocker; DRG—diagnois related group; HF—heart failure; LV—left ventricular; LVEF—left ventricular ejection fraction

clinical pathway is a lack of voluntary participation among key individuals. The additional paperwork involved in tracking outcomes and data regarding use of the pathway is seen as a burden to some health-care workers, but these documents may be used as a QI tool, and may serve to fulfill regulatory requirements. The paper format may affect the ability to effectively evaluate variances, link clinical processes with patient outcomes, and see real-time benefits.[17] Absence of documentation can lead to pathway discontinuity and inaccurate data. Continued education, frequent communication, and sharing of outcome data encourage participation with the pathway. Cost savings should be evaluated, and the information shared with the multidisciplinary team and hospital administrators. Automated pathways may be created to coincide with electronic medical record charting and to query outcome data in a more timely fashion.

▶ **BENEFITS OF A HEART FAILURE CLINICAL PATHWAY**

Pathways have been shown to decrease LOS and resource consumption.[8] They may help to define the patient care roles and responsibilities of health-care professionals, improve integration and communication in the health-care system, develop learning processes within an organization, reduce inpatient mortality, and improve patient clinical outcomes. They support risk management, utilization management, and the evaluation that is necessary for growth and improvement in any setting. Pathways can assist with documentation and validation of the desired outcomes.[12]

Clinical pathways address the complex needs of HF patients and are designed to increase the use of appropriate medications, consults, and education. Consumers may find clinical management pathways attractive due to better service, improved communication from providers, and superior outcomes. This information can be used as a marketing tool by health-care institutions. Increased patient satisfaction is related to a decrease in medical lawsuits, and in most cases, a patient's decision to sue results from weak attitudes or inferior communication skills by providers.[18]

Goals to be achieved by using a clinical pathway include decreasing, LOS, readmissions, and emergency rooms visits; documenting left ventricular dysfunction; prescribing appropriate medications; initiating nutrition consults; and scheduling a follow-up appointment with the HF team or the patient's health-care provider 1–2 weeks following discharge. Periodic review of pathways allows an opportunity to incorporate new advances in medical care and may provide a source of continuous medical education for providers.[7]

▶ OUTCOMES RELATED TO CLINICAL PATHWAYS

Preventing medical errors contributes to cost savings in health care and enhances patient outcomes. It is estimated that between 44,000 and 98,000 patients die annually due to medical errors in the United States.[19] Reducing variations in care practices by standardizing the patient's clinical path may be an effective tool to reduce the probability of medical errors.

▶ **Table 19-2** Expected outcomes of using clinical pathways in heart failure patients

- Reduce cost of care
  - Decrease length of stay
  - Reduce hospital charges
  - Reduce readmissions
  - Streamline procedures and tests
  - Promote early discharge planning
- Reduce variations in patient care
  - Promote use of evidence-based practices
  - Standardize patient care based on national guidelines
  - Ensure processes of care (i.e., daily weights, recording intake/output, etc.)
- Reduce mortality
- Enhance patient education
- Promote communication among patient care disciplines
  - Provide a "map" to outline each discipline's role each day

The high cost of health care has necessitated the adoption of cost-effective approaches in patient management. As an interdisciplinary instrument, clinical pathways move the patient care process through a sequence of clinical interventions toward desired outcomes (Table 19-2). These outcomes may include cost-efficient care and reduced variations in patient management.

Numerous authors have reported improved outcomes after the application of a clinical pathway for the management of HF patients. Cordoza and Aherns analyzed the use of a clinical pathway, looking at LOS, cost of care, mortality data, readmission statistics, and performance rates of care processes in a group of elderly HF patients admitted to the hospital.[8] They compared a random sample of hospitalized HF patients receiving usual care to a group of HF patients who were managed on a clinical pathway. There was a significant reduction in the LOS, variable cost, and readmission rate in the patients managed with the clinical pathway compared to the patients receiving usual care without a pathway. Mortality rate during hospitalization remained unchanged. Several processes of patient care were significantly improved among the patients on the clinical pathway, including early initiation of discharge planning, early mobilization of patients' activity, and providing basic HF education to patients. Additionally, documentation of daily weights, heparin prescription, and echocardiography were improved. Importantly, patients on the clinical pathway had more effective diuresis per patient than those who were not managed with a clinical pathway.

After implementation of a clinical pathway for HF patients Panella et al. reported a decrease in total hospital admissions, inpatient mortality, and LOS.[12] They also found a significant improvement in some predetermined quality indicators, such as left ventricular assessment, smoking cessation counseling, discharge instructions, and completion of clinical documentation. They did not, however, find a decrease in costs after implementing the pathway.

Ranjan et al. developed and implemented a clinical pathway for patients with HF in order to decrease hospital charges and maintain efficiency and quality of care.[20] After 2 years of using the pathway, they evaluated the effectiveness of the program. They found that LOS was reduced to under 4 days in 65% of the pathway patients compared to 42% of patients who were not using a clinical pathway. Hospital charges were significantly reduced, and use of angiotensin-converting enzyme inhibitors was greater in the patients on the clinical pathway. These improved outcomes held true for patients who had 2–4 comorbidities, and even in complicated patients with 5 or more comorbidities. The authors were able to demonstrate that duality of care was not compromised by reduced length of hospital stay in patients on the clinical pathway.

Several authors have reported improved outcomes in HF disease management programs in which the clinical pathway was only one component. Knox and Mischke described a program that incorporated inpatient education, an inpatient HF clinical pathway, an outpatient clinic, and cardiac home care using a home care clinical pathway.[14] They reported a 50% decrease in direct inpatient costs and a decrease in the LOS to 4 days, compared with 6.2 days before implementing the

program. Quality indicators also improved, such as documentation of daily weights, frequency of dietary consultation, documentation of left ventricular function, appropriate medication use, and scheduling follow-up care. Rauh et al. also reported improved outcomes after implementing an inpatient and outpatient HF program that utilized a clinical pathway.[21] They demonstrated a reduction in LOS, reduced 90-day readmission rate, and significantly reduced inpatient costs.

Not all authors have reported positive outcomes after implementing a clinical pathway for HF patients. Philbin et al. did not find statistically significant improvement in five quality-of-care markers after initiating a clinical pathway for the management of HF patients.[13] The etiology of HF and prescription of angiotensin-converting enzyme inhibitors was improved slightly, but documentation of left ventricular systolic function was reduced. Hospital LOS and hospital charges were not significantly reduced. The effects on mortality, hospital readmission, and quality of life after discharge were not significant.

▶ CLINICAL PATHWAYS IN THE OUTPATIENT SETTING

Clinical pathways can be useful in the outpatient setting, either in an outpatient clinic or in the home health setting. Standards of care for the management of chronic HF are clearly delineated and can easily be incorporated into a pathway (App. 19-C). Outpatient clinical management pathways can be useful to ensure that standards of care are followed by all providers, particularly those who do not specialize in HF management, such as primary care practices.

Hoskins et al. compared two groups of elderly home health patients with HF. An outpatient clinical pathway guided care in one group of patients, while the other group was given "usual" home health care.[22] They reported a 45% reduction in the rehospitalization rate among patients whose care was guided by a clinical pathway compared to patients who were not managed on a pathway.

	Phase 1 Initial consult and treatment	Phase 2 Ongoing treatment	Phase 3 Maintenance
I. Health care provider	First office visit with MD or hospital inpatient consult: history and physical	Vital signs & weight recorded by staff at each visit	Vital signs & weight recorded by staff at each visit
		Interim focused cardiac history and physical by NP, PA or MD	Interim focused cardiac history and physical by NP, PA or MD
		Medications reviewed	Medications reviewed
II. Consults	If indicated: Subspecialty consultation Home health and other services Heart Failure Clinic referral if: 1. New diagnosis of HF, pt requires education about lifestyle changes 2. Hospitalizations >2/year or rehospitalized within 3 months of discharge 3. Medications actively being titrated 4. Patient is non-compliant 5. Pt is NYHA class III or IV Refer to nursing staff for application for pharmaceutical assistance if appropriate.	If indicated: Subspecialty consultation Home health and other services Evaluate need for pharmaceutical assistance. Refer to nursing staff for application	1. Subspecialty consultation prm 2. Home health or hospice referral prm 3. Continue to evaluate need for pharmaceutical assistance. Refer to nursing staff for application
III. Medical and device therapy	Initiate or titrate: 1. ACEI or ARB (titrate to target dose maintaining systolic blood pressure 90–110 without orthostatic hypotension, if patient not on ACEI or ARB document reason) 2. Carvedilol, metoprolol XL, or bisoprolol 3. Diuretics (assess need and efficacy) 4. Aldosterone inhibitor (spironolactone or eplerenone) if K+ & renal function adequate 5. Digitalis if symptoms persist after ACEI and BB therapy or if tachycardic (if EF < 40% or atrial fibrillation; adjust if renal impairment) 6. Assess requirements for nitrate (ischemic cardiomyopathy, persistent PND/orthopnea despite optimal diuresis)	1. Assess need for medication adjustment, titrate ACEI/ARB or β-blocker 2. Initiate or discontinue meds as appropriate 3. Evaluate need for renewal of pharmaceutical assistance 4. Refer for device therapy if pt is appropriate candidate	Adjust medications as needed. Assess need for additional medications if necessary (i.e., antihypertensives, antiarrhythmic agents) Evaluate need for renewal of pharmaceutical assistance Refer for device therapy if pt is appropriate candidate

Appendix 19-C Heart failure outpatient clinical management pathway.

	Middle column	Right column
	7. Assess need for other vasodilators (ARB, hydralazine, calcium channel blocker) 8. Assess need for anticoagulation if atrial fib present 9. Assess need for antiarrhythmic therapy or cardioversion (if A. fib present) 10. Ensure that co-morbidities are properly addressed, i.e., diabetes, hyperlipidemia, anemia, thyroid abnormalities, depression, etc.	
IV. Diagnostic studies	1. Labwork as appropriate, including: CBC Electrolytes Magnesium Baseline BNP Liver profile Lipid profile PT, INR (if on Coumadin) Thyroid function studies if indicated Other screening labs/drug screen as indicated 2. Other procedures as appropriate: CXR 12-lead ECG Echo with doppler flow studies MUGA Consider stress thallium, cardiac catheterization or endomyocardial biopsy, as indicated Consider holter monitor or EP testing if indicated Collagen vascular studies, if indicated	1. Lab work as necessary: Electrolytes Magnesium Digoxin level BNP CBC, as indicated Iron studies, ferritin Protime/INR Lipids Liver profile 2. Other procedures as appropriate: - 12-lead ECG - Echo if significant change in patient's status 3. Consider stress thallium, cardiac catheterization if angina or suspicion of coronary event	1. Lab work as necessary 2. Echo if status changes 3. Review lab data trends
V. Nutrition	1. 2–4 gram sodium cardiac fitness diet or other fluid restriction requirement (2 liters/day for serum sodium < 130). 2. Diabetic, low cholesterol and low sodium dietary teaching as needed	1. Assess dietary compliance and continue dietary education. Provide written materials 2. Refer to dietician if appropriate	Continue to promote low sodium, low fat diet
VI. Activity	1. Advise patient of the benefits of aerobic activity and discuss initiation of a walking program increasing to 30–60 minutes daily, as tolerated 2. Discourage lifting, pushing or pulling weight over 25 lbs	1. Assess current level of activity and stress importance of aerobic activity 2. Refer to cardiac rehab program as appropriate	Continue to assess and promote physical activity program

Appendix 19-C   *(Continued)*

VII. **Patient** **education**	1. Assess knowledge base/educational needs of patient & family pertaining to: Causes of HF Medication, diet, activity Sexuality What to report to NP or MD: weight gain, edema, orthopnea, PND, exercise intolerance or frequent dry hacking cough Daily weight Importance of compliance! 2. Instruct patient/family and provide written teaching material on: Diet & fluid Exercise Medications Daily weights	1. Continue to review patient education material to include signs and symptoms of worsening heart failure 2. Continue to review medication actions, interactions and side effects 3. Review dietary recommendations 4. Continue to reinforce activity recommendations	1. Continue to review patient education material 2. Continue to review medication actions, interactions and side effects 3. Review dietary recommendations 4. Continue to reinforce activity recommendations
VIII. **Telephonic** **monitoring**	N/A	CHF Clinic follow-up: Medication adjustments Symptoms Problems Lab/diagnostic results & follow-up Phone-in prescriptions as needed	Continue telephonic follow-up and availability as needed

Appendix 19-C (*Continued*)

► SUMMARY

Over the last 20 years, there has been increasing emphasis on containing costs without compromising the quality of patient care. QI includes the use of clinical management pathways and disease management programs, and has improved patient outcomes.[13] Clinical management pathways are an overall QI plan to meet specific patient population needs in all settings, particularly HF. The use of clinical management pathways allows patients to receive better care through an organized method that coordinates the clinical processes and reduces variations in patient care practices.

► REFERENCES

1. Massie B, Shah N. Evolving trends in the epidemiologic factors of heart failure: rationale for preventive strategies and comprehensive disease management. *Am Heart J.* 1997;133:703–712.

2. American Heart Association. Heart Disease and Stroke Statistics: 2007 Update. Dallas, Texas: American Heart Association; 2007.

3. Koelling T, Chen R, Lubwama R, et al. The expanding national burden of heart failure in the United States: the influence of heart failure in women. *Am Heart J.* 2004;147:74–78.

4. O'Connell J, Bristow M. Economic impact of heart failure in the United States: time for a different approach. *J Heart Lung Transplant.* 1994;13:S107–S112.

5. DeFrances C, Hall M, Podgornik M. 2003 National Hospital Discharge Survey. Hyattsville, MD: U.S. Department of Health and Human Services; July 8, 2005.

6. Luttman J, Laffel G, Pearson S. Using program evaluation and review technique/critical path method to design and improve clinical processes. *Qual Manag Health Care.* 1995;3:1–13.

7. Cardozo L, Ahrens S, Steinberg J, et al. Implementing a clinical pathway for congestive heart failure: experiences at a teaching hospital. *Qual Manag Health Care.* 1998;7:1–12.

8. Cardozo L, Aherns S. Assessing the efficacy of a clinical pathway in the management of older patients hospitalized with congestive heart failure. *J Healthc Qual.* 1999;21:12–16.

9. Venner G, Seelbinder J. Team management of congestive heart failure across the continuum. *J Cardiovasc Nurs.* 1996;10:71–84.

10. Every N, Hochman J, Becker R, et al. Critical pathways. *Circulation.* 2000;101:461–465.

11. Edick V, Whipple T. Managing patient care with clinical pathways: a practical application. *Jour Nurs Care Qual.* 2001;15:16–31.

12. Panella M, Marchisio S, DiStanislao F. Reducing clinical variations with clinical pathways: do pathways work? *Int J Qual Health Care.* 2003;15:509–521.

13. Philbin E, Rocco T, Lindenmuth N, for the MIS-CHF Investigators. The results of a randomized trial of a quality improvement intervention in the care of patients with heart failure. *Am J Med.* 2000;109:443–449.

14. Knox D, Mischke L. Implementing a congestive heart failure disease management program to decrease length of stay and cost. *J Cardiovasc Nurs.* 1999;14:55–74.

15. Haffercamp-Venner G. Team management of congestive heart failure across the continuum. *J Cardiovasc Nurs.* 1996;10:71–84.

16. Kinsman L. Clinical pathway compliance and quality improvement. *Nurs Stand.* 2004;18:33–35.

17. Dykes P, Acevedo D, Boldrighini J, et al. Clinical practice guideline adherence before and after implementation of the Heart Failure Effectiveness & Leadership Team (HEARTFELT) intervention. *J Cardiovasc Nurs.* 2005;20:306–314.

18. Sage W, Hastings K, Berenson R. Enterprise liability for medical malpractice and health care quality improvement. *Am J Law Med.* 1994;20:14–28.

19. Weingart S, Wilson R, Gibberd R, et al. Epidemiology of medical error. *Br Med J.* 2000;320:774–777.

20. Ranjan A, Tarigopula L, Srivastava R, et al. Effectiveness of the clinical pathway in the management of congestive heart failure. *South Med J.* 2003;96:661–663.

21. Rauh R, Schwabauer N, Enger E, et al. A community hospital-based congestive heart failure program: impact on length of stay, admission and readmission rates, and cost. *Am J Manag Care.* 1999;5:37–43.

22. Hoskins L, Clark H, Schroeder M, et al. A clinical pathway for congestive heart failure. *Home Healthc Nurse.* 2001;19:207–217.

CHAPTER 20

Integrating Inpatient and Outpatient Heart Failure Management

Maryjane B. Giacalone, RN, NP/
Marc J. Semigran, MD

▶ OVERVIEW

Heart failure is a major public health problem and a growing economic burden, both in the United States and worldwide. There are approximately 1 million hospitalizations, 6 million hospital days, and anywhere from 3 to 15 million office visits for heart failure each year in the United States, and a similar number in the European Union.[1,2] The 30-day readmission rate after discharge for a heart failure hospitalization is approximately 25%, the highest rate of any health-care diagnosis-related group (DRG).[3,4] Furthermore, in the United States alone, $25.8 billion dollars are spent on direct and indirect heart failure costs.[1] Readmission for heart failure is one measure to view quality of care for the heart failure population, or to reassess its needs. Decreasing readmissions may help to control the costs; however, the inpatient and outpatient care required for these patients must be well-coordinated in order to achieve this goal.

A multivariate analysis of readmission rate among heart failure patients identified severity of illness and functional status as well as the presence of comorbidities such as depression and lack of social support as predictive of readmission of heart failure within 3 months.[5] Kassovsky et al. retrospectively evaluated unplanned readmissions for heart failure within 31 days of the index heart failure admission. In addition to age and history of revascularization, they found lack of readiness for discharge in the index hospitalization as a predictor of readmission.[6] Readiness for discharge was defined by a stable cardiac medication regimen for at least 24 hours; no evidence of deterioration of laboratory results, vital signs, or physical examination findings; and documented dietary education and postdischarge plans.

Integrating inpatient and outpatient care begins while the patient is hospitalized, with an assessment both at the beginning of and throughout the hospitalization of an individual patient's social and psychological issues that may affect compliance with a complex regimen. Identification of potential barriers to a patient's understanding of their illness, such as cognitive deficits or their ability to read and understand the language that is being used to communicate with them, is of basic importance. Assessment of financial considerations that may impede their compliance with medical and general care regimens remains important, as is the identification of community and governmental services that can be deployed to help overcome these and other barriers. An understanding of a patient's ethnic traditions can also assist in designing a long-term care plan that takes both their beliefs about health care and their medical program into consideration. Any barriers to adherence to self-care should be addressed prior to discharge.

The performance of this assessment while improving the patient's medical condition can be challenging, especially when issues of length of stay are also stressed. The use of multidisciplinary teams, in both inpatient and outpatient settings, can add to the effectiveness of an outpatient heart failure regimen.[7] A randomized controlled trial of multidisciplinary team care of heart failure patients transitioning from the inpatient to outpatient setting showed a significant decrease in readmission rates.[8] Such a team can also have a beneficial effect on an individual health-care provider's effectiveness and job satisfaction, although this has not been formally studied.

Medical Treatment

Guidelines have clearly outlined recommended medications for heart failure due to left ventricular systolic dysfunction.[2,9] The evidence for the benefits of treatment with angiotensin-converting enzyme (ACE) inhibitors, angiotensin receptor blockers (ARBs), β-blockers, hydralazine and nitrates, diuretics, anticoagulants, and heart failure device therapies are outlined, as are the appropriate patient subgroups in which they should be used. At this time, the guidelines for diastolic dysfunction are less extensive, emphasizing the treatment of the underlying cause such as hypertension, and the use of diuretics to minimize congestive symptoms. Importantly, the initiation of appropriate medical therapies to heart failure patients during hospitalization has been shown to improve the frequency of their use after the patient is discharged. The Initiation Management Predischarge process for Assessment of Carvedilol Therapy for Heart Failure (IMPACT-HF) trial demonstrated a higher rate of outpatient β-blocker utilization if therapy was started during inpatient hospitalization rather than following discharge.[10]

Insurance formulary restrictions on medications must be kept in mind when selecting among possible therapeutic options within a class of agents. Although short-acting medications are often used on inpatients for careful titration, they have the disadvantage of requiring multiple doses during the day. Adherence to medication treatment plans falls off quickly when patients are required to take medications more than twice daily. Adjusting medications to longer-acting preparations prior to discharge will help to promote adherence and could prevent readmission. Where these longer-acting preparations will result in higher costs to the patient, a discussion with the patient as to their preference can avoid discontinuation of an important therapy when the patient is faced with a high payment at their pharmacy after discharge. Some patients are willing to pay more in order to have the convenience of once- or twice-daily dosing. Enlisting the patient in decisions such as this helps to promote their ownership of the plan. If patients have no medication coverage and cannot afford medication, consultation with case managers, social workers, or financial counselors should be sought well before discharge.

Education

Assessment of patient's knowledge or predetermined misconceptions about their illness is an important start to the education process. Information about heart failure and its treatment should be geared toward the person's cognitive ability, ability to learn, and level of schooling. Understanding the pathophysiology of heart failure in appropriate lay terms can lay the basis for adherence to medical regimens. Health-care providers should teach patients about their heart failure in person, either alone or preferably with their families. A hospitalization creates an opportunity for education about heart failure, if only because of the focus that can be brought to bear by multiple professional caregivers and also because of the patients' increased motivation to take better care of themselves so as to avoid readmission. However, since patients' retention of much of what they are taught during an inpatient stay can be limited, having a family member present may help to fill in gaps once the patient has been discharged. In addition, outpatient reinforcement of

key educational messages may help patients to consolidate this important fund of knowledge. Written information about pathophysiology, medications, dietary restrictions, daily weights, and follow-up will also reinforce teaching, but it should be accompanied by direct contact with a health-care professional that can individualize a patient's learning and address questions and concerns.

For patients who cannot read, possible alternatives should be provided: videotaped information, a schedule of outpatient classes, consultation with an outpatient heart failure health advocate, and a telemanagement program or home health-care provider. These patients will benefit from earlier and more frequent follow-up after discharge to reinforce their learning and prevent adverse outcomes.

Heart failure patients are often older, and may be sensory-impaired or cognitively impaired. Hearing impairment can interfere with the effectiveness of teaching. Some patients are embarrassed and will nod in agreement rather than admit to being unable to hear teaching or discussions. If the patient has a hearing aid, make sure it is functional and that the patient is wearing it. If the patient is cognitively impaired and will be going home with family, several sessions of teaching time with the family should be arranged. In this way, if family members have digested the information and have questions or concerns, there is opportunity to address them.

Other important methods of learning occur through the regular inpatient routine. Recording daily weights during a hospitalization is extremely important as role modeling for patients and provides an opportunity to discuss how a patient should manage these results at home. Discussing dietary choices on menus and delivered food trays is a practical method of reinforcing sodium and fluid restrictions. Evaluation of exercise tolerance in the hospital can be an occasion to discuss exercise schedules at home as well as symptoms and how to manage them. Interpreters should be available when necessary for assessment and educational encounters, as well as for discharge teaching.

Sodium Restriction

Education on sodium restriction should include reasons why it is necessary, including the adverse effects of lack of compliance on quality of life. A review of foods high in sodium, typical 24-hour dietary recall, how to read nutritional labels, and how to eat out in various restaurants will provide a basis on which the patient can function. Having the patient recall their dietary choices for the 24–48 hours prior to admission can be particularly instructive and offer an opportunity to explore alternatives that are palatable.

Different ethnic preferences need to be addressed in dietary considerations. If certain (high sodium) dishes are important to a person's identity, the dietitian should be consulted for assistance in finding a way to adapt that food in a healthy way if possible, and to emphasize the role of that food in the total daily dietary sodium allotment as a means of permitting its use in a limited quantity.

Meals on Wheels or other food programs for elders and indigent patients may not be as low in sodium as desirable. The monitoring of daily weights and close follow-up with health-care providers should be strongly considered in these cases.

When patients seem overwhelmed by the amount of dietary education, or are upset with a perceived large dietary change, it may take some time and compromise to reach healthier dietary habits. Ultimately good dietary habits provide positive reinforcement. In the interim, however, it may be useful to invoke the "80/20" rule used in business management: 20% of what you do causes 80% of the problem. A good dietary history may provide information about significant culprits that the patient is willing to eliminate, moving the patient closer to an ideal regimen.

Daily Weights

Assessment and treatment of a heart failure patient's volume status is often guided by the measurement of daily weights. Discussion of daily weights should assure that the patient has a working scale at home; if not, the patient should be instructed to have family members or friends purchase one prior to the patient's discharge. Hospital staff should determine that the patient can get on the scale and can read the results. For those who cannot afford them on their own, case managers may be able to explore other mechanisms for obtaining scales. Some heart failure programs have included the provision of scales to patients who cannot afford them as a routine part of the discharge planning process. Patients should be taught to weigh themselves at the same time each day and to keep a log of their weights. Making sure that daily weights are done in the hospital is an extremely important method of teaching patients by role modeling and by discussing the interpretation. Finally, patients should be taught the use of a sliding scale diuretic regimen or be given parameters for when to call their provider.

Fluid Restriction

For some patients, fluid restriction is necessary, and often difficult. Patients need to be taught in terms that are available to them in the real world, such as 2-liter bottles and ounces, not in milliliters (rare) and ccs/cubic centimeters (almost never). A 24-hour recall can be a starting place. The total daily allotment of fluid can be apportioned among meals and an in-between meal allocation so that patients can avoid consuming the entire allowed amount prior to the end of the day. Providing coaching with meals that are delivered to inpatients may help to clarify that soup and gelatin are considered fluids. In the hospital and at home, patients can visually keep track of their fluid intake by filling a 21 soda bottle or milk jug with an equivalent amount of fluid. Hard candies or frozen grapes can be offered to help to alleviate thirst.

Symptom Recognition

During the hospitalization, while more intense observation is available, providers should try to determine the particular constellation of symptoms for that patient. For example, an older thin female with diastolic dysfunction with some right-sided heart failure may have a 1-lb weight gain, mild bloating, and mild ankle edema that are relieved with mild diuretic adjustment. Other patients may need to recognize that the development of dyspnea with personal grooming or while washing dishes is indicative of a need to augment their diuretic regimen. Teaching symptom recognition and stressing specific signs may help the patient retain the information after discharge. Helping patients recognize their symptoms may lead to earlier treatment and prevention of hospitalization.

Exercise

Exercise can be an important component of both inpatient and outpatient treatment plans for patients. Long periods of immobilization can be deleterious to patients; symptoms associated with deconditioning can be confused with symptoms of congestion. Increases in activity can be encouraged once symptoms are better controlled; some concrete methods of determining a patient's readiness to increase activity and initiate an exercise program include the ability to speak without dyspnea, a resting heart rate less than 120 beats/min, or the occurrence of no more than moderate fatigue with activities of daily living.[11] While increasing activity, the rating of perceived exertion (RPE) scale can be used to evaluate level of exertion. Often patients can benefit from working with a physical therapist after a moderate period of inactivity within the hospital, and this can occur on both an inpatient and an outpatient basis. Enrollment in a cardiac rehabilitation program can help to facilitate the development of an outpatient exercise program, but one must ensure that the program's staff is oriented to the needs of a heart failure

patient, which may differ from those of patients with ischemic heart disease.

Social Support

The level of social support available to patients may be a factor in their recovery and ability to stay out of the hospital. As previously noted, the amount of information to be absorbed during hospitalization can be overwhelming for one person; the presence of family or companions at key points during the education process can be important in providing a source for missed information. Enlisting family or community resources prior to discharge can also assist in maintaining a heart failure patient's well-being afterward, as these patients often suffer from fatigue, an energy limitation that limit their ability to care for themselves. Simple activities such as shopping, food preparation, filling pillboxes, or refilling medications may not be manageable for some patients. Depression, which is a predictor of readmission for heart failure, is exacerbated by a lack of social support. Supplemental supports to be evaluated prior to discharge include the Visiting Nurse Association (VNA), and home health aides as well as governmental or nongovernmental elder services programs. In a multidisciplinary approach, both social workers and case managers provide invaluable assistance in finding support and guidance for patients. Even informal social support offered to the patient by the inpatient caregivers has been shown to be effective in decreasing the 3-month readmission rate.[5]

Comorbid Illnesses

Diabetes and depression are both associated with worsening heart failure. Hospitalization is an opportunity to address and improve care for both of these conditions. Renal failure can greatly complicate the treatment and prognosis of a patient with heart failure, making diuresis more difficult and exacerbating prerenal azotemia that can occur with a diminished cardiac output.[12,13] Consultation with a nephrologist may assist in the treatment of reversible causes of renal dysfunction as well as identify the occasional patient for whom dialysis may be necessary for control of their volume status.

Other Factors

There are certain drugs that can cause worsening heart failure symptoms. These include nonsteroidal anti-inflammatory drugs (NSAIDS) and thiazolidinediones (rosiglitazone and pioglitazone). Patients are advised against taking NSAIDS as they cause renal sodium retention. A 2002 review of thiazolidinediones by the U.S. Food and Drug Administration (FDA) advised against this class of drugs in Class III and IV heart failure and cautioned careful observation of other patients with heart failure. Cephalosporin therapy can decrease the effectiveness of loop diuretics, and a patient should be cautioned to monitor their weight closely during the period for which they are prescribed. Smoking cessation counseling should be provided or reinforced.

Heart Failure Severity

The amount of outpatient support a patient will require is often predicted by assessment of heart failure severity. The New York Heart Association (NYHA) classifications essentially are measures of functional status and have traditionally reflected HF severity. Patients with NYHA Class I or II functional capacity may benefit from outpatient education and uptitration of medication to evidence-based target levels. Patients with Class III or IV heart failure usually require closer and more frequent attention.[14] Patients who are being evaluated for heart transplant are likely to be connected to a heart failure specialist team for management. Some patients are on chronic infusion therapy; their discharge preparation is more involved. Patients with ventricular assist devices for destination therapy should be followed in a formal ventricular assist device (VAD) program.

Those with end-stage heart failure benefit from thoughtful discussions about end-of-life issues, comfort measures, and preferences for treatment. Studies have shown that a person's priorities and preferences for end-of-life treatment may vary or evolve over time.[15] Many hospitals offer consultation from palliative care services that can help provide patients and clinicians with decision-making options. Hospice services, either inpatient or at home, are an option for further care. While eligibility for hospice usually includes likelihood of death within a 6-month time frame, the results from the Supplemental Benefit of ARB in Hypertensive Patients with Stable Heart Failure Using Olmesartan (SUPPORT) trial demonstrated the difficulty in predicting timing of death, with as many as 77% of patients meeting hospice admission criteria alive 6 months later.[16,17] Thus providers must be flexible as they offer a prognosis. Hospice also usually precludes use of advanced medical therapy, such as intravenous inotropes. However, distinctions in the availability of advanced therapies as opposed to palliative care in the hospice setting are evolving, allowing patients to receive the medical comfort and social support traditionally available through hospice care, while at the same time letting them receive sophisticated medical treatments (Abelson, R "A chance to pick hospice, and still hope to live." *The New York Times,* published 2/10/07).

▶ INTEGRATION TO OUTPATIENT CARE

Too often, there is a gap between inpatient and outpatient care. Referral to appropriate follow-up care and thoughtful communication from inpatient to outpatient clinicians is critical.[18] A recent meta-analysis of over 3000 patients age 65 or older with heart failure found that comprehensive discharge planning combined with postdischarge support leads to a reduction in readmission risk of 25%, improved quality of life, and a reduction in the patients' medical care expenses.[19] Possible follow-up for patients includes primary care practice, general or heart failure cardiologist, general or specialized VNA services, specialized heart failure clinics, disease management programs, and cardiac rehabilitation. In this section, the potential issues that need to be addressed to facilitate coordination of a patient's inpatient care with an appropriate outpatient medical support program will be discussed.

Communication

Communication is vital in a variety of areas. Written communication with the patient consisting of clear discharge instructions for medications and their timing, diet, and follow-up plans reinforce verbal teaching. Discharge summaries are often the primary source of communication with primary care or referring physicians. The quality and timeliness of discharge summaries are important for outpatient care. Several factors have been noted to be important in transfer of information: discharge medications, recent laboratory values, ejection fraction, and timeliness of discharge summary preparation.[20] Continuation and uptitration of evidence-based medications can also be emphasized through discharge summaries. Often, there are multiple providers, increasing the complexity of effective communication. Timely dissemination of data to all providers is important.

Harrison et al. have identified "intersector linkages" in the transition from hospital to home for heart failure patients.[21] These linkages emphasize consistency in educational efforts and communication between the hospital nursing staff and home care nurses during the vulnerable period immediately after discharge, and are compared with a traditional model for the transition from inpatient to outpatient care in Table 20-1. Improvement in quality of life and reduced emergency room visits resulted.

As noted, the immediate postdischarge period is critical. Home care nurses and/or follow-up phone calls to patients can answer questions, ensure that prescriptions have been filled, and essentially put out any preventable fires. Although Medicare currently requires patients to be homebound for continuous visiting nurse visits, usually an initial evaluation visit can be arranged. In some areas, VNAs have clinicians who have specialized heart failure expertise. Discharge planners or case managers in hospitals should be able to identify availability for a particular patient.

▶ **Table 20-1** Interventions to improve the transition from inpatient to outpatient care in heart failure patients

1. Hospital primary nurse assigned on admission
2. Home care notified of admission
3. Evidence-based education program
4. Education booklet to be used at home reviewed with patient prior to discharge
5. Written referral to home care on discharge
6. Nursing transfer letter to be received by home care nurse
7. Phone outreach within 24 hours of discharge
8. Phone advice from hospital nurse
9. Ongoing community nurse consultation with hospital nurse
10. Community nurse visits scheduled at a minimum of two visits in the first 2 weeks after discharge

Source: Adapted from Harrison MB, Browne GB, Roberts J, et al. Quality of life of individuals with heart failure: a randomized trial of the effectiveness of two models of hospital-to-home transition. *Med Care.* 2002;40:271–282.

Disease Management Programs

As noted in Chap. 18, disease management programs have been shown to be very helpful for managing patients with chronic disease. This is especially true for heart failure patients, where disease management results in reduced emergency room visits, readmissions, and mortality and improved quality of life.[22,23] These programs come in many shapes and sizes; studies are often done on small numbers and the variability among the interventions makes them difficult to compare or categorize or meta-analyze. Programs are usually based on telephone contact with nurses, pharmacists, or specially trained personnel, and may include home nurse visits or clinic appointments after discharge. Importantly, such programs often comprise the critical link between the inpatient and outpatient environments, thus promoting better continuity of care.

Telephone contact programs vary in their content and approach:

- Coaching: primarily education, problem solving, and encouragement to maintain advised treatment regimen.
- Clinical evaluation ± treatment: with assessment of symptoms, weights, and medications and education; nurse caller either reports back to physician with results of encounter or first adjusts medications (usually diuretics) according to standing orders and then reports to referring provider.

Home visits have been done by specialized nurses or nurse practitioners who have been able to perform clinical assessments and possibly make changes in the field. Additionally, they can assess home situations and dietary and medication adherence in ways probably more reliable than self-reporting. If available, this approach may be preferable for frail at-home elders, patients with frequent readmissions, and those whose compliance is questioned. Office visits to specialized heart failure clinics can provide opportunity to educate, assess, adjust treatment regimens, and provide access to other members of the multidisciplinary team: nutritionists, physical therapists, social workers.

Advantages of formalized programs include skilled clinicians; an approach to evidence-based medicine with protocols directing the uptitration of medications to optimal dosages; access to nutrition specialists with knowledge of diverse ethnic backgrounds; and collaborative associations with access to physician specialists. Communication among all clinicians and with patients is key to caring for these patients. Programs of greater intensity in terms of visit frequency and assessment are preferable for persons with Class III or IV symptoms. Although they have been shown to reduce hospitalizations and emergency room visits, heart failure disease management programs, or any intensive follow-up, are not without cost.[23] Insurance coverage needs to be considered. Some programs are sponsored by insurance agencies and CMS may assist in payment for certain programs.[24]

Inotropic Support

Patients who are dependent upon inotropic infusions require close follow-up. Specialized infusion companies, often in collaboration with visiting nurses, or outpatient heart failure clinics provide assessment and care of infusion issues. These patients will also benefit from more intensive outpatient management.

Ventricular Assist Devices

Patients who have had mechanical circulatory devices placed have a very different set of requirements.[25] Transition to home requires medical stability and intensive therapy to resolve possible major reconditioning issues. The hospital-based program provides education for community resource personnel, such as EMTs, police and fire department personnel, and local emergency room staff.

► SUMMARY

Caring for heart failure patients and implementing the care described is too large a task for one person. Current practice demands make it difficult to provide the amount of time and effort necessary to provide adequate assessment, education, and treatment. Multidisciplinary teams are extremely important in providing quality care to heart failure patients. Assuring a smooth intersection between the inpatient and outpatient arenas should help to provide a stable course for patients, without backsliding on important gains made during hospitalization and preventing rehospitalization. It should also increase satisfaction among patients and all providers.

► REFERENCES

1. Thom T, Haase N, Rosamond W, et al. Heart disease and stroke statistics—2006 update: a report from the American Heart Association Statistics Committee and Stroke Statistics Subcommittee. *Circulation.* 2006;113:e85–e151.

2. Hunt SA, Abraham WT, Chin MH, et al. ACC/AHA guidelines for evaluation and management of chronic heart failure in the adult-2005. *Circulation.* 2005;112:e154–e235.

3. Armola RR, Topp R. Variables that discriminate length of stay and readmission within 30 days among heart failure patients. *Lippincotts Case Manag.* 2001;6:246–255.

4. Dicker RC. Introducing the Medicare quality of care surveillance system. Quality Resume, No. 1. Baltimore: Health Care Financing Administration, 1997.

5. Schwarz KA, Elman CS. Identification of factors predictive of hospital readmissions for patients with heart failure. *Heart Lung.* 2003;32:88–99.

6. Kassovsky MP, Sarasin FP, Perneger TV, et al. Unplanned readmissions of patients with congestive heart failure: do they reflect in-hospital quality of care or patient characteristics? *Am J Med.* 2000;109:386–390.

7. Grady KL, Dracup K, Kennedy G, et al. Team management of patients with heart failure: A statement for healthcare professionals from the cardiovascular nursing council of the American Heart Association. *Circulation.* 2000; 102:2443–2456.

8. McDonald K, Ledwidge M, Cahill J, et al. Heart failure management: multidisciplinary care has intrinsic benefit above the optimization of medical care. *J Card Fail.* 2002;8:142–148.

9. Adams KF, Lindenfeld J, Arnold JMO, et al. HFSA 2006 comprehensive heart failure practice guideline. *J Card Fail.* 2006;12:e1–e122.

10. Gattis WA, O'Connor CM, Gallup DS, et al. Predischarge initiation of carvedilol in patients hospitalized for decompensated heart failure: results of the initiation management predischarge: process for assessment of carvedilol therapy in heart failure (IMPACT-HF) trial. *J Am Coll Cardiol.* 2004;43:1534–1541.

11. Cahalin LP. Exercise training in heart failure: inpatient and outpatient considerations. *AACN Clin Issues.* 1998;9:225–243.

12. Dries DL, Exner DV, Domanski MJ, et al. The prognostic implications of renal insufficiency in asymptomatic and symptomatic patients with left ventricular systolic dysfunction. *J Am Coll Cardiol.* 2000;35:681–689.

13. Butler J, Forman DE, Abraham WT, et al. Relationship between heart failure treatment and development of worsening renal function among hospitalized patients. *Am Heart J.* 2004;147:331–338.

14. Hauptman PJ, Masoudi FA, Weintraub WS, et al. Variability in the clinical status of patients with advanced heart failure. *J Card Fail.* 2004; 10:397–401.

15. Steinhauser KE, Christakis NA, Clipp EC, et al. Factors considered important at the end of life by patients, family, physicians, and other care providers. *JAMA.* 2004;484:2476–2482.

16. Lynn J, Arkes HR, Stevens M, et al. Rethinking fundamental assumptions: SUPPORT's implications for future reform. Study to Understand Prognoses and Preferences and Risks of Treatment. *J Amer Geriatr Soc.* 2000;48 (5 Suppl):S214–S221.

17. Fox E, Landrum-McNiff K, Zhong Z, et al, for the SUPPORT Investigators. Evaluation of prognostic criteria for determining hospice eligibility in patients with advanced lung, heart, or liver disease. *JAMA.* 1999;282:1638–1645.

18. Walblay AM. Heart failure management across the continuum: a communication link. *Outcomes Manag.* 2004;8:39–44.

19. Phillips CO, Wright SM, Kern DE, et al. Comprehensive discharge planning with post-discharge support for older patients with congestive heart failure: a meta-analysis. *JAMA.* 2004;291:1358–1367.

20. Van Walraven C, Rokosh E. What is necessary for high-quality discharge summaries? *Am J Med Qual.* 1999;14:160–170.

21. Harrison MB, Browne GB, Roberts J, et al. Quality of life of individuals with heart failure: a randomized trial of the effectiveness of two models of hospital-to-home transition. *Med Care.* 2002;40:271–282.

22. Gonseth J, Guallar-Castillon P, Banegas JR, et al. The effectiveness of disease management programmes in reducing hospital re-admission in older patients with heart failure: a systematic review and meta-analysis of published reports. *Eur Heart J.* 2004;25:1570–1595.

23. Berg GD, Wadhwa S, Johnson AE. A matched-cohort study of health services utilization and financial outcomes for a heart failure disease-management program in elderly patients. *J Am Geriatr Soc.* 2004;52:1655–1661.

24. CMS urges States to adopt disease management programs, agency will match state costs. February 26, 2004. Available at *http://www.cms.hhs.gov/apps/media/press_releases.asp.* Accessed April 11, 2007.

25. Thoratec VAD & IVAD Community Living Guide. Available at *http://thoratec.com/medical-professionals/pdf/files/101467C_Thorate_VAD_Community_Living_ENGLISH.pdf.* Accessed April 11, 2007.

CHAPTER 21

What Is a Heart Failure Clinic?

Gregg C. Fonarow, MD, FACC

Heart failure (HF) remains a major public health problem, affecting 5 million patients in the United States.1 HF is the leading cause of hospitalization for persons 65 years of age and rates of hospital readmission within 6 months range from 25% to 50%.1,2 It also poses a substantial economic burden with annual direct costs for care of HF patients estimated to be between $20 and $56 billion.1–3 The personal burden of HF includes debilitating symptoms, functional limitations, frequent rehospitalizations, and a very high mortality rate.2 With alarming hospitalization rates, declining quality of life, significant morbidity, and high mortality rates among patients with HF, it has become obvious that there are substantial opportunities for improvements in the inpatient and outpatient management of HF.

Care for patients with chronic HF ideally integrates inpatient and outpatient health-care delivery with a goal of reducing symptoms, improving functional capacity, decreasing the need for hospitalization, and prolonging life. A number of studies have documented substantial underuse of evidence-based guideline-recommended HF therapies and marked variation in the quality of care judged by specific performance measures and in patients receiving conventional care.2,5,6 Moreover, patient behavioral factors, such as nonadherence to diet and medications, and economic and social factors frequently contribute to disease progression, frequent hospitalizations, and diminished quality of life.2,6 The traditional model of care delivery is thought to contribute to frequent hospitalizations in HF patients because in these brief, episodic encounters, little attention may be paid to the common, modifiable factors that precipitate many hospitalizations.6–8 Many overburdened primary care and cardiology practices have not fully integrated the treatment recommendations from randomized clinical trials and HF practice guidelines into routine clinical practice. Unfamiliarity with medications, doses for HF, and device indications or concerns regarding potential side effects may lead to underutilization of beneficial therapies such as angiotensin-converting enzyme (ACE) inhibitors, β-blockers, aldosterone antagonists, and HF device therapy. Education of patients and family members regarding pharmacologic and nonpharmacologic therapies such as diet and exercise requires significant staff time and commitment. Close tracking of relevant clinical and laboratory data by health-care providers may not be practical except for groups of patients with similar diagnoses.[8] As such, there has been much interest in identifying effective methods to improve the quality of care for HF patients, while reducing the substantial economic costs associated with HF.

Concentrated HF programs may be able to provide more focused care that could improve quality of care and patient outcomes and decrease hospitalizations, thus decreasing costs. Based on early reports of success with HF clinics, there has been a growing recognition of the role these programs can play in improving the management of patients with HF. In 1994, the Cardiology Preeminence Roundtable published a detailed assessment of HF patient management and highlighted the benefits on the quality of HF care and potential financial benefits of the HF clinic model.[8] Since that time, there have been numerous studies, reviews, meta-analyses, workshops, and symposiums focused on strategies to improve the quality of care while also reducing total health-care costs and hospital readmissions for patients with HF. The general aims of HF disease management strategies are to successfully impact quality-of-care measures such as use of evidence-based therapies, measurement of left ventricular function, and provision of patient education and clinical outcome measures such as rehospitalization rates, patients' functional status, quality of life, patient satisfaction, and medical costs. HF disease management programs also aim to achieve improved quality and outcomes at lower cost than that of conventional HF care. HF clinics are very well suited to meet all these aims.

A number of HF disease management programs centered around the HF clinic model of care have been developed and have provided assessments of their impact on quality of care and clinical outcomes. HF patients who were cared for in these programs were shown to have improved utilization of evidence-based therapies, significantly fewer rehospitalizations, lower health-care costs, improved functional and symptom status, and better quality of life compared with HF patients treated with conventional care. While each of these HF clinics for which data have been reported have had slightly different management emphasis, outcome focus, and utilization of health-care team members, there are a number of common elements to these programs. This chapter will review the impact that such programs can have on HF patients' quality of care and clinical outcomes, the components of a HF clinic, patient management and educational approaches utilized, and highlight the individual patient care processes that may favorably impact HF patient outcomes.

▶ HEART FAILURE CLINIC MODELS

There are several components of HF clinic programs frequently highlighted as being important to improving outcomes (Table 21-1). These program components include the following: optimization of HF medical therapy, assessment and management of patient comorbidities, close monitoring of volume status, use of a flexible diuretic regimen, comprehensive HF education in the hospital and outpatient setting to patients and their family members, hospital discharge and continuity of care planning, increased outpatient access to health care professionals, and long-term coordinated follow-up of patients.[9-11] Early descriptions of HF clinics frequently assessed their impact on patient care and clinical outcomes by comparing patients during the period before and the period after their care was assumed by the HF clinic. Other studies retrospectively compared patients managed in HF clinics to those undergoing care in a conventional practice setting. Subsequently, prospective randomized clinical trials have also

▶ **Table 21-1** Heart failure clinic components

- Multidisciplinary team: heart failure specialists, advance practice nurses, home nursing, pharmacists, medical social workers, nutritionists, administrative personnel
- Detailed assessment of heart failure etiology, potential reversible causes, and related risks
- Optimization of heart failure medical therapy
- Evaluation of need for heart failure device therapy
- Assessment and management of patient comorbidities
- Close monitoring of volume status and use of a flexible diuretic regimen
- Comprehensive heart failure education in the hospital and outpatient setting to patients and their family members
- Meticulous tracking of clinical status, laboratories, and diagnostic testing
- Hospital discharge and continuity of care planning
- Increased outpatient access to health-care professionals
- Long-term coordinated follow-up of patients
- Access to clinical trials and experimental therapies

assessed the impact of such programs. A number of these studies will be discussed in this section (Table 21-2).

Cintron and colleagues assessed the impact of a HF clinic utilizing advance practice nurses with 15 patients with New York Heart Association (NYHA) Class III–IV HF symptoms (mean age 65 years).[12] Outcomes were measured pre- and postintervention and included medical costs, patient satisfaction, and inpatient hospital time. Key aspects of this HF clinic model studied included frequent scheduled outpatient clinic visits (average 18 visits/year), patient education (medications, weight control, and diet), emphasis on family support and the home situation, and increased health-care provider availability. Postintervention data obtained at 24 months revealed a 60% reduction in rehospitalizations, 85% reduction in hospital days, decreased medical costs, and significantly increased patient satisfaction.

A HF clinic described by Lasater enrolled 41 patients with HF and assessed the impact on outcomes.[13] This clinic also utilized advance practice nurses working in close conjunction with physicians, social worker, and dieticians. Patients were seen on a weekly basis for 4 weeks. The nurses provided patient education regarding the diuretic

regimen and weighing daily (providing scales when necessary), performed physical assessments and adjusted diuretics, monitored medication compliance, and assisted with financial constraints. Outcomes were measured pre- and postintervention. At 1 year, patients demonstrated increased knowledge of their medical regimen. There were also reductions in hospitalization rates and average hospital length of stay.

Assessing the impact of a physician-directed, nurse-coordinated clinic on 134 HF patients (mean age 52 years), Hanumanthu et al. measured outcomes 12 months pre- and postintervention. Patients were medically managed by HF specialty cardiologists in conjunction with advance practice nurses.[10] One year after referral to the HF clinic, patients had a 53% reduction in annual hospitalization rate (decrease in total cardiovascular and HF), substantially higher diuretic dosing, significantly improved peak VO_2 on exercise testing, and improved quality-of-life scores. Smith et al. enrolled 21 patients (mean age 61 years) with NYHA Class II–III HF symptoms into a HF clinic.[14] Clinic visits were frequent (average 10 visits/6 months), and patients were seen by either the physician or advance practice nurse. Patients received detailed education about HF, diet, daily weights, and the importance

▶ **Table 21-2** Selective studies of heart failure clinics

Reference	Sample	Study design	Intervention	Components of intervention	Outcomes*
Cintron et al., 1983[12]	• 15, NYHA III–IV, mean age 65 years • Sex of patients not indicated although study conducted at a Veteran's Administration hospital so likely exclusively men • Puerto Rico	Within subjects preintervention, postintervention comparison with mean follow-up of 24 months	Heart failure clinic staffed with nurse practitioners	• Nurse practitioner managed • Frequent follow-up via clinic visits • Education reinforced at each visit: medication, weight control, diet • Assessment of home situation • Family support • Increased availability of nurse practitioner ("walk-ins" encouraged) • Cardiologist consultation for unstable patients	• 60% reduction in rehospitalizations • 85% reduction in hospital days • Reduction in total medical costs of $8009 per patient
Lasater 1996[13]	• 41 HF patients • United States	Within subjects preintervention, postintervention comparison with mean follow-up of 6 and 12 months	Heart failure clinic staffed by advanced practice nurses	• Four weekly visits with an experienced hospital staff nurse • Direct access to physician consultation, social worker, dietitian • Patient education regarding diuretic regimen and importance of daily weights • Scales provided as needed • Diuretics adjusted based on physical assessment	• 4% decrease in readmission rate • Mean hospital length of stay decreased 1.6 days • Increased knowledge of medical regimen demonstrated at 1 year

Source	Sample	Design	Intervention	Outcomes
Hanumanthu et al., 1997[10]	• 134, NYHA not indicated, mean age 52 ± 12 • 71% • United States	Within subjects preintervention, postintervention comparison with follow-up of 12 months	Physician-directed, nurse coordinated comprehensive heart failure clinic • Medication compliance monitored • Assistance with financial constraints • Heart failure/transplant physician-directed • Nurse coordinators assisted with inpatient and outpatient management • Team exclusively managed heart failure patients • Optimization of medical therapy • Periodic meetings with home health care agency and hospice program to integrate care	• 53% reduction in annual hospitalization rate • 63% reduction in heart failure rehospitalizations • Increased peak VO_2
Fonarow et al., 1997[9]	• 214, NYHA III and IV, mean age 52 ± 10 years • 81% male • United States	Within subjects preintervention, postintervention comparison with follow-up of 6 months	Heart failure cardiologist directed, advanced practice nurse, follow-up, comprehensive inpatient and outpatient management program • Heart failure cardiologist directed • Follow-up by heart failure cardiologist, advanced practice nurse, and referring physician • Optimization of drug therapy in hospital and during follow-up • Comprehensive patient and family/caregiver education by heart failure clinical nurse specialist about daily weights and flexible diuretic regimen, diet,	• 85% reduction in rehospitalizations • Improvement in functional status • Lower costs

(Continued)

281

Reference	Sample	Study design	Intervention	Components of intervention	Outcomes[*]
Smith et al., 1997[14]	• 21, mean NYHA 2.6 ± 0.5, mean age 61 years • 100% male • United States	Within subjects preintervention, postintervention comparison with follow-up of 6 months	Physician or nurse practitioner comprehensive care in heart failure clinic	medications, smoking and alcohol abstinence, home exercise instruction, warning signs of worsening heart failure, and prognosis • Weekly follow-up at heart failure clinic until stable with education reinforced • Phone follow-up after medication changes and if indicated • Care provided by physician or nurse practitioner • Optimization of medical therapy • Identification and management of etiology of heart failure • Patient education about diet, medications, compliance, daily weights and flexible diuretic regimen, alcohol abstinence • Nurse practitioner available by phone • Increased access to clinic (without appointment) for worsening symptoms or medication needs	• 86% reduction in heart failure hospitalizations • Improved quality of life • Improved functional status • More patients on optimal medications and doses

| Cline et al., 1998[15] | • 190, mean NYHA 2.6 ± 0.7, mean age 75.6 ± 5.3 years
• 52.3% male
• Sweden | Randomized control trial with follow-up of 12 months | Nurse-directed outpatient clinic | • Before hospital discharge, patient and family education about heart failure and pharmacologic and nonpharmacologic aspects of its treatment
• Medication organizer given
• Patients receive guidelines for self-management of diuretics
• One-hour information visits for patient and family at home after discharge
• Easy access to a nurse-directed outpatient clinic with one prescheduled visit at 8 months; nurses available by phone and could see patients at short notice
• Encouragement to contact nurses at clinic for any problems or questions or concerns | • Time to first admission 33% longer in intervention group
• 59% increase in number of days hospitalized compared to 12-month period before start of study in control group versus no increase in intervention group
• 36% fewer hospitalizations in intervention group (but nonsignificant at P = 0.08)
• Trend toward mean annual reduction in health-care costs (P = 0.07) |

(Continued)

▶ **Table 21-2** Selective studies of heart failure clinics (*Continued*)

Reference	Sample	Study design	Intervention	Components of intervention	Outcomes[*]
Dahl & Penque, 2000[16]	• 1192 nonrandomized patients (583 before program, 609 after program initiated) • Pretreatment group mean age 72 years, 95% Caucasian • Post-treatment group mean age 75 years, 96% Caucasian • United States	Post-test only design with nonequivalent groups	Advanced practice nurse-directed inpatient heart failure program	• Advanced practice nurse coordinated inpatient care • Intensive patient education • Heart failure medical orders reviewed with primary physician in reference to clinical guidelines • Multidisciplinary services as needed • Home health care plan • High-risk patients telephoned after discharge	• 36% reduction in hospital deaths • Increased use of ACE inhibitors • Decreased readmission rates • Shorten length of stay

[*]Results are statistically significant unless otherwise indicated; NYHA = New York Heart Association functional class

of compliance. Patients had access to the advance practice nurse via the phone for questions or could see them during the day without an appointment. Outcomes were measured pre- and postclinic intervention. After 6 months, patients had a greater than 80% reduction in HF hospitalizations and emergency medical center visits, reported improved quality of life, and increased exercise time, and more patients were placed on the appropriate HF medications and dosages.

In one of the first prospective, randomized trial of HF clinics, Cline et al. assessed outcomes in 190 patients (mean age 75 years) assigned to either "routine clinical practice" or a HF cardiologist staffed, nurse-coordinated outpatient HF clinic.[15] Patients in the intervention group received extensive education on HF, pharmacologic and nonpharmacologic therapies, self-management of diuretics; had easy access to the advance practice nurse over the phone or in the clinic; and saw the HF cardiologist at 1 and 4 months after hospital discharge. At 1-year follow-up, time to readmission was 33% longer and the number of hospitalized days was fewer in the intervention group, and a higher percentage of these patients were treated with ACE inhibitors.

Using a retrospective design, Dahl and Penque evaluated an advanced practice nurse directed HF clinic program on 1192 nonrandomized patients (583 patients before the existence of the program and 609 patients after program initiation).[16] Patients in the program group had an advance practice nurse coordinating their inpatient care, providing intensive patient education, addressing clinical guidelines with the patients' physician, ordering additional multidisciplinary services as needed, developing a home health-care plan, and providing clinical phone call follow-up and HF clinic visits to high-risk patients postdischarge. Patients in the advance practice nurse-directed care program had a 36% reduction in hospital deaths, significantly greater use of ACE inhibitors, decreased total 90-day readmission rates, and a significantly shorter length of stay.

The UCLA Heart Failure Clinic Experience

The impact of one of the first organized HF management programs based on the HF clinic model based at the UCLA Medical Center has been studied in detail. At UCLA, our comprehensive HF management program incorporates a systematic approach to evidence-based medical therapy, extensive patient education about diet, exercise, and self-care methods, and meticulous tracking of patients including regular contact between the patient and the HF team. Patients are evaluated and managed by HF specialty cardiologists in conjunction with HF trained advance practice nurses. The hospital-based clinic provides HF disease management on both an inpatient and outpatient basis, ensuring continuity of education and care. This program was one of the first to develop a flexible diuretic program with patients being educated as to how to adjust their diuretic dosing based on daily weight.

The study population at the UCLA Medical Center that validated this HF clinic approach consisted of patients with severe HF referred to the Ahmanson-UCLA Cardiomyopathy Center as potential candidates for heart transplantation, between 1991 and 1994.[9] All patients included in this study had congestive NYHA Class III or IV HF symptoms for at least 6 months prior to referral. This analysis was confined to patients who were determined to be potential candidates for heart transplantation.[9] At the time of referral, patients underwent a detailed initial assessment including review of all available medical records. The number of hospitalizations, precipitating symptoms, and admission diagnoses for all hospitalizations in the 6 months prior to referral were determined by patient interview and confirmed by review of the discharge summaries.

After initial assessment of the patients HF etiology, comorbidities and related risks, prior HF management, and possible eligibility for transplantation, 214 patients underwent formal evaluation for transplantation. Meticulous attention was paid to initiating and adjusting evidence-based medications for HF and any of the patients' other related risks (such as diabetes, atherosclerosis, and atrial fibrillation). Patients who were hospitalized at the time of referral or whom remained significantly symptomatic despite empiric HF medical therapy underwent pulmonary artery catheter guided therapy as previously described.[17] Oral ACE inhibitors were initiated or reinitiated and titrated to initially match the hemodynamics achieved on intravenous therapy and then adjusted to "target" doses. Other patients had empiric adjustments of their HF medications. The regimen of loop diuretics was adjusted to achieve and then maintain the patient's daily weight to within 2 lb of the weight at which optimal hemodynamics were achieved or the "dry" weight assessed clinically. Patients and their family members received comprehensive education taught individually by one of the HF advanced practice nurses and tailored to that patient's educational level and educational needs, as described previously. The verbal instruction was reinforced with a HF patient education booklet provided to each patient. A flexible diuretic regimen was utilized. Patients were instructed to monitor and record their daily weights. The loop diuretic dose is doubled for 2 lb or more weight gain and if the patient responds with an increase in urine output additional potassium supplementation is taken. Patients were instructed to call the advance practice nurse if they did not respond or were having to more frequently double the diuretic dosing. Dietary guidelines included a 2 g sodium restriction and a 2 L fluid restriction. Complete abstinence from smoking and alcohol was emphasized. A home-based walking exercise regimen was utilized. Patients and families were also advised of the uncertain prognosis, resources for patient and caregiver support, and advance directives. They were given detailed instruction regarding warning symptoms of worsening HF or other complications such as arrhythmias or embolic events.

Patients were followed by the HF cardiologist and advance practice nurse in the HF clinic setting, in conjunction with their referring physician(s). Posthospital discharge phone calls were made by the advance practice nurses within 3 days of discharge and weekly during the initial month after discharge, less often after stability was demonstrated. Patients were seen twice a month at the HF center until criteria for clinical stability were met.[9] Patients were interviewed regarding symptoms and examined for any signs of fluid retention. The patient education program was reinforced during each visit and the weight charts and exercise program specifically reviewed by the advance practice nurse and cardiologist. Diuretic regimens were adjusted for frequent weight gain or physical examination signs of volume overload or when postural hypotension or low jugular venous pressure suggested excessive diuresis. HF medications were closely tracked and doses adjusted for symptomatic hypotension, changes in renal function, or as otherwise indicated. All hospitalizations were recorded regardless of cause or precipitating factor. At 6 months, patients underwent detailed reassessment with review of all hospitalizations, determination of NYHA class, and repeat cardiopulmonary exercise testing. Patients with a major improvement in exercise performance, defined as an increase in peak oxygen uptake ≥ 2 mL/kg/min to ≥ 12 mL/kg/min, who also met criteria for clinical stability, were taken off the heart transplant list.[18]

During the study period, 214 patients were followed in the HF clinic and met the entry criteria. Baseline characteristics for the 214 study patients included left ventricular ejection fraction of 0.21 ± 0.07 and HF symptom duration of 18 ± 29 months (all at least 6 months). Peak oxygen uptake within 6 weeks of referral was 11.0 ± 4.0 mL/kg/min. ACE inhibitors had been prescribed prior to referral in 165 patients (77.1%) at an average dose of 95 ± 120 mg (captopril equivalent dosing). The patient's referring physician was an internist or family physician in 12.1% of patients and a cardiologist in 87.8%. Redesign of the medical regimen included initiation of an ACE inhibitor in an additional 18% of patients, for a total of 95% of patients on an

ACE inhibitor. Average net diuresis was 4.2 ± 4.6 l. Compared to the time of referral, the mean daily dose in patients receiving ACE inhibitors increased by 98%.

During reassessment at 6 months, patients had significant improvement in subjective and objective indices of functional status. NYHA Class improved significantly for the 179 patients alive without transplantation at 6 months (P <0.001), with 48.6% of patients classified as Class I or II. The improvement remained significant (P <0.01) when the 35 patients dying or undergoing transplantation were included and ranked as Class IV for reassessment. Repeat cardiopulmonary exercise testing was available in 121 of the 179 patients (68%), with increased oxygen consumption from 11.0 ± 3.6 to 15.2 ± 4.4 mL/kg/min (P <0.001) and comparable improvement in anaerobic threshold. Based on improved exercise capacity and demonstrated clinical stability, 30% of patients were removed from the active transplant list with subsequent 18-month survival of 92% without death or relisting for transplantation.[9]

The improved functional status was reflected in the decreased hospitalization rate after referral. In the 6 months prior to referral, 429 hospitalizations for HF occurred in the study population. In the 6 months after discharge as transplant candidates, there were 63 hospitalizations, an 85% reduction (P <0.0001). Although only admissions attributed directly to HF were included from the prereferral period, all 63 rehospitalizations after referral were included as potentially related to the redesign of therapy. During the 6 months, only 25.7% of the 214 patients required any hospitalizations, compared to 91.6% in the prior 6 months. Of the nine deaths, six occurred suddenly, two were attributed to pump failure, and one was noncardiac. Actuarial survival was 95.8% at 6 months, with 89.2% of patients without death or urgent transplantation.

HF clinic management was associated with a substantial reduction in hospital-related medical costs. The average cost of rehospitalization at UCLA was $9178 (range $2890 to $38930), comparable to estimates previously published

by O'Connell and Bristow for the U.S.[3] For the whole group, the cost of rehospitalization after referral thus was estimated to be $578,000, compared to $3,937,000 prior to referral. The hospitalization costs are considered to dominate overall costs of HF. No attempt was made to track the total outpatient costs, shared between the HF clinic and referring physicians, but these have been estimated in previous literature to be about $4238 per patient per year.[8,19,20] The additional burden of these candidates constituted half of a full-time equivalent HF advanced practice nurse, or about $490 dollars per patient for the 6 months. Further management costs included office administration for the coordination of communication between the HF team, referring physicians, and visiting nurses. These costs are hard to isolate for transplant candidates within the much larger volume of an active regional HF program. Any outpatient costs, however, were dwarfed by the costs of rehospitalization, which were reduced by approximately $15,700 per patient over the 6 months after referral.

This study demonstrates that the clinical improvement following referral to a clinic-based comprehensive HF management program translates into a major improvement in patients' clinical and functional status, with reduction in hospitalization rates and thus the cost of HF. Together these studies lend support to the concept that the concentrated care and expertise in a HF center provides more focused care and as a result improves patient outcomes, decreases hospitalizations, and decreases total medical costs.

▶ META-ANALYSES OF HEART FAILURE DISEASE MANAGEMENT PROGRAMS

McAlister and colleagues reviewed randomized trials of HF disease management programs published through 1999.[21] This analysis included programs based on multidisciplinary teams providing direct specialized follow-up in a HF clinic setting, programs using home-based nursing care, and those using telephone contact for coordinated primary care. This analysis concluded that studies using multidisciplinary teams providing direct specialized follow-up care, when pooled together, resulted in statistically significantly reduced hospitalization and health-care costs. In marked contrast, studies that used telephone contact to coordinate primary care services seemed to have no effect. Since 1999, several more randomized trials have been published and an updated analysis by McAlister and colleagues was published.[22] HF disease management strategies that incorporated follow-up by a specialized multidisciplinary team (either in a clinic or a nonclinic setting) reduced mortality (risk ratio [RR] 0.75, 95% confidence interval [CI] 0.59 to 0.96), HF hospitalizations (RR 0.74, 95% CI 0.63 to 0.87), and all-cause hospitalizations (RR 0.81, 95% CI 0.71 to 0.92). In addition, 15 of the 18 trials reported that their disease management interventions were cost-saving, with the other three trials reporting cost neutrality. Strategies that employed telephone contact and advised patients to attend their primary care physician in the event of deterioration reduced HF hospitalizations, but not mortality or all-cause hospitalizations. Another meta-analysis including 18 trials published between 1993 and 2003 confirms that, overall, HF clinic and nonclinic disease management interventions directed at recently hospitalized patients with HF significantly reduce rehospitalizations and health-care costs with a trend toward lower all-cause mortality rates.[23] The authors concluded that if applied on a national basis, multidisciplinary disease management strategies for HF have the potential to prevent 84,000 readmissions with an estimated reduction in Medicare payments of $424 million per year.[23]

► COMPONENTS OF A HEART FAILURE CLINIC

HF clinics are organized in a variety of ways as evidenced in examples discussed previously. Some of the most successful clinic models are organized to provide care utilizing a multidisciplinary team approach.[24] Cardiologists with expertise in HF evaluate and manage patients in conjunction with advance practice nurses. The advance practice nurses may have training as either clinical nurse specialists or nurse practitioners. The advance practice nurse has multiple roles which incorporate HF patient education, dietary counseling, social support assessment, review of medications, exercise counseling, discharge planning, and ongoing assessment of clinical stability. Some programs are organized to incorporate dietitians, pharmacists, and medical social workers to provide these functions or augment the services provided by the advance practice nurses. A program may include home health nursing directly or coordinate care with outside home nursing agencies. Ideally, HF programs are set up to follow patients on both an inpatient and outpatient basis, thus improving continuity of care.[24] These clinics may be hospital or outpatient practice based with regard to their organizational and financial structure.[24] Many HF clinics have developed in conjunction with heart transplantation programs or were organized to conduct research and clinical trials in HF management.[7,24]

The components that are integrated into the HF clinic model are illustrated below with an overview of the process of patient evaluation, education, and management. Patients with HF referred to a HF specialty clinic usually undergo a detailed evaluation. A comprehensive history and review of any available medical records by both the cardiologist and advance practice nurse occur to define the etiology of the patient's HF, identify contributing causes and comorbidities, review treatments and responses, and define the patients' physiologic state. Physical examination by the cardiologist together with the advance practice nurse takes place on the initial visit and each subsequent visit with close assessment of volume status and documentation of physical findings. Diagnostic testing is reviewed and the need for further testing assessed. Evaluation of left ventricular function by echocardiography is indicated, if it has not yet been performed or assessed in the prior year. Functional status is not only assessed by the patient's history, but more objective testing such as cardiopulmonary exercise testing or the 6-minute walk test. The physician-advance practice nurse team also evaluates the patient's understanding of their disease, compliance history with medications, diet, and fluids. Patients are also evaluated to determine if there is a reversible cause of HF, such as coronary artery disease with significant ischemia and/or hibernating myocardium or uncorrected valvular heart disease.[2] Such patients would potentially benefit from surgical therapies such as revascularization or valve replacement. For patients with severe symptoms and/or a high risk of mortality, heart transplantation is considered.[2] Assessment of sudden death risk is made for each patient as well as eligibility for HF device therapy. Eligible patients without contraindications are referred to an electrophysiologist for implantation of an implantable cardioverter-defibrillator and/or cardiac resynchronization therapy, unless specific contraindications exist or the patient declines device placement.

After initial assessment, the HF cardiologist and advance practice nurse devise a medical and nonpharmacologic treatment plan.[24] Patients receive detailed information regarding the nature and severity of their disease, warning signs of worsened HF, medications and potential side effects, and the short-term and long-term follow-up plans. Arrangements for further testing, additional patient education, and medical follow-up are made. The assessment and treatment plans are also communicated to other physicians that may be involved in the patient's care.

HF clinics have the potential to improve the utilization and dosing of beneficial medical therapies.[24] There is marked practice variation in the management of patients with HF. This variation is often the result of a failure of general practice to incorporate the advances in clinical management that are supported by clinical trials. Despite overwhelming clinical trial evidence demonstrating that the use of ACE inhibitors and β-blockers reduce hospitalizations, improve

functional status, and prolong life in patients with HF, these evidence-based, guideline-recommended therapies are prescribed to less than half the patients with symptomatic HF in many practice settings.[25] Additional therapies for HF such as aldosterone antagonists are slow to be integrated into the care of patients in conventional practice settings.

A standardized approach to pharmacologic therapy for patients with HF may improve patient outcomes if it results in a greater utilization of available beneficial therapies and reduces utilization of therapies that are detrimental. HF clinics frequently incorporate such a standardized approach.[24] Evidence-based HF therapies are initiated as described in detail in HF clinical guidelines.[2] Treatment regimens are updated when new information from clinical trials becomes available. The initiation and monitoring of the medications can be enhanced with the multidisciplinary resources of the HF clinic. There is a greater focus on ensuring initiation of evidence-based therapies and studies have documented increased utilization of therapies such as ACE inhibitors, β-blockers, and aldosterone antagonists in HF clinics.[7] The advanced practice nurse and/or pharmacist can describe in detail the indications and potential side effects and discuss this with patients and their family members.

Many HF medications require titration over time and careful monitoring of the patient's clinical response. ACE inhibitors are initiated at lower starting doses and the dose is titrated upwards over time. Monitoring of serum potassium, blood urea nitrogen (BUN), and creatinine during initiation and titration of HF medications allows early identification of potential abnormalities before being clinically manifested.[24] β-Blockers are initiated at low dose in stabilized patients with NYHA Class I to IV HF, with uptitration occurring at 2–4-week intervals.[2] Patients may require 3–5 titration steps before target doses are achieved. To enhance the safety of initiating β-blockers, patients are closely monitored for signs of volume overload and bradycardia.[2] During initiation of aldosterone antagonists, adjustments are frequently necessary in the loop diuretic dosing and potassium supplementation. Additionally, these patients require meticulous monitoring of renal function and serum potassium levels. HF clinics are organized to closely track patients' medications and dosing regimens, thus facilitating the titration of medications and ensuring appropriate laboratory testing. Medications that can result in complications or that can worsen outcome in patients with HF such as nonsteroidal anti-inflammatory agents (NSAIDS) can be avoided.[2] Potential drug interactions, for example the effect of amiodarone on raising digoxin levels and the degree of anticoagulation, may be more readily recognized and addressed prospectively.

Many HF programs are designed to encounter patients when they are first hospitalized with HF. When the patient is initially hospitalized for HF, opportunities exist to begin the optimization of medical therapy and provide intensive patient education. The readmission rate for HF has been reported to be as high as 28–52% within 90 days.[26,27] Deficiencies in HF inpatient care as defined by explicit process criteria have been shown to be associated with a higher rate of rehospitalization and increased death rates following hospital discharge.[28] Members of the HF clinic, specifically the advance practice nurse, can work in conjunction with the inpatient physicians and nurses to develop pathways to expedite patient care and begin the education process. The transition from inpatient hospitalization to outpatient management is a critical period where medication errors are frequently made. Educating patients as to how their medical regimen has been altered during hospitalization poses a challenge, especially if left to hospital staff nurses. The HF advance practice nurse can provide this education in a comprehensive fashion by reviewing what new medications are now in the regimen and creating a simplified medication schedule for the patient. Involving the HF clinic team members in the inpatient setting creates a situation that will minimize medication errors and improve care, as these members will

also be the ones following and tracking the HF patients on an outpatient basis.[24]

Tracking patients' symptoms, functional status, weights, medications, compliance, laboratory monitoring, and diagnostic tests over time poses a major challenge. In general, conventional clinical practices are not able to provide this type of monitoring.[8] HF clinics utilize a variety of tracking methods to closely follow patients. For example, specialized tracking sheets and computerized monitoring programs can track patients' weights, NYHA Functional Class, medications and doses, diagnostic parameters such as left ventricular ejection fraction, degree of mitral regurgitation, left ventricular end-diastolic dimension, and laboratories, that is, serum sodium, potassium, BUN, creatinine, and B-type natriuretic peptide (BNP) levels.[24] These tracking programs make trends easy to follow and significant changes can be readily identified. With close monitoring, changes in a patient's condition can be identified early and alterations in management made *before* the patient has deteriorated to the point of requiring hospitalization.

Patients with HF and atrial fibrillation, left ventricular thrombus, or prior systemic embo-lization require systemic anticoagulation, unless contraindications exist.[2] Monitoring of anticoagulation with the advance practice nurse following standardized protocols can improve this process of care, as has been demonstrated in general anticoagulation clinics.[29] Approximately two-thirds of patients with HF also have coronary artery disease, and thus these patients would benefit from lipid management and other secondary prevention measures.[2] Many studies have shown lipid-lowering medications are underutilized in conventional practice settings, with only 10–20% of patients with coronary artery disease at goal for low-density lipoprotein (LDL) cholesterol.[25] The initiation and titration of lipid-lowering medications to achieve National Cholesterol Education Program goals of LDL cholesterol of <100 mg/dL (or <70 mg/dL) can be facilitated by the HF clinic staff. Thus, as seen for lipid centers as well, higher treatment rates can readily be achieved.

Patient compliance is a key issue in HF management and a major determinant of clinical outcomes.[30] HF clinics are oriented toward the assessment and optimization of patient compliance. In addition to the direct education provided by team members, specific patient educational materials are also provided by these programs to reinforce and enhance the education provided to patients and family members.[24] The educational components that can favorably impact patient care have been described in other chapters.

Individual Variables That Impact Outcome

The clinical studies reviewed in this chapter demonstrate that providing HF specialty care in the HF clinic model can have a significant and favorable impact on patient outcomes. The design of these studies does not isolate the discrete contributions of the many program components and patient care interventions, each of which could have variable degrees of impact on patient outcomes. Many of these components of care are provided at relatively low marginal cost by HF clinics so determining the individual impact of each variable may not be that essential, with the net effect being so favorable.

Increased utilization of HF medications is one of the variables that may contribute to the improved outcomes of patients managed in an HF clinic. As mentioned previously, medical therapies that have been demonstrated by major trials to be effective in HF have been found to be underutilized outside of HF clinics.[25] In the studies detailed earlier in the chapter, the number of patients referred to the HF clinic on ACE inhibitors and β-blockers was quite variable. There are multiple reasons why HF patients are not treated with evidence-based therapies; often concerns about side effects and the impact ACE inhibitors and β-blockers may have on the patient's blood pressure limit the use of these medications. Many studies showed that patients managed in a HF clinic were more likely to be treated with ACE inhibitors and β-blockers, as well as being more likely to be treated with target doses.[7] In the UCLA HF clinic study, there was an increase from 77% to 95% in ACE inhibitor utilization. In addition, patients on ACE inhibitors had an increase of 98% in average daily dose equivalents, which may have been a major component in clinical improvement.[9] Additional studies have demonstrated increased use of β-blockers and aldosterone antagonists. Increased utilization of these medications in patients followed in a HF failure clinic would have a highly favorable impact on functional status, hospitalization rates, as well as survival.

Improved volume status management and early adjustment of the diuretic regimen is another variable that likely contributes to reduced hospitalization rate seen with HF failure clinic programs. There is limited information regarding the optimal dosing of diuretics, but HF clinics often dose diuretics to maintain a dry weight determined by physical examination by clinicians with extensive HF management experience.[2] Further outpatient modifications of the diuretic regimen are made in clinical assessment at follow-up visits, with the specific goal of maintaining freedom from congestion.

In addition to the flexible diuretic regimen, patients receive detailed instruction regarding all of the patient education issues described in the ACC/AHA HF Practice Guidelines.[2] Specific instructions are given to the patient and family regarding sodium restriction and, in most cases, fluid restriction as well.[26] Specific explanations of each medication's action and side effects are given by the advanced practice nurse in the hospital and again at follow-up visits. This vigilance in instruction may help to decrease the rate of noncompliance, which was described in 54% of patients with HF and was implicated in 53% of readmissions in a group of elderly patients with HF.[31,32] The impact of educational programs for improvement of compliance has been shown for HF and other chronic illnesses.[30,33]

While exercise and other purposeful activity are routinely recommended at most HF clinics, prior to referral many patients have received specific instructions to avoid exercise and stress.[30] Lack of activity contributes to the deconditioning and sense of helplessness that often accompanies advanced HF. In addition to improving patients' attitude and feeling of self-worth, exercise has been shown to improve functional capacity and decrease symptoms.[30,34,35] There may be additional long-term benefit resulting from improvement of autonomic balance.[35] HF clinics emphasize cardiac rehabilitation or a self-supervised program of progressive walking, whereby patients report the frequency, duration, and exercise distance at each visit.[26] Better access to local cardiac rehabilitation programs for more formal training perhaps in conjunction with strength training may yield greater benefit.

HF clinics may also benefit HF patients by improving communication between patients and the health-care team. In the HF clinic model, there is regular communication between patient and HF team members. HF clinics utilize frequent phone contact with patients, and some programs also include home health nursing visits. In conventional care, patient/physician-nurse interaction may be triggered only by symptoms of deterioration. In the UCLA program, phone calls were initially made by the advance practice nurses within 3 days of discharge and weekly during the initial month after discharge, then less often after stability was demonstrated.[9] While it is not possible to identify which early interventions averted subsequent hospitalizations, the aggregate effect has been a marked reduction in hospitalization rates. HF often inspires reactions of despair and frustration from clinicians caring primarily for healthier and less demanding populations.[30] Patients may derive confidence from regular personal contact with a team that is dedicated to their chronic disease.

In studies that assessed HF clinics' impact on medical costs, most showed substantial reductions. Any increased costs associated with the HF clinic itself have been offset by the reduction in hospitalizations. In the UCLA study, the cost of inpatient care was reduced by approximately half during the 6 months after referral, even if the initial hospitalization at the time of referral was included as part of postreferral care. For the 179 patients alive without transplantation after 6 months from referral, the estimated hospitalization cost was $1.4 million compared to $3.2 million in the preceding 6 months.[9] The lower inpatient medical costs for patients followed by HF clinic medical staff reflects an economy of scale resulting from an organized approach to optimization of therapy for discharge. It has been estimated that outpatient care for advanced HF costs about $4238 per patient per year.[19] Salaries plus benefits for the HF advance practice nurses vary greatly between regions, with a standard case load of 100–150 patients with Class III–IV HF. The cost per patient of the additional outpatient administrative and nursing salary costs of a heart center do not approach the cost of a single hospitalization for HF. The relationship between costs and charges remains murky in most hospital accounting systems. The actual costs of program management are easier to calculate over a time interval than per patient. Despite concerns regarding cost calculations, however, the magnitude of the decrease in hospitalization rate compared to a broad range of administrative costs would yield a clear cost saving from referral to the HF clinic. However, the financial benefits for a HF clinic for patients at higher risk for hospitalization such as those with advanced HF, recent hospitalizations, the elderly, and the underserved/vulnerable may not be generalizable to lower risk HF patients.[36,37] It must also be acknowledged that even with a similar focus, different HF clinics may substantially differ in their ability to implement change and improve health-related outcomes. It is also essential for each HF clinic to closely track the quality of care being provided and health relative outcomes for the patients being followed, adhering to principles set forth by the American Heart Association for disease management programs (Table 21-3).[38]

▶ **Table 21-3** American Heart Association's guiding principles of disease management

- The main goal of disease management should be to improve the quality of care and patient outcomes.
- Scientifically derived, peer-reviewed guidelines should be the basis of all disease management programs. These guidelines should be evidence-based and consensus-driven.
- Disease management programs should help increase adherence to treatment plans based on the best available evidence.
- Disease management programs should include consensus-driven performance measures.
- All disease management efforts must include ongoing and scientifically based evaluations, including clinical outcomes.
- Disease management programs should exist within an integrated and comprehensive system of care in which the patient-provider relationship is central.
- To ensure optimal patient outcomes, disease management programs should address the complexities of medical comorbidities.
- Disease management programs should be developed for all populations and should particularly address members of the underserved or vulnerable populations.
- Organizations involved in disease management should scrupulously address potential conflicts of interest.

Source: Faxon DP, Schwamm LH, Pasternak RC, et al. Improving quality of care through disease management: principles and recommendations from the American Heart Association's Expert Panel on Disease Management. *Circulation.* 2004;109:2651–2654.

▶ SUMMARY

Improved clinical status and decreased hospitalizations have now been shown for patients with HF cared for in the setting of a HF clinic. As health care becomes more complex, there are growing data to support the concept that the persistence of Class III or IV HF is itself sufficient indication for referral to a HF clinic. These patients with moderate-severe symptoms are best managed in this setting. Patients with milder HF also appear to benefit from the comprehensive approach to patient management provided by a HF clinic. The need remains for additional testing of best practices and sharing of information on successful HF clinic components. Health-care providers, insurers, and policy makers should now recognize the value of HF clinics. With the cost and complexity of HF patient care, the HF clinic is ideally suited to provide care that improves quality and clinical outcomes at substantially lower total medical costs compared to care in the conventional practice setting.

▶ REFERENCES

1. 2004 Heart and Stroke Statistical Update. Dallas, TX: American Heart Association; 2004.
2. Hunt SA, Abraham WT, Chin MH, et al. ACC/AHA 2005 Guideline Update for the Diagnosis and Management of Chronic Heart Failure in the Adult—Summary Article. *Circulation.* 2005;112: 1825–1852 and *J Am Coll Cardiol.* 2005;46: 1116–1143.
3. O'Connell JB, Bristow MR. Economic impact of heart failure in the United States: time for a different approach. *J Heart Lung Transplant.* 1993;13:S107–S112.
4. Jencks SF, Cuerdon T, Burwen DR, et al. Quality of medical care delivered to Medicare beneficiaries. *JAMA.* 2000;284:1670–1676.
5. Havaranek EP, Wolfe P, Masoudi FA, et al. Provider and hospital characteristics associated with geographic variation in the evaluation and management of elderly patients with heart failure. *Arch Intern Med.* 2004;164: 1186–1191.
6. Moser DK, Mann DL. Improving outcomes in heart failure: It's not unusual beyond usual care. *Circulation.* 2002;105:2810–2812.

7. Rich MW, Nease RF. Cost-effectiveness analysis in clinical practice: the case of heart failure. *Arch Intern Med.* August 9–23, 1999; 159 (15): 1690–1700.

8. Advisory Board Company. Beyond Four Walls. Cost effectiveness management of chronic congestive heart failure. 1994. Washington D.C.

9. Fonarow GC, Stevenson LW, Walden JA, et al. Impact of a comprehensive heart failure management program on hospital readmission and functional status of patients with advanced heart failure. *J Am Coll Cardiol.* 1997;30:725-32.

10. Hanumanthu S, Butler J, Chomsky D, Davis S, Wilson JR. Effect of a heart failure program on hospitalization frequency and exercise tolerance. *Circulation.* 1997;96:2842–2848.

11. West JA, Miller NH, Parker KM, et al. A comprehensive management system for heart failure improves clinical outcomes and reduces medical resource utilization. *Am J Cardiol.* 1997;79:58–63.

12. Cintron G, Bigas C, Linares E, et al. Nurse practitioner role in a chronic congestive heart failure clinic: In hospital time, costs and patient satisfaction. *Heart & Lung.* 1993;12:237–240.

13. Lasater M. The effect of a nurse managed CHF clinic on patient readmission and length of stay. *Home Healthc Nurse.* 1996;14(5):351–356.

14. Smith L, Fabbri S, Pai R, et al. Symptomatic improvement and reduced hospitalization for patients attending a cardiomyopathy clinic. *Clin Cardiol.* 1997;20:949–954.

15. Cline CM, Israelsson BY, Willenheimer RB, et al. Cost effective management program for heart failure reduces hospitalization. *Heart.* 1998;80:442–446.

16. Dahl J, Penque S. The effects of an advanced practice nurse-directed heart failure program. *Nurse Pract.* 2000;25:61–77.

17. Fonarow GC, Chelimsky-Fallick C, Stevenson LW, et al. Effect of direct vasodilation with hydralazine versus angiotensin-converting enzyme inhibition with captopril on mortality in advanced heart failure: the Hy-C trial. *J Am Coll Cardiol.* 1992;19:842–850.

18. Stevenson LW, Steimle AE, Fonarow G, et al. Improvement in exercise capacity of candidates awaiting heart transplantation. *J Am Coll Cardiol.* 1995;25:163–170.

19. Schulman K, Mark D, Califf R. Outcomes and costs within a disease management program for advanced congestive heart failure. *Am Heart J.* 1998;135(6):S285–S292.

20. Rajfer SI. Perspective of the pharmaceutical industry on the development of new drugs for heart failure. *J Am Coll Cardiol.* 93;22: 198A–200A.

21. McAlister FA, Lawson FME, Teo KK, et al. A systemic review of randomized trials of disease management programs in heart failure. *Am J Med.* 2001;110:378–384.

22. McAlister FA, Stewart S, Ferrua S, et al. Multidisciplinary strategies for the management of heart failure patients at high risk for admission: a systematic review of randomized trials. *J Am Coll Cardiol.* 2004;44:810–819.

23. Phillips CO, Wright SM, Kern DE, et al. Comprehensive discharge planning with postdischarge support for older patients with congestive heart failure: a meta-analysis. *JAMA.* 2004;291:1358–1367.

24. Fonarow GC, Walden JW, Livingston N. *The Clinic Model of Heart Failure Care. The Heart Failure Handbook.* Aspen Publishers, 2000, 301–315.

25. Sueta CA, Chowdhury M, Boccuzzi SJ, et al. Analysis of the degree of undertreatment of hyperlipidemia and congestive heart failure secondary to coronary artery disease. *Am J Cardiol.* 1999;83:1303–1307.

26. Brophy JM, Deslauriers G, Boucher B, et al. The hospital course and short term prognosis of patients presenting to the emergency room with decompensated congestive heart failure. *Can J Cardiol.* 1993;9:219–224.

27. Rich MW, Beckham V, Wittenberg C, et al. A multidisciplinary intervention to prevent the readmission of elderly patients with congestive heart failure. *N Engl J Med.* 1995;333: 1190–1195.

28. Kahn KL, Rogers WH, Rubenstein LV, et al. Measuring quality of care with explicit process criteria before and after implementation of the DRG-based prospective payment system. *JAMA.* 1990;264:1969–1973.

29. Chiquette E, Amato MG, Bussey HI. Comparison of an anticoagulation clinic with usual medical care: anticoagulation control, patient outcomes, and health care costs. *Arch of Int Med.* 1998;158:1641–1647.

30. Dracup K, Baker DW, Dunbar SB, et al. Management of heart failure. II. Counseling,

education, and lifestyle modifications. *JAMA*. 1994;272:1442–1446.

31. Ghali JK, Kadakia S, Cooper R, et al. Precipitating factors leading to decompensation of heart failure. *Arch Intern Med*. 1988; 148:2013–2016.

32. Vinson JM, Rich MW, Sperry JC, et al. Early readmission of elderly patients with congestive heart failure. *J Am Geriatr Soc*. 1990;38: 1290–1295.

33. Mullen PD, Green LW, Persinger GS. Clinical trials of patient education for chronic conditions: a comparative meta-analysis of intervention types. *Prev Med*. 1985;14:753–781.

34. McKelvie RS, Teo KK, McCartney N, et al. Effects of exercise training in patients with congestive heart failure: a critical review. *J Am Coll Cardiol*. 1995;25:789–796.

35. Coats AJ, Adamopoulos S, Radaelli A, et al. Controlled trial of physical training in chronic heart failure: exercise performance, hemodynamics, ventilation, and autonomic function. *Circulation*. 1992;85:2119–2131.

36. DeBusk RF, Miller NH, Parker KM, et al. Care management for low-risk patients with heart failure: a randomized, controlled trial. *Ann Intern Med*. 2004;141:606–613.

37. Wagner EH. Deconstructing heart failure disease management. *Ann Intern Med*. 2004; 141:644–646.

38. Faxon DP, Schwamm LH, Pasternak RC, et al. Improving quality of care through disease management: principles and recommendations from the American Heart Association's Expert Panel on Disease Management. *Circulation*. 2004;109:2651–2654.

CHAPTER 22

Putting It All Together: Optimizing the Management of Chronic Heart Failure Patients

WILLEM J. REMME, MD, PHD

▶ INTRODUCTION

Over the years, heart failure has become one of the most dramatic developments in medicine, exemplified by fast increasing incidence worldwide, its debilitating nature, enormous cost aspects, and a mortality rate which surpasses many other diseases, including most cancers.

Changing lifestyles leading to more cardiovascular disease, a better treatment of ischemic syndromes resulting in more patients alive albeit with an impaired cardiac function, and the general population getting older and, hence, at higher cardiovascular risk result in a high prevalence of heart failure, particularly in the elderly.

To cope with a situation such as this requires full awareness of size and severity of the problem, not only by the doctor or nurse directly involved in heart failure care, but also by the health-care authorities who sanction the means for improved care and research into better forms of treatment, as well as the patient, his family, and indeed the general public, who may force health-care authorities into this.

Accordingly, heart failure management encompasses far more than the prescription of the correct medication or performing the appropriate diagnostic techniques, important as they are.

Extensive educational programs for the public, health-care officials, paramedical personnel, primary care physicians, and specialists involved in heart failure patient care form an integral part when it comes to improving heart failure management.

In addition, a better understanding of the need for primary and secondary preventive measures, the importance of screening programs, structured HF management pathways, including nurse-led outpatient and home care and HF clinics, and the role of nonpharmacological therapies, for example, devices and exercise programs, is mandatory if we want to contain this major medical problem.

Obviously, the doctor, whether primary care physician, internist, geriatrician, or cardiologist, has a pivotal position in the management of heart failure patients and should be well educated about how to provide appropriate care. Guidelines on diagnosis and treatment of heart failure exist in many countries worldwide and do provide the intellectual means to optimize HF management in the individual patient.

This chapter aims, with a view on the most recent HF guidelines, at painting a picture of how, with currently available information, optimal HF care may be achieved.[1-3]

▶ HOW TO DETECT HEART FAILURE

The characteristic signs and symptoms of heart failure are by no means specific. Although orthopnea and nocturnal dyspnea may suggest a high likelihood of heart failure, the more common symptoms such as dyspnea on effort and tiredness are less specific, certainly in the elderly. Also, typical signs of heart failure like ankle edema or rales can often be explained by other causes, particularly in women or the elderly, whereas other, potentially more specific signs such as a third heart sound or an elevated jugular pressure demand a certain level of diagnostic experience.

Nevertheless, these signs and symptoms should alert the physician, and when presenting in clinically meaningful combination and/or against the background of cardiovascular disease, should prompt additional investigations including an electrocardiogram (ECG), chest x-ray, and, if available, B-type natriuretic peptide (BNP) or NT-proBNP. An abnormal ECG is common in heart failure, but does not have much predictive value. In contrast, a normal ECG makes heart failure unlikely. A chest x-ray should always be part of the initial workup and may suggest heart failure when cardiomegaly or pulmonary congestion is present, particularly when typical signs and symptoms and an abnormal ECG are present. On its own, its predictive value is too low and should not be considered sufficient for the diagnosis.

There is accumulating evidence that natriuretic peptides have strong prognostic value in heart failure.[4] Their potential to monitor treatment is questionable, though. In particular, the effect of β-blockade is not consistently reflected by reductions in natriuretic peptide levels. In the CARMEN study, carvedilol alone significantly reversed cardiac remodeling, but this was not accompanied by decreased BNP levels.[5] In contrast, whereas enalapril alone did not decrease cardiac volumes in that study, it did lead to a significant reduction in BNP. Natriuretic peptides are particularly useful to exclude heart failure, as in untreated patients a normal value strongly suggests the absence of heart failure.[6] In particular, if the ECG and natriuretic peptides are normal, it is unlikely that heart failure is present, and the doctor is well advised to consider other explanations for the patient's complaints.

In all other cases, however, cardiac function needs to be evaluated. Heart failure should never be diagnosed based on clinical signs and symptoms alone. Unfortunately, this is still practiced by many primary care physicians, as indicated by the SHAPE study.[7] In this survey carried out in 2003 of more than 4000 primary care physicians in nine European countries, 75% would still diagnose heart failure based on signs and symptoms alone and 22% believed the response to diuretics necessary to confirm the diagnosis. Only a minority would request an echocardiogram to ascertain cardiac dysfunction.

Echocardiography is the preferred method for the assessment of cardiac function, allowing for the measurement of both systolic and diastolic function noninvasively. The most important measurement here is the left ventricular (LV) ejection fraction to distinguish patients with LV systolic dysfunction from those with preserved LV systolic function. The latter is not equivalent to diastolic LV dysfunction. To diagnose heart failure due to diastolic LV dysfunction in patients with typical signs and symptoms of heart failure and a (near) normal LV ejection fraction, relaxation abnormalities, diastolic distensibility, or diastolic stiffness needs to be present.

The combined assessment of mitral annular velocities and transmitral blood flow velocities may allow one to assess different filling patterns inherent with mild, moderate, and severe diastolic dysfunction, that is, impaired relaxation, pseudonormal filling, and restrictive filling, respectively.[8,9]

How important the diagnosis of diastolic heart failure really is, is uncertain as prospective data in controlled studies are lacking. Most heart failure patients have a certain degree of diastolic dysfunction together with systolic dysfunction, and the management of both conditions does not differ much (see the following paragraphs).

In cases where echocardiography cannot be performed, LV function may be determined by nuclear angiography, contrast angiography, or cardiac magnetic resonance imaging (MRI). The latter provides well-reproducible information on cardiac volumes, size, wall motion, and myocardial mass, but is not readily available in many places worldwide.

Other investigations may be useful to detect underlying causes of heart failure or suggest alternative diagnoses, but are not really necessary to define whether heart failure is present or not. Thus, exercise testing should not routinely be performed to diagnose heart failure, although exercise capacity is likely to be reduced in heart failure. It may be useful, though, like stress echocardiography or scintigraphy, to detect myocardial ischemia. Similarly, coronary angiography should not be performed routinely when angina is not present, but may be considered when, in acute or worsening heart failure, patients do not react sufficiently to therapy to detect significant, treatable coronary disease. Similarly, cardiac catheterization, including angiography, should be considered when treatment effect is inappropriate and the underlying cause is unclear and to consider the need for valve repair in severe mitral or aortic disease.

Essential hematological and biochemical evaluations during diagnosis include hemoglobin, hematocrit, renal function tests (creatinine clearance, serum urea), electrolytes, liver function tests, serum glucose, and urine analysis. Anemia and renal dysfunction are important prognostic indicators, which may cause or contribute to worsening heart failure, and are targets of specific therapies (see Chap. 10). Severe renal dysfunction and electrolyte disorders may be limiting factors in therapies such as angiotensin converting enzyme (ACE) inhibitors, angiotensin receptor antagonists, and aldosterone antagonists. The presence of diabetes should be evaluated routinely, but thyroid function on indication only. A flowchart of diagnostic steps and necessary or supporting components of heart failure diagnosis are given in Fig. 22-1 and Tables 22-1 and 22-2, respectively.

▶ HEART FAILURE THERAPY— WHAT IS AVAILABLE

ACE Inhibitors

Irrespective of the severity of heart failure, patients should receive an ACE inhibitor. This includes asymptomatic left ventricular dysfunction. Patients usually tolerate ACE inhibition well

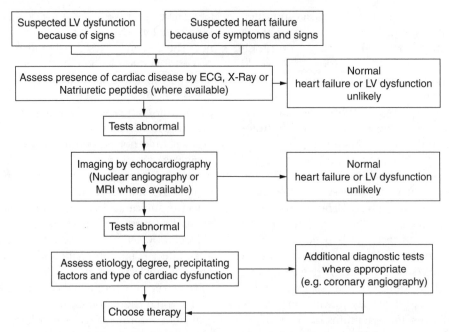

Figure 22-1 Algorithm of procedures to be followed in the diagnosis of heart failure and evaluation of underlying mechanisms as proposed by the ESC. (Reproduced with permission from Ref 3.)

and there are few absolute contraindications (bilateral renal artery stenosis and angioedema during previous ACE inhibitor use). Relative contraindications may include severe renal dysfunction, severe hypotension, and persistent hyperkalemia despite non-potassium-sparing diuretic therapy. If there are no signs of fluid overload, ACE inhibitors are to be administered before diuretic therapy, with fluid overload together with diuretics.[1] Whereas ACE inhibitors should be uptitrated starting with low dosages, it is important to continue until the dosages have been reached, which when used in large randomized controlled trials (RCT) have been shown to improve mortality and morbidity. All too often, ACE inhibitor uptitration is stopped too early at insufficient dose levels, that is, those that were not studied in RCTs and for which there is no indication of efficacy. A survey of European primary care physician (PCP) practices in 1999 indicated that overall doses prescribed were approximately 50% of the target

dose levels of ACE inhibitors suggested by available European guidelines on heart failure treatment.[10,11] A recent survey, also amongst European PCPs, did not indicate any improvement in PCP prescription practice, as less than 50% of the PCPs would reach target doses.[7] One contributing reason for undertreatment may be that many PCPs overestimate the risk of side effects with ACE inhibitors and this overestimation may undermine doctors' accurate assessment of the benefit-risk ratio, potentially increasing the likelihood of not starting or inappropriately stopping treatment.[10] Changes in blood pressure and increases in serum creatinine are usually small with ACE inhibition in normotensive patients without severe heart failure, and symptomatic hypotension is uncommon. This overestimation of the risk of side effects with ACE inhibitors very likely contributes to the PCPs' preference of diuretics as first-line treatment of heart failure, also in patients without overt signs of fluid overload.

▶ **Table 22-1** Assessments to be performed routinely to establish the presence and likely cause of heart failure

Assessments	The diagnosis of heart failure			Suggests alternative or additional diagnosis
	Necessary for	Supports	Opposes	
Appropriate symptoms	*		* (If absent)	
Appropriate signs		*	† (If absent)	
Cardiac dysfunction on imaging (usually echocardiography)	*		* (If absent)	
Response of symptoms or signs to therapy		*	* (If absent)	
ECG			* (If normal)	
Chest x-ray		If pulmonary congestion or cardiomegaly	† (If normal)	Pulmonary disease
Full blood count				Anemia/secondary polycythemia
Biochemistry and urinalysis				Renal or hepatic disease/diabetes
Plasma concentration of natriuretic peptides in untreated patients (where available)		† (If elevated)	† (If normal)	

* = of great importance; † = of some importance
Source: Reproduced with permission from Ref. 3.

The recent SHAPE survey found that 39% of European PCPs would start treatment with a diuretic and only 43% would always (in >90% of their patients) use an ACE inhibitor for the treatment of heart failure.[5] In contrast, 64% of European internists and geriatricians and 82% of European cardiologists would always prescribe an ACE inhibitor for heart failure.[12]

Diuretics

Diuretics are obviously essential for symptomatic treatment when fluid overload is clinically manifest as peripheral edema or pulmonary congestion, as they may quickly diminish symptoms such as dyspnea and improve exercise tolerance. However, there are no RCTs with diuretics with regard to their effect on mortality and, indeed, symptoms. As diuretic treatment may lead to adverse effects such as neurohormonal activation, renal dysfunction, and hyponatremia, diuretics should be used in a flexible way as adjunctive therapy to ACE inhibition, β-blockade, and possibly low-dose aldosterone antagonists and angiotensin receptor blockade (ARB).[3] Nevertheless, diuretics are used as first-line therapy without ACE inhibition by a sizeable percentage of PCPs (39%) and by 18% of internists and geriatricians in Europe.[7,12] If a patient's symptoms improve following diuretic treatment, its use should always be reconsidered and reduced or even stopped as patients are apparently free of fluid overload and free of symptoms.

▶ **Table 22-2** Additional tests to be considered to support the diagnosis or to suggest alternative diagnoses

Assessments	The diagnosis of heart failure		Suggests alternative or additional diagnosis
	Supports	Opposes	
Exercise test	* (If impaired)	† (If normal)	
Pulmonary function tests			Pulmonary disease
Thyroid function tests			Thyroid disease
Invasive investigation and angiography			Coronary artery disease, ischemia
Cardiac output	† (If depressed at rest)	† (If normal; especially during exercise)	
Left atrial pressure	† (If elevated at rest)	† (If normal; in absence of therapy)	

* = of some importance; † = of great importance
Source: Reproduced with permission from Ref. 3.

Potassium-sparing diuretics should only be considered if despite ACE inhibition and/or ARBs hypokalemia persists (and its use interrupted or permanently stopped when normokalemia resumes), under careful control of electrolytes.

1964 INTERNSHIP STAN ZEEMAN M P

β-Blockade in Heart Failure

The greatest recent advance in heart failure therapeutics is the finding that β-blockers further reduce morbidity and mortality when added to an ACE inhibitor. This evidence became apparent from 1996 onwards and international guidelines produced since then clearly mandate the use of β-blockade in addition to ACE inhibitors and diuretics in all symptomatic heart failure patients.[1,2,13–16] β-Blockers are also indicated in asymptomatic LV dysfunction after a myocardial infarction (MI).[17]

Nevertheless, uptake of β-blockade for the treatment of heart failure by the medical community has been slow and hesitant, particularly by noncardiologists. Whereas in a survey

carried out in 1998 amongst PCPs. β-blocker use was as low as 6%, the recent SHAPE survey indicated that still only 5% of European PCPs would always (in >90% of patients) and 35% (in >50%) prescribe a β-blocker, whereas 11% of PCPs would never prescribe a β-blocker.[7,10] Overall, 35% would not prescribe a β-blocker to a patient who had mild symptoms on treatment with an ACE inhibitor and a diuretic. The main risks of treatment with β-blockers were thought to be bronchospasm, heart block, cold extremities, worsening of heart failure, and hypotension, which were also given as a reason for stopping β-blocker therapy by 66%, 58%, 18%, 31%, and 25%, respectively. Most PCPs said they would not prescribe a β-blocker for patients with a bradycardia or asthma/chronic obstructive pulmonary disease. Overall, 35% said they would not prescribe a β-blocker to a patient who had mild symptoms on treatment with an ACE inhibitor.

Of interest, this is not much better among internists and geriatricians. In the same SHAPE survey, only 39% would prescribe a β-blocker in >50% of their patients, compared to 73% of cardiologists.[12]

Which β-Blocker?

At present, four β-blocking drugs have been shown to improve survival and/or lead to clinical benefit, at least including a reduction in cardiovascular hospitalizations: bisoprolol, metoprolol succinate, carvedilol, and nebivolol.[13–16,18] Bisoprolol and metoprolol succinate are β_1 selective blockers without and nebivolol with vasodilating properties. Carvedilol, on the other hand, has a more profound antiadrenergic effect, including β_1 and α_2 and β_1 antagonistic properties. Moreover, it has antioxidative and antiendothelin effects. Together, these properties suggest a better

therapeutic profile in heart failure. Indeed, in the only head-to-head comparison with another β-blocker, metoprolol tartrate, carvedilol displayed a more profound improvement in survival and reduced the occurrence of death and hospitalizations for heart failure more than metoprolol during long-term treatment.[19] As it also had a significant effect on all vascular modes of death (Fig. 22-2) and on myocardial infarction and stroke, a vascular component in its mode of action seems likely, possibly the result of its alpha-1 blocking properties. Suggestions that the better effect of carvedilol was due to a more profound effect on heart rate and blood pressure and/or to dose differences were recently shown unfounded.[22]

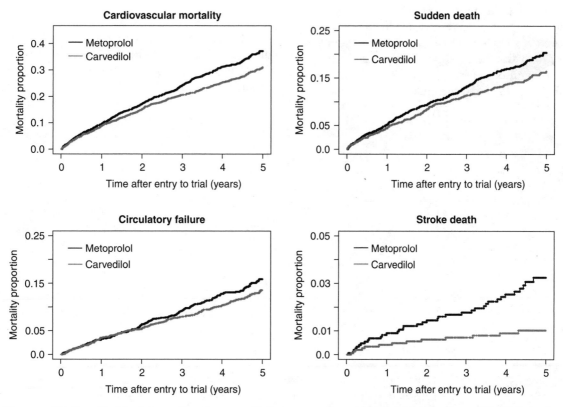

Figure 22-2 Survival benefit of carvedilol over metoprolol tartrate in the COMET study. Carvedilol significantly better protects against cardiovascular death, sudden death, and death due to stroke than metoprolol tartrate. (Adapted from Torp-Pederson et al. AHJ. 2005;149: 370–376.)

β-Blockade or ACE Inhibition in Mild Heart Failure–Which One First?

All large β-blocker trials were conducted on top of ACE inhibition. As a consequence, guidelines would advocate the use of ACE inhibitors as a first step (with or without a diuretic), followed by β-blockade if symptoms persist; that is, as patients would become asymptomatic β-blockade would not be advocated in conditions where chronic heart failure was not caused by an MI. Typically based on historical grounds (the ACE inhibitor being the first to be explored in heart failure), one may wonder whether this assumption is correct. In view of its pharmacological profile in relation to early mechanisms in cardiac remodeling and heart failure, a β-blocker such as carvedilol may well be as good or possibly better than an ACE inhibitor. The CARMEN study indicated that carvedilol alone had a better long-term effect on remodeling in mild heart failure than enalapril alone, although the combination proved to be superior (Fig. 22-3).[5] In the latter arm of the study, carvedilol was uptitrated first and appeared well tolerated. The results of

CARMEN suggest that in cases where ACE inhibition is contraindicated carvedilol is a good alternative, but that, whenever possible, both drugs should be combined from the start of treatment to achieve the best effect on remodeling. Sliwa et al. subsequently reported in a smaller, single-center study that the order of administration favored carvedilol.[23] Both CARMEN and the study of Sliwa et al indicate that β-blockade (with carvedilol) may be the first rather than the second step, particularly in patients with an elevated heart rate.[24] CIBIS III examined the effect of bisoprolol as first-line treatment as compared to enalapril and determined that it was as safe and efficacious to start bisoprolol first.

Aldosterone Antagonists

Aldosterone plays a pivotal role in the pathophysiology of several cardiovascular syndromes, including heart failure. Aldosterone synthase and the mineralocorticoid receptor are produced in close proximity in organs such as

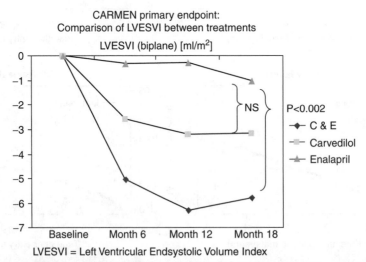

Figure 22-3 A comparison of the effect of combined treatment with carvedilol and enalapril versus that of carvedilol alone or enalapril alone on cardiac remodeling. The combined therapy results in greater reversal of left ventricular volumes as compared to enalapril alone and to a lesser extent to carvedilol alone.(Reproduced with permission from Ref 5.)

the heart, vascular tissue, and the brain. As such, aldosterone acts not only as an endocrine hormone following suprarenal production, but also as a paracrine neurohormone. Of importance, its production is greatly stimulated in the cardiovascular system following an acute myocardial infarction and in the failing heart.[25] Among its multiple actions are fibrosis of the heart and vessels, myocardial hypertrophy, cytokine activation, endothelial dysfunction, vascular inflammation, increased cardiac norepinephrine uptake, sodium reabsorption, and potassium and magnesium excretion, which together may lead to hypertension, ischemia, arrhythmias, and heart failure. As many other stimuli than angiotensin II result in aldosterone activation, ACE inhibition or angiotensin II receptor blockade (ARB) do not suppress aldosterone production. To block the untoward effects of the neurohormone, aldosterone receptor antagonists are required. Spironolactone binds to mineralocorticoid receptors, but also to glucocorticoid receptors and has progestational and antiandrogenic actions. Eplerenone has a greater specificity for mineralocorticoid receptors and fewer progestational and antiandrogenic actions. Both drugs have clear antiremodeling effects in postinfarct and heart failure models,

reduce oxyradicals formation, improve endothelial function, and prevent cardiovascular fibrosis. Spironolactone significantly improved survival in advanced heart failure in addition to ACE inhibition and β-blockade, and reduced cardiovascular and heart failure hospitalizations in the RALES study.[26] In EPHESUS, eplerenone had similar effects on mortality in postinfarct heart failure patients with LVSD, and reduced sudden death in particular (Fig. 22-4).[27] Again, effects were present, and in fact better, when administered in addition to ACE inhibition and β-blockade, a clear demonstration of the importance to block the 3 major neurohormonal systems simultaneously with combined targeted therapy. Of importance, this combined therapy was generally well tolerated, hypotension not being a major issue. Hyperkalemia did occur in both RALES and EPHESUS in patients receiving aldosterone antagonists in addition to ACE inhibition, as to be expected. However, serious hyperkalemia was not an issue in RALES and occurred in 1.6% of eplerenone patients in EPHESUS, but not leading to excess deaths. This small increase in serious hyperkalemia was offset by a 4.7% absolute decrease in serious hypokalemia in these patients, very likely having contributed to the reduction in sudden death

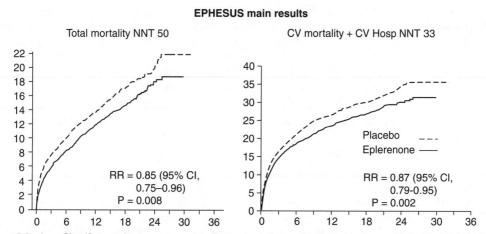

Figure 22-4 Significant improvement of survival in patients with heart failure following acute myocardial infarction with eplerenone, a selective aldosterone antagonist, in addition to optimal therapy including ACE inhibitors and β-blockers. (From Ref 27.)

in patients treated with eplerenone. Although hyperkalemia was not a major issue in RALES and EPHESUS due to adherence to a strict titration scheme, an increase in hospitalizations for hyperkalemia due to a surge in spironolactone use following publication of the RALES results was recently reported.[28] Most likely this is due to a less careful approach in spironolactone administration and patient selection in usual clinical care as compared to controlled study conditions. Based on the trial results, aldosterone antagonists are recommended in patients with heart failure post-MI and in advanced heart failure in addition to ACE inhibition and β-blockade. Although it is very likely that these agents will be beneficial in patients with mild heart failure, this will be clarified in an upcoming large multinational study in patients with New York Heart Association (NYHA) Class II heart failure (EMPHASIS-HF).

Angiotensin Receptor Blockers

ARBs are advocated in patients who are intolerant to ACE inhibitors.[1-3] In the CHARM–Alternative study, candesartan significantly reduced cardiovascular death or hospitalizations for heart failure.[30] Whereas this makes sense and is not very surprising, there are seemingly good reasons to expect a better effect from an ARB than an ACE inhibitor in heart failure treatment. Studies have indicated that during long-term ACE inhibition the initial decrease in circulating angiotensin II levels diminishes over time, possibly the result of alternative pathways to form angiotensin II from its precursor, for example, by way of chymases. However, and in contrast to the consistent beneficial effects of ACE inhibitors, β-blockers, and aldosterone antagonists in heart failure, the potential positive effects of ARBs in chronic heart failure have been more difficult to demonstrate. In ELITE 2, the first large controlled study in heart failure, which compared ACE inhibition (captopril) head to head with an ARB (losartan), monotherapy with the ARB did not prove better than the ACE inhibitor.[31] If anything, there was a tendency to a worse outcome

with losartan, although side effects were less. Subsequent meta-analyses also including smaller studies indicated equal efficacy in terms of survival and reduced morbidity.[32] Nevertheless, in post-MI patients with LV systolic dysfunction or heart failure, again a diverse pattern emerged with less efficacy of the ARB as compared to ACE inhibition in one and no inferiority in another study.[33,34]

Further studies concentrated on a combined ACE inhibitor and ARB effect, comparing this combination to ACE inhibition alone. The obvious idea behind this is that the combination would take care of a possible ACE inhibitor escape effect on angiotensin II levels, at the same time preserving the effect of ACE inhibition on bradykinin, an essential modulator of cardiac remodeling and a strong vasodilator. The Val-HeFT study compared the ARB valsartan plus ACE inhibition to ACE inhibition alone.[35] The first primary endpoint, survival, did not improve with the combination, but there were fewer heart failure hospitalizations. In contrast, in the CHARM–Added study, candesartan plus ACE inhibition significantly reduced the combination of cardiovascular death or heart failure hospitalizations by 15% compared to ACE inhibition alone and reduced LV function.[36] However, in both Val-HeFT and CHARM–Added there was a higher rate of discontinuation due to renal impairment, hyperkalemia, and hypotension in the combination arms, indicating a need for careful monitoring. In heart failure or LV dysfunction post-MI, there was similar efficacy in the combination and single component arms, but again a higher incidence of side effects.[34] Despite a lack of homogeneous efficacy in the above studies, possibly caused by relatively low dosages in several studies, the most recent guidelines are relatively mild, suggesting that ARBs are used as an alternative to ACE inhibitors, if intolerant, or can be considered in combination with ACE inhibitors in patients who remain symptomatic despite accepted therapy including ACE inhibitors and β-blockers.[3,31,33] Concerns regarding a negative interaction with β-blockade raised by earlier studies could not be confirmed in later trials.

Digitalis Glycosides

Digitalis glycosides are prescribed less and less, although they are still favored by PCPs and in Eastern European countries. Their use is primarily in atrial fibrillation (preferably together with β-blockade) for heart rate control, and in more advanced heart failure in patients with sinus rhythm for symptom control. The DIG study did not indicate a positive effect on survival, but hospitalizations and heart failure hospitalizations were reduced.[37] This study, performed before the introduction of β-blockade and aldosterone antagonism for the treatment of heart failure, leaves much doubt about the efficacy of glycosides in the presence of these drugs. Both efficacy and adverse effects may be less when plasma levels are relatively low.[38]

Vasodilators

With the exception of African Americans, there is no specific role for direct-acting vasodilators in heart failure. The combination of nitrates and hydralazine, better than placebo, is less effective than ACE inhibition in the overall population, although a recent study indicated a significant better effect in African Americans.[39–41] Other vasodilators, including nitrates and long-acting calcium antagonists such as amlodipine and felodipine, which do not lead to beneficial effects but also are not harmful in the setting of heart failure, may be considered for concomitant treatment of angina and hypertension.[42]

Antiarrhythmic Agents or Implantable Cardioverter Defibrillators

In terms of antiarrhythmic agents, only β-blockers (class II drugs) have been shown to reduce sudden death in heart failure. Amiodarone may be effective against supraventricular and ventricular arrhythmias; it does not affect death in heart failure, at least not in mild-moderate chronic

heart failure. In the SCD-HeFT study, amiodarone was not better than placebo in NYHA II patients on ACE inhibition and β-blockade (approximately 70%) but relatively low numbers on aldosterone antagonists, but was significantly better in NYHA Class III patients.[43] Conversely, simple shock-only implantable cardioverter defibrillator (ICD) prevented death better in mild heart failure, but not in NYHA Class III compared to placebo. Nevertheless, if the overall population was considered, amiodarone proved no better than placebo, but ICD did. The place of amiodarone in death prevention is unclear and there appears no reason for routine use in chronic heart failure. However, the agent may be effective in restoring sinus rhythm in atrial fibrillation (with or without electrical cardioversion) and has the advantage of not being negatively inotropic. Besides SCD-HeFT, other data from large controlled studies supported by meta-analyses including smaller studies indicate an important role of ICDs in symptomatic heart failure patients due to significant LV dysfunction, despite optimal background therapy including β-blockade, in order to reduce the occurrence of sudden death.[43,44] Also, ICD is effective in post-MI patients with LV systolic dysfunction, but not necessarily symptomatic heart failure.[45] Thus far, the efficacy has not been well established in NYHA Class IV chronic heart failure. Moreover, a greater use of aldosterone antagonists, effective against sudden death, may impact on the efficacy of ICD. Which patient is a good candidate for ICD needs further evaluation, also in light of cost.

Pacemaker therapy for CHF—The Role of Cardiac Resynchronization Therapy

Cardiac dyssynchrony is a common feature in heart failure, particularly advanced cases. Resynchronization with multiple-lead biventricular pacing improves cardiac function, symptoms, and exercise capacity in the course of several months.[46,47] An important part of symptomatic improvement may relate to reduction of mitral insufficiency as contraction sequence improves. Two large trials have focused on the long-term effect of cardiac resynchronization therapy (CRT) on mortality and morbidity. COMPANION selected patients with NYHA Class III–IV heart failure, LV ejection fraction ≤35%, and a QRS width 120 msec to optimal pharmacological therapy only, CRT, or CRT with ICD.[48] Both CRT arms significantly reduced the primary endpoint (time to death or all-cause hospitalization) compared to placebo, although there was no difference between the arms. All cause death was only significantly reduced by the CRT–ICD combination.

In CARE-HF, patients with similar entry criteria, and also LV end diastolic dimension ≥30 mm, were randomized to medical therapy alone or with CRT.[49] There was a significant 37% relative risk reduction in the primary endpoint (all-cause death or cardiovascular hospitalization) and a 36% relative risk reduction in all-cause death in the CRT arm. These significant clinical effects were supported by hemodynamic improvement, less mitral insufficiency, and a reduction in LV end-diastolic volume. Based on the results of COMPANION and CARE-HF, the new European Society of Cardiology (ESC) guidelines indicate that CRT can be considered in patients with NYHA Class III–IV with reduced LV function and ventricular dyssynchrony (QRS width ≥120 msec), who remain symptomatic despite optimal medical therapy.[3]

Devices and Surgery

The surgical approaches to chronic heart failure can be divided into revascularization procedures, mitral valve surgery, LV restoration procedures, and heart transplantation.

Although symptomatic relief is observed in individual patients with symptomatic ischemic heart disease, the lack of prospective data from large controlled trials does not allow the use of bypass surgery in the average heart failure patient, also as heart failure patients have a considerably increased operative mortality risk.

Mitral valve surgery may significantly improve symptoms, particularly in patients with large ventricles and severe mitral insufficiency. Whether survival improves is unknown, however.

Left ventricular restoration attempts to reduce wall stress by reducing cardiac volumes or restricting further dilatation. Thus far, aneurysmectomy can be advocated in patients with sufficiently large aneurysms. In contrast, results of other procedures including cardiomyoplasty or the so-called Batista procedures have been disappointing and are not to be recommended as yet.

In addition to these procedures, several new techniques have been developed, including the myosplint and the Acorn external cardiac support device, both of which aim at reducing wall stress by restricting enlargement of the left ventricle.[50,51] Initial data are encouraging, but the outcomes of larger prospective trials are awaited.

Heart transplantation has gradually become a successful mode of treatment in end-stage cardiac failure despite optimal medical treatment, with a 5-year survival of approximately 75%. The main problems are shortage of donor hearts, early rejection, long-term consequences of immunosuppressive therapy, and new progressive coronary disease.

Although novel pharmacological therapies have resulted in patients improving to such an extent that they can be removed from the transplant list, bridging with ventricular assist devices or artificial hearts is often considered necessary. Despite the fact that at present assist devices are still external and prone to complications such as infections, they are often used for relatively long periods due to the scarcity of donor hearts.[52] Studies with fully implantable devices are currently in progress.

▶ WHEN TO TREAT AND HOW

Heart Failure Due to LV Systolic Dysfunction

Attention should be paid to treatable underlying causes of heart failure and to reasons for heart failure worsening.

In asymptomatic patients, ACE inhibition, and in post-MI patients, a β-blocker added to ACE inhibition, is mandatory. In mild symptomatic heart failure without signs of fluid retention, ACE inhibitors and β-blockers suffice, but diuretics should be added when fluid retention is present. It is important not to leave a time delay between, prescribing the ACE inhibitor and the β-blocker; the sequence of administration depends on the individual patient. If patients are intolerant to ACE inhibitors an ARB should be given. Patients with heart failure post-MI should receive an aldosterone antagonist in addition to ACE inhibitors and β-blockade. In other cases, an ARB may be added when patients remain symptomatic or worsen. However, in NYHA Class III patients who have improved from NYHA Class IV, an aldosterone antagonist would be the first choice and the addition of an ARB may be considered if symptoms persist. Potassium-sparing diuretics are usually not necessary, particularly when low-dose spironolactone may already be part of the treatment package. Digoxin should be considered in atrial fibrillation and continued in sinus rhythm if patients do improve from severe-to-milder heart failure. In worsening patients, it may be useful to prescribe a combination of different diuretics, that is, loop diuretics and thiazides, if increasing doses of a loop diuretic are not sufficient. At this stage, the usefulness of mitral valve operation may be considered, or cardiac transplantation. The latter should always be considered in end-stage heart disease with or without bridging procedures such as assist devices or interim support with intravenous inotropic agents. Figure 22-5 displays the use of pharmacological therapy as proposed by the ESC.[3]

Heart Failure with Preserved LV Systolic Function or Diastolic Dysfunction

Currently there are few data from controlled studies indicating how heart failure due to

	For survival/morbidity *Mandatory therapy*	For symptoms *Supportive therapy*
NYHA I	Continue ACE inhibitor/ARB if ACE inhibitor intolerant Continue aldosterone antagonist if post-MI Add beta-blocker if post-MI	Reduce/stop diuretic
NYHA II	ACE inhibitor as first-line therapy ARB if ACE inhibitor intolerant Add beta-blocker Add aldosterone antagonist if post-MI	+/- diuretic depending on fluid retention
NYHA III	Continue ACE inhibitor Add ARB or only ARB if ACE inhibitor intolerant Continue beta-blocker Add aldosterone antagonist	+ diuretics + digitalis If still symptomatic
NYHA IV	Continue ACE inhibitor/ARB Beta-blocker Aldosterone antagonist	+ diuretics + digitalis + consider temporary inotropic support

Figure 22-5   Algorithm of mandatory and supportive therapy of chronic heart failure due to systolic left ventricular dysfunction as proposed by the ESC. (Reproduced with permission from Ref 3.)

diastolic dysfunction or with preserved LV systolic function should be treated. Basically, suggested therapies conform to those of patients with systolic LV dysfunction. Of importance is to detect and correct underlying mechanisms, for example, ischemia (β-blockers, nitrates, calcium antagonists), to reduce heart rate to lengthen the diastolic period and improve diastolic coronary perfusion (β-blockers, verapamil-type calcium antagonists), and to correct hypertension if present and reduce cardiac hypertrophy (ACE inhibitors, ARB, and possibly dihydropyridine type calcium antagonists). ACE inhibitors directly improve relaxation and cardiac distensibility. Verapamil has shown improvement in hypertrophic cardiomyopathy and ARB reduced hospitalization for heart failure in CHARM–Preserved.[53,54] Of importance, although it may often be necessary to prescribe diuretics as pulmonary fluid retention occurs easily in rigid hypertrophied hearts, they may reduce preload extensively and lead to hypotension.

▶ THE ROAD TO OPTIMAL HEART FAILURE MANAGEMENT AND CARE

In the last few decades, significant improvements in heart failure diagnosis and, particularly, therapy have been achieved. Nevertheless, many patients are undermanaged, and many heart failure patients may even be undetected. Particularly nonspecialist doctors are insufficiently aware of the seriousness of heart failure and the necessity for early detection and management. Education is clearly needed. However, even with fast improvements in this respect and appropriate perception of optimal heart failure management of all caregivers involved, there are also important logistical aspects to be taken care of. The heart failure patient typically is an example of a chronically disabled patient with the potential to quickly change from a stable to an unstable condition, leading to (repeat) hospitalizations or (sudden) death.

To prevent this, continuous control by a specialized heart failure team is necessary. There are ample examples in the literature showing that a well-structured system of supervision and patient care may significantly reduce hospitalization frequency.[55,56] Which of the different models used is the best is unclear. However, a system employing specialized heart failure nurses would appear to be effective and cost-efficient. The extent to which this form of care is set up depends on whether all patients or only selected patient groups are involved and the availability of the necessary funds. In this respect, the awareness and perception of heart failure in all its aspects should not only be a matter for health-care providers, be it doctors, nurses, or other paramedical personnel and patients, but also for the general public and, in particular, the health-care authorities.[57]

▶ REFERENCES

1. Remme WJ, Swedberg K, for the Task Force for the Diagnosis and Treatment of Chronic Heart Failure. Guidelines for the diagnosis and treatment of chronic heart failure. *Eur Heart J.* 2001;22:1527–1560.
2. Hunt SA, Baker DW, Chin MH, et al. ACC/AHA guidelines for the evaluation and management of chronic heart failure in the adult: executive summary: a report of the American College of Cardiology/American Heart Association Task Force on Practice Guidelines. *J Am Coll Cardiol.* 2001;38:2101–2113.
3. The Task Force for the Diagnosis and Treatment of Chronic Heart Failure of the ESC. Guidelines for the diagnosis and treatment of chronic heart failure: executive summary (update 2005). *Eur Heart J.* 2005;26:1115–1140.
4. De Lemos JA, McGuire DK, Drazner MH. B-type natriuretic peptide in cardiovascular disease. *Lancet.* 2003;362:316–322.
5. Remme WJ, Riegger G, Hildebrandt P, et al, on behalf of the CARMEN investigators. The benefits of early combination treatment of carvedilol and an ACE-inhibitor in mild heart failure and left ventricular systolic dysfunction. The Carvedilol and Ace-inhibitor Remodelling Mild heart failure EvaluatioN trial (CARMEN). *Cardiovasc Drugs Ther.* 2004;18:57–66.

6. Cowie MR, Wood DA, Coats AJ, et al. Survival of patients with a new diagnosis of heart failure: a population based study. *Heart.* 2000; 83:505–510.

7. Remme WJ, Cline C, Cohen-Solal A, et al. Inadequate perception of heart failure is associated with underuse of diagnostic and therapeutic strategies in heart failure by the primary care physician: Results from SHAPE, a major European survey. *J Am Coll Cardiol.* 2004;43 (Supplement A):222A.

8. Myreng Y, Smiseth OA, Risoe C. Left ventricular filling at elevated diastolic pressures: relationship between transmitral Doppler flow velocities and atrial contribution. *Am Heart J.* 1990;119:620–626.

9. Sohn DW, Chai IH, Lee DJ, et al. Assessment of mitral annulus velocity by Doppler tissue imaging in the evaluation of left ventricular diastolic function. *J Am Coll Cardiol.* 1997;30:474–480.

10. Hobbs FDR, Jones MI, Allan TF, et al. European survey of primary care physician perceptions on heart failure diagnosis and management (Euro-HF). *Eur Heart J.* 2000;21:1877–1887.

11. The Task Force of the Working Group on Heart Failure of the European Society of Cardiology. Guidelines for the treatment of heart failure. *Eur Heart J.* 1997;18:736–753.

12. Remme WJ, Zannad F, Rauch B, et al. Awareness of recommended heart failure management among specialists. Do internists, geriatricians and cardiologists differ?—Results of SHAPE. *J Am Coll Cardiol.* 2005;45(Supplement A):11A.

13. Packer M, Bristow MR, Cohn JN, et al. The effect of carvedilol on morbidity and mortality in patients with chronic heart failure. *N Engl J Med.* 1996;334:1349–1355.

14. The Cardiac Insufficiency Bisoprolol Study II (CIBIS-II): a randomised trial. *Lancet.* 1999; 353:9–13.

15. Effect of metoprolol CR/XL in chronic heart failure: Metoprolol CR/XL Randomised Intervention Trial in Congestive Heart Failure (MERIT-HF). *Lancet.* 1999;353:2001–2007.

16. Packer M, Coats AJ, Fowler MB, et al. Effect of carvedilol on survival in severe chronic heart failure. *N Engl J Med.* 2001;344:1651–1658.

17. The CAPRICORN Investigators. Effect of carvedilol on outcome after myocardial infarction in patients with left-ventricular dysfunction: the CAPRICORN randomised trial. *Lancet.* 2001;357:1385–1390.

18. Flather MD, Shibata MC, Coats AJ, et al. Randomised trial to determine the effect of nebivolol on mortality and hospital admissions in elderly patients with heart failure (SENIORS). *Eur Heart J.* 2005;26:215–225.

19. Poole-Wilson PA, Swedberg K, Cleland JG, et al, Carvedilol Or Metoprolol European Trial Investigators. Comparison of carvedilol and metoprolol on clinical outcomes in patients with chronic heart failure in the Carvedilol Or Metoprolol European Trial (COMET): randomised controlled trial. *Lancet.* 2003;362: 7–13.

20. Remme WJ, Cleland JG, Di Lenarda A, et al. Carvedilol better protects against vascular events than metoprolol in heart failure: Results from COMET. *J Am Coll Cardiol.* 2007;49(to be published).

21. Remme WJ, Cleland JG, Torp-Pedersen C, et al. Consistent survival benefit of carvedilol over metoprolol irrespective of baseline characteristics of heart failure patients—Mode of death evaluation in COMET. *J Am Coll Cardiol.* 2005;45(Supplement A):155A.

22. Metra M, Torp Pedersen Ch, Cleland JGF, et al. Influence of heart rate, blood pressure and beta-blocker dose on outcome and the differences in outcome between carvedilol and metoprolol in patients with chronic heart failure: results from the COMET trial. *Eur Heart J.* 2005;26:2259–2268.

23. Sliwa K, Norton GR, Kone N, et al. Impact of initiating carvedilol before angiotensin-converting enzyme inhibitor therapy on cardiac function in newly diagnosed heart failure. *J Am Coll Cardiol.* 2004;44:1825–1830.

24. Remme WJ, Riegger G, Ryden L, et al. Does baseline heart rate determine the effect of carvedilol on ventricular remodeling in heart failure? Results of the CARMEN trial. *Eur Heart J.* 2003;24(Abstract supplement):711.

25. Mizuno Y, Yoshimura M, Yasue H, et al. Aldosterone production is activated in failing ventricle in humans. *Circulation.* 2001;103: 72–77.

26. Pitt B, Zannad F, Remme WJ, et al. The effect of spironolactone on morbidity and mortality in patients with severe heart failure. *N Engl J Med.* 1999;341:709–717.

27. Pitt B, Remme WJ, Zannad F, et al. Eplerenone, a selective aldosterone blocker, in patients with

left ventricular dysfunction after myocardial infarction. *N Engl L Med.* 2003;348:1309–1321.

28. Juurlink DN, Mamdani MM, Lee DS, et al. rates of hyperkalaemia after publication of the Randomised Aldactone Evaluation Study. *N Engl J Med.* 2004;351:543–551.

29. Bozkurt B, Agoston I, Knowlton AA. Complications of inappropriate use of spironolactone in heart failure: when an old medicine spirals out of new guidelines. *J Am Coll Cardiol.* 2003;41:211–214.

30. Granger GB, McMurray JJ, Yusuf S, et al. Effects of candesartan in patients with CHF and reduced left ventricular systolic function intolerant to angiotensin-converting-enzyme inhibitors; the CHARM-alternative trial. *Lancet.* 2003;362: 772–776.

31. Pitt B, Poole Wilson PA, Segal R, et al. Effect of losartan compared with captopril in patients with symptomatic heart failure: randomized trial: the Losartan Heart Failure Survival Study ELITE II. *Lancet.* 2000;355:1582–1587.

32. Jong P, Demers C, McKelvie RS, et al. Angiotensin receptor blockers in heart failure: meta-analysis of randomized controlled trials. *J Am Coll Cardiol.* 2002;39:463–470.

33. Dickstein K, Kjekshus J. Effect of losartan and captopril on mortality and morbidity in high-risk patients after acute myocardial infarction: the OPTIMAAL randomized trial. Optimal Trial in Myocardial Infarction with Angiotensin II Antagonist Losartan. *Lancet.* 2002;360:752–760.

34. Pfeffer MA, McMurray JJ, Velazques EJ, et al. Valsartan, Captopril, or both in myocardial infarction complicated by heart failure, left ventricular dysfunction, or both. *N Engl J Med.* 2003;349:1893–1906.

35. Cohn JN, Tognoni G. A randomized trial of the angiotensin-receptor blocker valsartan in CHF. *N Engl J Med.* 2001;345:1667–1675.

36. McMurray JJ, Ostergen J, Swedberg K, et al, Effects of candesartan in patients with CHF and reduced left-ventricular systolic function taking angiotensin-converting-enzyme inhibitors: the CHARM-Added trial. *Lancet.* 2003;362:767–771.

37. The Digitalis Investigation Group. The effect of digoxin on mortality and morbidity in patients with heart failure *N Engl J Med.* 1997;336: 525–533.

38. Rathore SS, Curtis JP, Wang Y, et al. Association of serum digoxin concentration and outcomes in patients with heart failure. *N Engl J Med.* 2002;289:871–878.

39. Cohn JN, Archibald DG, Phil M, et al. Effect of vasodilator therapy on mortality in chronic congestive heart failure. Results of a veterans administration cooperation study. *N Engl J Med.* 1986;314:1547–1552.

40. Cohn JN, Johnson G, Ziesche S, et al. A comparison of ennalapril with hydralazine—isosorbide dinitrate in the treatment of chronic congestive heart failure. *N Engl J Med.* 1991; 325:303–310.

41. Taylor AL, Ziesche S, Yancy C, et al. Combination of isosorbide dinitrate and hydralazine in blacks with heart failure. *N Engl J Med.* 2004;351: 2049–2057.

42. Cohn JN, Ziesche S, Smith R, et al. Effect of the calcium antagonist felodipine as supplementary vasodilator therapy in patients with CHF treated with enalapril: V-HeFT III. Vasodilator –Heart Failure Trial (V-HeFT) Study Group. *Circulation.* 1997;96:856–863.

43. Bardy GH, Lee KL, Mark DB, et al. Amiodarone or an implantable cardioverter defibrillator for congestive heart failure. *N Engl J Med.* 2005;352:225–237.

44. Nanthakumar K, Epstein AE, Kay GN, et al. Prophylactic implantable cardioverter-defibrillator therapy in patients with left ventricular systolic dysfunction: a pooled analysis of ten primary prevention trials. *J Am Coll Cardiol.* 2004; 44:2166–2172.

45. Moss AJ, Zareba W, Hall WJ, et al. Prophylactic implantation of a defibrillator in patients with myocardial infarction and reduced ejection fraction. *N Engl J Med.* 2002;347:877–883.

46. Linde C, Leclercq C, Rex S, et al. Long-term benefits of biventricular pacing in congestive heart failure: results from the MUltisite STImulation in Cardiomyopathy (MUSTIC) study. *J Am Coll Cardiol.* 2002;40:111–118.

47. Abraham WG, Fisher WG, Smith AL, et al. Cardiac resynchronisation in chronic heart failure. *N Engl J Med.* 2002;346:1845–1853.

48. Bristow MR, Saxon LA, Boehmer J, et al. Cardiac resynchronisation therapy with or without an implantable defibrillator in advanced chronic heart failure. *N Engl J Med.* 2004;350:2126–2128.

49. Cleland JG, Daubert JC, Erdmann E, et al. The effect of cardiac resynchronisation on morbidity and mortality in heart failure. *N Engl J Med*. 2005;352:1539–1549.

50. Guccione JM, Salahieha A, Moonly SM, et al. Myosplint decreases wall stress without depressing function in the failing heart: a finite element model study. *Ann Thorac Surg*. 2003;76: 1171–1180.

51. Oz MC, Konertz WF, Kleber FX, et al. Global surgical experience with the Acorn cardiac support device. *J Thorac Cardiovasc Surg*. 2003;126: 983–991.

52. Rose EA, Geleyns AC, Moskowitz AJ, et al. Long–term mechanical left ventricular assistance for end-stag heart failure. *N Engl J Med*. 2001;345:1435–1443.

53. Bonow RO, Dilsizian V, Rossing DR, et al. Verapamil-induced improvement in left ventricular diastolic filling and increased exercise tolerance in patients with hypertrophic cardiomyopathy: short- and long-term effects. *Circulation*. 1985: 72:853–864.

54. Yusuf S, Pfeffer MA, Swedberg K, et al. Effects of candesartan in patients with CHF and preserved left-ventricular ejection fraction: the CHARM-Preserved Trial. *Lancet*. 2003; 362: 777–781.

55. Stewart S, Marley JE, Horowitz JD. Effects of a home-based intervention amongst patients with congestive heart failure discharged from acute hospital care. *Arch Intern Med*. 1998; 158: 1067–1072.

56. Stromberg A. Nurse-led heart failure clinics improve survival and self-care behaviour in patients with heart failure: results from a prospective, randomised trial. *Eur Heart J*. 2003;24:1014–1023.

57. Remme WJ, McMurray JJV, Rauch B, et al. Public awareness of heart failure in Europe: first results from SHAPE (Study of Heart failure Awareness and perception in Europe). *Eur Heart J*. 2005;26:2413–2421.

Index

Page numbers followed by *f* or *t* denote figures or tables, respectively.